PET/MR Imaging: Current and Emerging Applications

Lale Umutlu
Ken Herrmann
Editors

PET/MR Imaging: Current and Emerging Applications

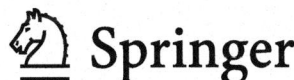 Springer

Editors
Lale Umutlu
Department of Diagnostic
and Interventional Radiology
and Neuroradiolgy
University Hospital Essen
Essen
Germany

Ken Herrmann
Department of Nuclearmedicine
University Hospital Essen
Essen
Germany

ISBN 978-3-030-09904-6   ISBN 978-3-319-69641-6   (eBook)
https://doi.org/10.1007/978-3-319-69641-6

Printed on acid-free paper

This Springer imprint is published by the registered company Springer International Publishing AG part of Springer Nature
The registered company address is: Gewerbestrasse 11, 6330 Cham, Switzerland

To my parents and my sister—my bastion of calm and support. Lale

Preface

PET imaging was developed as early as the 1970s and started clinical adoption in the 1990s. However, only the introduction of hybrid PET/CT significantly impacted disease detection, staging, restaging, and monitoring of oncologic and inflammatory diseases. With increasing adoption and improvement of MR imaging, the idea to integrate PET and MR scanners into one scanner system was born. After overcoming defying technical and methodological challenges, this notion has come to an end with the introduction of commercially available integrated PET/MR systems into clinical imaging in 2010. Despite the short time since the first introduction, PET/MR imaging has already demonstrated its high diagnostic value for an innumerous amount of applications. Apart from its utilization as an alternative diagnostic tool to PET/CT for local or whole-body staging, integrated PET/MRI epitomizes the endeavor of precision diagnostics and medicine, incorporating simultaneous assessment of noninvasive biomarkers based on multiparametric imaging comprising morphologic, functional, and metabolic features.

The aim of this book is to give an overview as well as dedicated display of current and emerging applications of PET/MR imaging including technical and methodological aspects as well as oncological and inflammatory disease imaging. The combination of nuclear medicine specialists and radiologists as authors, who are also dedicated hybrid imagers, is designed to allegorize and conjoint all aspects of hybrid imaging.

Lale Umutlu
Ken Herrmann

Contents

Current and Emerging Applications

Lale Umutlu and Ken Herrmann

1.1 From Current...

After the majority of the initial studies on PET/MRI focused on technical and methodological issues such as attenuation correction (Wagenknecht et al. 2013; Martinez-Möller et al. 2009), the research interest shifted towards the assessment of its clinical diagnostic capability as well as its potential for multiparametric tissue imaging over time (Eiber et al. 2014; Beiderwellen et al. 2014; Wang et al. 2017). Over the past 7 years innumerous studies evaluated its diagnostic performance for a large variety of different application fields, with an emphasis on oncologic applications including whole-body, dedicated head and neck, lung, liver and prostate imaging as well as non-oncologic applications, by means of inflammatory and neurodegenerative disease imaging (Beiderwellen et al. 2013; Buchbender et al. 2012; Heusch et al. 2014; Nensa et al. 2014a, b; Platzek et al. 2017; Ruhlmann et al. 2016; Wetter et al. 2014; Eiber et al. 2016a; Rischpler et al. 2015; Catalano et al. 2016).

Comparable to the implementation of any new imaging technique, the focus of research, its application and the overall understanding of PET/MRI have shown an evolving character. The majority of early clinical PET/MRI trials investigated its diagnostic performance in comparison to the gold-standard of hybrid imaging, by means of PET/CT, as well as to conventional imaging (MRI), with a focus on clinical viability assessment (Beiderwellen et al. 2013; Buchbender et al. 2012; Heusch et al. 2014; Erfanian et al. 2017; Grueneisen et al. 2014, 2015a; Sekine et al. 2017). Overwhelmed by the infinite matrix for MR sequence options and potentially elicited by the insecurity of utilizing a new imaging technology for clinical care, the majority of early trials comprised overly long MR protocols, which resulted in extensive examination times of >90 minutes (Drzezga et al. 2012, Schulthess et al. 2014). The majority of the initiated studies yielded foreseeable results, in terms of the general comparability of PET/MRI to PET/CT for whole-body staging with a favorable performance of PET/MRI regarding soft-tissue lesions (e.g. liver metastases) (Fig. 1.1) and metastases as well as its inferiority towards PET/CT considering lung nodules (Beiderwellen et al. 2013; Sawicki et al. 2016, 2017). However, the excessively long examination times rendered PET/MRI as an "ineffective, cost-intensive" research tool, incompatible for clinical usage. Adding potential patient discomfort (due to long examination times) into the

L. Umutlu (✉)
Department of Diagnostic and Interventional Radiology and Neuroradiology, University Hospital Essen, Essen, Germany
e-mail: Lale.Umutlu@uk-essen.de

K. Herrmann
Department of Nuclear Medicine, University Hospital Essen, Essen, Germany

© Springer International Publishing AG 2018
L. Umutlu, K. Herrmann (eds.), *PET/MR Imaging: Current and Emerging Applications*,
https://doi.org/10.1007/978-3-319-69641-6_1

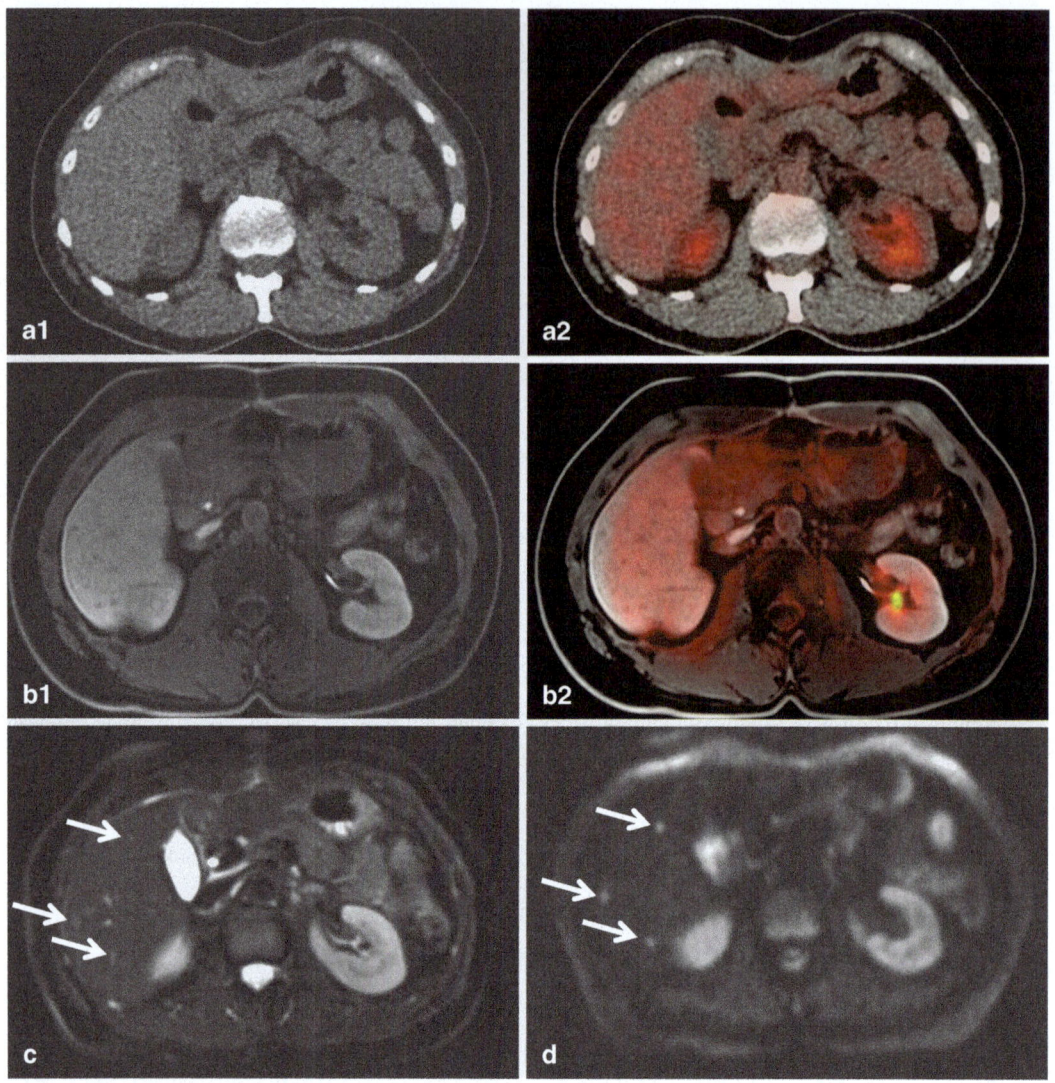

Fig. 1.1 Figure 1 shows a patient with a leiomyosarcoma. While the liver metastases do not show an increased FDG-uptake and are not visible in low-dose PET/CT (**a**1,**a**2) or non-enhanced T1-weighted PET/MR imaging (**b**1,**b**2), (fatsaturated) T2 weighted TSE imaging (**c**) and DWI (**d**) revealed three small liver metastases in the right liver lobe (arrows)

mixture of potentially negative impact on the clinical implementation of PET/MR imaging, a new era of investigations on optimized workflow management was born. One of the very first optimization strategies was proposed by Martinez-Möller indicating a differentiation of (whole-body imaging) protocols in accordance to the clinical indication (Martinez-Möller et al. 2012). Based on the categorization into (a) prior imaging results present versus (b) no prior results present, the authors proposed the application of different PET/MR imaging protocols to complement existing prior data as well as to further deepen the diagnostics if needed (e.g. add dedicated liver sequences in case of unclear liver lesions). Starting out with Martinez-Möller, an innumerous amount of different workflow optimization proposals were published within time (Von Schulthess et al. 2014; Ishii et al. 2016; Barbosa et al. 2015). While MR imaging is known to generally suffer from insufficient standardization of sequences and protocols, inherent to the complex and diverse nature of the technique, the conclusion derived from the majority of the early PET/MR studies disclosed the need to omit MR sequences that offer redundant information and aspire indication- and time-sensitive protocols. A workflow optimization proposal that aimed to significantly shorten the examination time of PET/MRI was introduced by Grueneisen et al. (2015b). This so-called "FAST" protocol is premised on a 4 minute PET per bed position protocol, that comprises T2 weighted HASTE imaging and diffusion-weighted-imaging as well as post-PET post-contrast T1 weighted VIBE imaging, reducing the total examination time to 27.8 ± 3.7 min, while preserving a comparable diagnostic performance to extensive protocols and PET/CT. Intrigued by the successful implementation of a significantly shorter workflow protocol, the urge for further protocol abbreviation was triggered. Diffusion-weighted imaging has been proven of high diagnostic value in exclusive MR imaging as an additional tool for identification of tumors and metastatic sites,

revealing restricted diffusivity due to enhanced tissue density. However, its PET-comparable utilization as a "searching tool" for the identification of tumorous lesions leaves its additional diagnostic value in a PET/MR setting disputable. Hence, based on study results demonstrating the insignificant improvement of diagnostic performance based on DWI in a whole-body PET/MRI setting, Kirchner et al. introduced an ultra-fast PET/MRI protocol, further abbreviating and equating the examination time to PET/CT levels (18.5 ± 1 versus 18.2 ± 1 for PET/CT, respectively) (Kirchner et al. 2017). Despite the distinctly abbreviated protocol, based on the omission of the DWI sequence, while entailing a T2 HASTE sequence within a 2 min PET per bed position and a post-PET post-contrast T1 weighted VIBE sequence, the ultra-fast PET/MRI protocol enabled equal diagnostic performance to PET/CT (Fig. 1.2). While Kirchner et al. preserved the high-resolution morphologic imaging feature of MRI, Kohan et al. introduced a protocol of similar shortage yet restricting the anatomic correlation to a 3D T1-weighted spoiled gradient echo

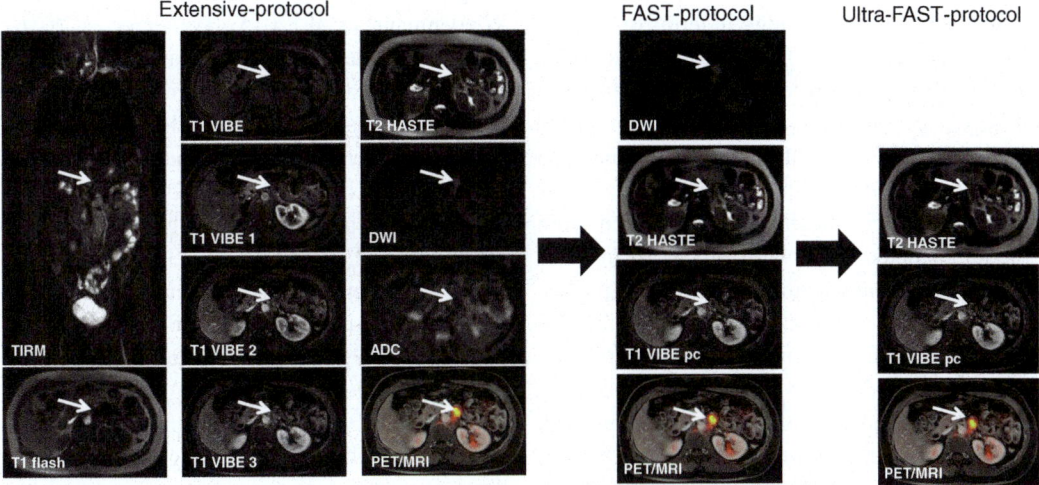

Fig. 1.2 Comparison of an extensive protocol (appr. 50 min acquisition time) to a FAST-protocol (27.8 min) and an Ultra-FAST protocol (18.5 min) demonstrating the feasibility and diagnostic capability of time-sensitive imaging protocols. Arrows mark a lymph node metastasis that can be equally well depicted in the ultra-fast protocol as the extensive protocol, offering redundant MR information

sequence designed for attenuation correction and hence, downgrading the diagnostic level of PET/MRI to low-dose PET/CT levels (Kohan et al. 2013). Although initial results were promising in terms of comparable diagnostic performance for N staging in lung cancer to PET/CT, the trade-off of reducing the examination time to a minimum of 13.5 min while forsaking any kind of high-resolution morphologic correlation seems to come at a very-high and questionable price.

1.2 ...To Emerging Application Fields of PET/MR Imaging

While the clinical viability of PET/MRI as a comparable diagnostic tool to PET/CT may be considered a "current application", it is well recognized that PET/MRI enables a platform of emerging imaging techniques that are in their emerging steps and yet to be fully exploited. These enticing and emerging applications range from multiparametric PET/MRI imaging utilizing radiomic analyses to enhance tumor characterization and understanding of tumor biology on the MRI side as well as new-generation tracers on the PET side, that bear the potential to uplift hybrid imaging to new diagnostic and potentially theranostic levels.

So far, precision oncology in terms of personalized cancer care was focused on the genomic based molecular characterization of tumor tissue derived from biopsy sampling. With an incrementally noticeable shift towards personalized diagnostics and treatment approaches, the demands towards imaging have exceeded from sole tumor detection towards advanced in vivo tumor mapping and characterization and predictive parameters. Hence, while the ability to provide accurate assessment of tumor location and extent remains to be of utmost importance and the prime skill of any diagnostic method, more in-depth understanding of tumor features and biology has gained an important role within the past few years. Expanding exclusive morphologic MRI by the combined analysis of morphologic and physiological properties based on diffusion-weighted imaging, dynamic contrast-enhanced imaging (DCE) and MR spectroscopy via multiparametric MR imaging have not only improved the staging performance of MR imaging but also leveraged it to advanced levels of understanding of tumor biology (An et al. 2015; Delongchamps et al. 2011; Bonekamp et al. 2011; Watanabe et al. 2011). While multiparametric MR has emerged to be the first-line diagnostic method in a number of indications (e.g. prostate imaging), the inclusion of complementary metabolic data based on PET/MRI has been shown to further enhance its diagnostic power. In a comparative study performed by Lee et al., PET/MRI was demonstrated to provide better sensitivity, accuracy and diagnostic value for detection and localization of prostate cancer when compared to sole multiparametric MRI (Lee et al. 2017). Apart from enhancing its staging performance, the combined assessment of morphologic, functional and metabolic tissue data renders the potential for advanced (tumor) tissue characterization. A number of recent trials have investigated the diagnostic and predictive power of non-invasive biomarkers derived from integrated PET/MRI scans for improved cancer detection, diagnosis, prediction of prognosis and treatment response, revealing promising results on the added value of multiparametric PET/MR imaging (Wang et al. 2017; Georg et al. 2017; Wiedenmann et al. 2015;, Pinker et al. 2016). Based on the demand to extract a large number of quantitative features solely from imaging datasets, the increasingly acknowledged potential of radiomic analyses and machine learning algorithms may facilitate a new platform for advanced tumor phenotyping and decoding based on multiparametric- PET/MRI (Fig. 1.3) (Gillies et al. 2016; Kumar et al. 2012; Parmer et al. 2015).

While the most distinct difference between PET/CT and PET/MRI clearly lies in the potential of multi-functional MR imaging, the continuous developmental work on new tracers also bears the potential to uplift PET/MR imaging onto a more disease-specific and personalized diagnostic level. Two newly introduced probes, that have recently gained major attention, are 18F-PSMA-1007 and 68Ga-Pentixafor (Kesch et al. 2017; Herrmann et al. 2015; Werner et al. 2017). These

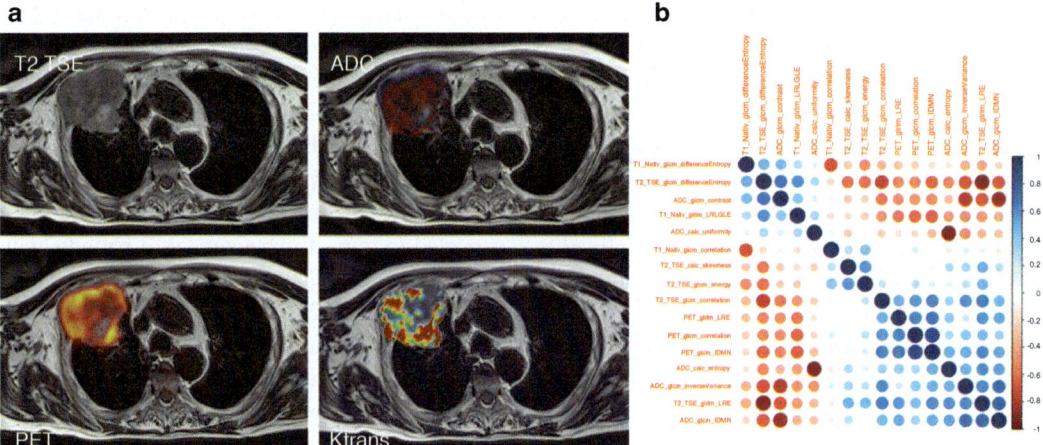

Fig. 1.3 (**a**) Multiparametric 18F-FDG-PET/MRI dataset of a patient with a pancoast tumor of the right hemithorax. (**b**) shows the corresponding correlation matrix of radiomic features for the assessment of the association between variables within the feature space

new-generation probes are not only expected to improve the diagnostic performance of hybrid imaging (may it be PET/CT or PET/MRI), but also to potentially facilitate theranostic approaches.

PET/MRI for prostate imaging has emerged to be one of the major application fields, showing benefits in terms of superiority of hybrid imaging over conventional imaging as well as of PET/MRI over PET/CT in terms of the combined assessment of metabolic data and high-resolution MR imaging of the prostate. Starting out with 11C-/18F-Choline imaging and shifting to 68Ga-PSMA over time, 18F-PSMA-1007 is the newest introduction into the family of metabolic prostate imaging (Schwarzenböck et al. 2017). Overcoming specific limitations of 68Ga, in terms of yielding a longer half-life and a fast non-urinary background clearance, which reduces the known and diagnostically challenging "halo"-effect (caused by tracer accumulation in the bladder and consecutive overlapping uptake), 18-F-PSMA-1007 has demonstrated its diagnostic power based on its outstanding tumor uptake and excellent sensitivity, specificity and accuracy rates >92% for lesion detection in initial trials (Kesch et al. 2017). Apart from 18F-PSMA-1007, the role of chemokines in tumor progression and metastasis development has gained major atten-

tion in the hybrid community within the last few years. Being involved in the growth of a large number of tumor entities (including breast cancer, ovarian cancer, melanoma and lung cancer) the altered expression of chemokines and their receptors may be utilized for display of tumorous lesions. A special focus was put on the molecular display of the chemokine receptor 4 (CXCR4)/chemokine ligand (CXCL 12) axis as it is known to play a critical role in the regulation of primary and metastatic tumor growth, resulting in an increased proliferation and survival of CXCR4-positive tumor cells (Mueller et al. 2001). As high CXCR4 expression is known to be associated with tumor dissemination, a novel CXCR4 probe by means of 68Ga-Pentixafor was introduced for molecular mapping of CXCR4 density. Initial studies on patients with advanced multiple myeloma showed promising results, yielding excellent specificity and high contrast in 68Ga-Pentixafor PET imaging as well as complementary and additional information when compared to 18F-FDG PET imaging (Philipp-Abbrederis et al. 2015).

Apart from the high diagnostic performance that both new-generation probes delivered, they also seem to enable the transition from an exclusively diagnostic to a theranostic approach.

Recent feasibility trials have investigated and demonstrated the potential of different theranostic concepts, involving 177Lu-DOTATATE, 177Lu-PSMA and 177Lu-Pentixather (Barrio et al. 2016; George et al. 2015; Werner et al. 2015; Herrmann 2016). In one of the first in vivo, in-human studies of CXCR4-directed endoradiotherapy with 177Lu- and 90Y-labeled Pentixather Herrmann et al. investigated its therapeutic effect in patients with intra- and extramedullary manifestations of multiple myeloma. The successful results of this preliminary study indicate that CXCR4-targeted radiotherapy with pentixather is a promising novel treatment option (in line with cytotoxic chemotherapy and autologous stem cell transplantation) for patients with advanced multiple myeloma (Fig. 1.4) (Herrmann et al. 2016). Another application field of hybrid imaging that

has become an attractive diagnostic and therapeutic target is the prostate specific membrane antigen. While the utilization of PSMA directed ligands labeled with ^{68}Ga is now established in prostate cancer hybrid imaging, recent trials have demonstrated its potential as therapeutic when labeled with [177]Lu. Hence, PSMA ligands are expected to impact management of patients with prostate cancer (Barrio et al. 2016; Fendler et al. 2017; Lütje et al. 2017).

All in all, secluding this chapter and the first 7 years of integrated PET/MR imaging, it is safe to conclude that, while PET/MRI has started off strong in demonstrating its clinical viability and extensive source for research applications, only the tip of the iceberg has been scratched so far and the true potential is yet to be exploited in upcoming years.

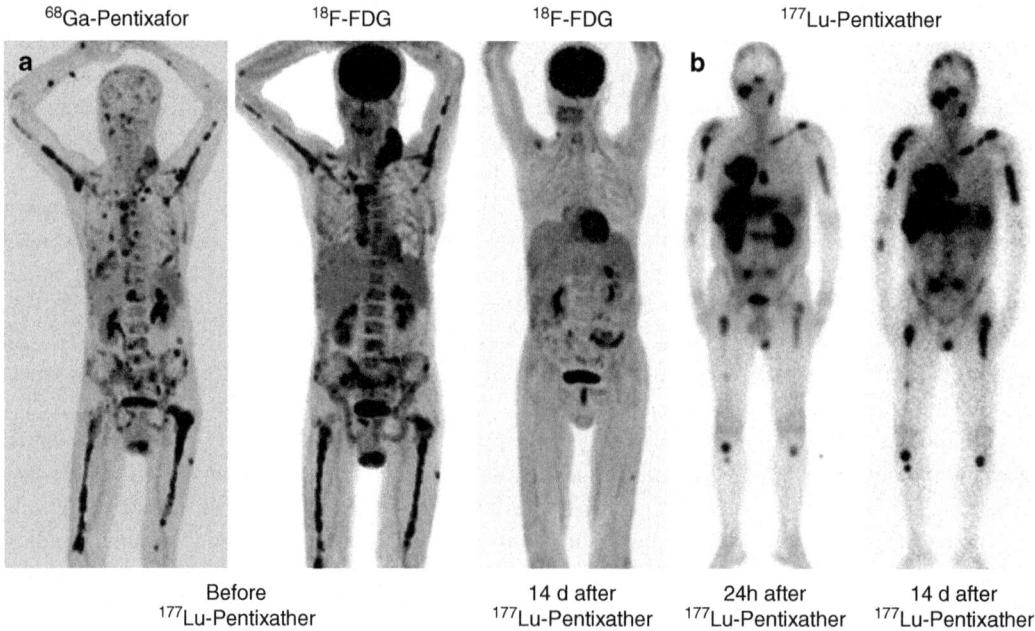

[68]Ga-Pentixafor　　[18]F-FDG　　[18]F-FDG　　[177]Lu-Pentixather

Before
[177]Lu-Pentixather

14 d after
[177]Lu-Pentixather

24h after
[177]Lu-Pentixather

14 d after
[177]Lu-Pentixather

Fig. 1.4 (a) In patient 3 before pentixather therapy, maximum-intensity projections of ^{68}Ga-pentixafor and ^{18}F-FDG PET/CT indicate high CXCR4 expression in multiple extra- and intramedullary ^{18}F-FDG-avid myeloma lesions. Corresponding ^{18}F-FDG PET/CT image 2 weeks. after ^{90}Y-pentixather shows complete metabolic response. (b) Scintigraphic images of patient 1 at 24 h and 15 d after 15.2 GBq of ^{177}Lu-pentixather confirm binding to CXCR4 target. Visual difference in tumor-to-background ratios is due to reduced background uptake at later time point and longer emission times due to lower count rates

References

An YS, Kang DK, Jung YS, et al. Tumor metabolism and perfusion ratio assessed by 18F-FDG PET/CT and DCE-MRI in breast cancer patients: correlation with tumor subtype and histologic prognostic factors. Eur J Radiol. 2015;84:1365–70.

Barbosa Fde G, von Schulthess G, Veit-Haibach P. Workflow in simultaneous PET/MRI. Semin Nucl Med. 2015;45:332–44.

Barrio M, Fendler WP, Czernin J, et al. Prostate specific membrane antigen (PSMA) ligands for diagnosis and therapy of prostate cancer. Expert Rev Mol Diagn. 2016;16:1177–88.

Beiderwellen K, Gomez B, Buchbender C, et al. Depiction and characterization of liver lesions in whole body [18F]-FDG PET/MRI. Eur J Radiol. 2013;82:e669–75.

Beiderwellen K, Huebner M, Heusch P, et al. Whole-body [(1)(8)F]FDG PET/MRI vs. PET/CT in the assessment of bone lesions in oncological patients: initial results. Eur Radiol. 2014;24:2023–30.

Bonekamp D, Jacobs MA, El-Khouli R, et al. Advancements in MR imaging of the prostate: from diagnosis to interventions. Radiographics. 2011;31:677–703.

Buchbender C, Heusner TA, Lauenstein TC, et al. Oncologic PET/MRI, Part 1: tumors of the brain, head and neck, chest, abdomen, and pelvis. J Nucl Med. 2012;53:928–38.

Catalano OA, Gee MS, Nicolai E, et al. Evaluation of quantitative PET/MRI enterography biomarkers for discrimination of inflammatory strictures from fibrotic strictures in Crohn disease. Radiology. 2016;278:792–800.

Delongchamps NB, Rouanne M, Flam T, et al. Multiparametric magnetic resonance imaging for the detection and localization of prostate cancer: Combination of T2-weighted, dynamic contrast-enhanced and diffusion-weighted imaging. BJU Int. 2011;107:1411–8.

Drzezga A, Souvatzoglou M, Eiber M, et al. First clinical experience with integrated whole-body PET/MR: comparison to PET/CT in patients with oncologic diagnoses. J Nucl Med. 2012;53:845–55.

Eiber M, Takei T, Souvatzoglou M, Mayerhoefer ME, et al. Performance of whole-body integrated 18F-FDG PET/MR in comparison to PET/CT for evaluation of malignant bone lesions. J Nucl Med. 2014;55:191–7.

Eiber M, Weirich G, Holzapfel K, Souvatzoglou M, Haller B, Rauscher I, et al. Simultaneous 68Ga-PSMA HBED-CC PET/MRI improves the localization of primary prostate cancer. Eur Urol. 2016;70:829–36.

Erfanian Y, Grueneisen J, Kirchner J, et al. Integrated 18F-FDG PET/MRI compared to MRI alone for identification of local recurrences of soft tissue sarcomas: a comparison trial. Eur J Nucl Med Mol Imaging. 2017. https://doi.org/10.1007/s00259-017-3736-y.

Fendler WP, Rahbar K, Herrmann K, et al. 177Lu-PSMA radioligand therapy for prostate cancer. J Nucl Med. 2017. https://doi.org/10.2967/jnumed.117.191023. pii: jnumed.117.191023, [Epub ahead of print]

Georg P, Andrzejewski P, Baltzer P, et al. Changes in tumor biology during chemoradiation of cervix cancer assessed by multiparametric MRI and hypoxia PET. Mol Imaging Biol. 2017. https://doi.org/10.1007/s11307-017-1087-5. [Epub ahead of print].

George GPC, Pisaneschi F, Nguyen QD, et al. Positron emission tomographic imaging of CXCR4 in cancer: challenges and promises. Mol Imaging. 2015;14:7290201400041. https://doi.org/10.2310/7290.2014.00041.

Gillies RJ, Kinahan PE, Hricak H. Radiomics: images are more than pictures, they are data. Radiology. 2016;278:563–77.

Grueneisen J, Beiderwellen K, Heusch P, et al. Simultaneous positron emission tomography/magnetic resonance imaging for whole-body staging in patients with recurrent gynecological malignancies of the pelvis: a comparison to whole-body magnetic resonance imaging alone. Investig Radiol. 2014;49:808–15.

Grueneisen J, Schaarschmidt BM, Heubner M, et al. Implementation of FAST-PET/MRI for whole-body staging of female patients with recurrent pelvic malignancies: a comparison to PET/CT. Eur J Radiol. 2015a;84:2097–102.

Grueneisen J, Nagarajah J, Buchbender C, et al. Positron Emission tomography/magnetic resonance imaging for local tumor staging in patients with primary breast cancer: a comparison with positron emission tomography/computed tomography and magnetic resonance imaging. Investig Radiol. 2015b;50:505–13.

Herrmann K, Lapa C, Wester HJ, et al. Biodistribution and radiation dosimetry for the chemokine receptor CXCR4-targeting probe 68Ga-pentixafor. J Nucl Med. 2015;56:410–6.

Herrmann K, Schottelius M, Lapa C, et al. First-in-human experience of CXCR4-directed endoradiotherapy with 177Lu- and 90Y-labeled pentixather in advanced-stage multiple myeloma with extensive intra- and extramedullary disease. J Nucl Med. 2016;57:248–51.

Heusch P, Nensa F, Schaarschmidt B, et al. Diagnostic accuracy of whole-body PET/MRI and whole-body PET/CT for TNM staging in oncology. Eur J Nucl Med Mol Imaging. 2014;42:42–8. https://doi.org/10.1007/s00259-014-2885-5.

Ishii S, Hara T, Nanbu T, et al. Optimized workflow and imaging protocols for whole-body oncologic PET/MRI. Jpn J Radiol. 2016;34:754–62.

Kesch C, Vinsensia M, Radtke JP, et al. Intra-individual comparison of 18F–PSMA-1007-PET/CT, multi-parametric MRI and radical prostatectomy specimen in patients with primary prostate cancer – a retrospective, proof of concept study. J Nucl Med. 2017. https://doi.org/10.2967/jnumed.116.189233. pii: jnumed.116.189233, [Epub ahead of print]

Kirchner J, Sawicki LM, Suntharalingam S, et al. Whole-body staging of female patients with recurrent pelvic malignancies: ultra-fast 18F-FDG PET/MRI compared to 18F-FDG PET/CT and CT. PLoS One. 2017;12:e0172553.

Kohan AA, Kolthammer JA, Vercher-Conejero JL, et al. N staging of lung cancer patients with PET/MRI using a three-segment model attenuation correction algorithm: initial experience. Eur Radiol. 2013;23:3161–9.

Kumar V, Gu Y, Basu S, et al. Radiomics: the process and the challenges. Magn Reson Imaging. 2012;30:1234–48.

Lee MS, Cho JY, Kim SY, et al. Diagnostic value of integrated PET/MRI for detection and localization of prostate cancer: comparative study of multiparametric MRI and PET/CT. J Magn Reson Imaging. 2017;45:597–609.

Lütje S, Slavik R, Fendler W, et al. PSMA ligands in prostate cancer - Probe optimization and theranostic applications. Methods. 2017.; pii: S1046–2023(16)30344–9. doi: 10.1016/j.ymeth.2017.06.026. [Epub ahead of print] Review

Martinez-Möller A, Eiber M, Nekolla SG, et al. Workflow and scan protocol considerations for integrated whole-body PET/MRI in oncology. J Nucl Med. 2012;53:1415–26.

Martinez-Moller A, Souvatzoglou M, Delso G, et al. Tissue classification as a potential approach for attenuation correction in whole-body PET/MRI: evaluation with PET/CT data. J Nucl Med. 2009;50:520–6.

Muller A, Homey B, Soto H, et al. Involvement of chemokine receptors in breast cancer metastasis. Nature. 2001;410:50–6.

Nensa F, Beiderwellen K, Heusch P, Wetter A. Clinical applications of PET/MRI: current status and future perspectives. Diagn Interv Radiol. 2014a;20:438–47.

Nensa F, Poeppel TD, Krings P, Schlosser T. Multiparametric assessment of myocarditis using simultaneous positron emission tomography/magnetic resonance imaging. Eur Heart J. 2014b;35:2173.

Parmar C, Grossmann P, Bussink J, Lambin P, Aerts HJ. Machine Learning methods for Quantitative Radiomic Biomarkers. Sci Rep. 2015;5:13087. https://doi.org/10.1038/srep13087

Phillip –AK, Herrmann K, Knop S, et al. In vivo molecular imaging of chemokine rexept or CXCR4 expression patients with advanced multiple myeloma. EMBO Mol Med. 2015;7:477–87. 10.15252/emmm.201404698

Pinker K, Andrzejewski P, Baltzer P, et al. Multiparametric [18F]Fluorodeoxyglucose/ [18F]Fluoromisonidazole positron emission tomography/magnetic resonance imaging of locally advanced cervical cancer for the non-invasive detection of tumor heterogeneity: a pilot study. PLoS One. 2016;11:e0155333.

Platzek I, Beuthien-Baumann B, Schramm G, et al. FDG PET/MRI in initial staging of sarcoma: Initial experience and comparison with conventional imaging. Clin Imaging. 2017;42:126–32.

Rischpler C, Langwieser N, Souvatzoglou M, et al. PET/MRI early after myocardial infarction: evaluation of viability with late gadolinium enhancement transmurality vs. 18F-FDG uptake. Eur Heart J Cardiovasc Imaging. 2015;16:661–9.

Ruhlmann V, Ruhlmann M, Bellendorf A, et al. Hybrid imaging for detection of carcinoma of unknown primary: A preliminary comparison trial of whole-body PET/MRI versus PET/CT. Eur J Radiol. 2016;85:1941–7.

Sawicki LM, Deuschl C, Beiderwellen K, et al. Evaluation of $_{68}$Ga-DOTATOC PET/MRI for whole-body staging of neuroendocrine tumours in comparison with $_{68}$Ga-DOTATOC PET/CT. Eur Radiol. 2017. https://doi.org/10.1007/s00330-017-4803-2. [Epub ahead of print]

Sawicki LM, Grueneisen J, Buchbender C, et al. Evaluation of the outcome of lung nodules missed on 18F-FDG PET/MRI compared with 18F-FDG PET/CT in patients with known malignancies. J Nucl Med. 2016;57:15–20.

Schwarzenböck SM, Rauscher I, Bluemel C, et al. PSMA ligands for PET-imaging of prostate cancer. J Nucl Med. 2017. https://doi.org/10.2967/jnumed.117.191031. pii: jnumed.117.191031, [Epub ahead of print]

Sekine T, Barbosa FG, Delso G, et al. Local resectability assessment of head and neck cancer: positron emission tomography/MRI versus positron emission tomography/CT. Head Neck. 2017. https://doi.org/10.1002/hed.24783.

Von Schulthess GK, Veit-Haibach P. Workflow considerations in PET/MR imaging. J Nucl Med. 2014;55(Supplement 2):19S–24S.

Wagenknecht G, Kaiser H-JJ, Mottaghy FM, et al. MRI for attenuation correction in PET: methods and challenges. Magn Reson Mater Phys Biol Med. 2013;26:99–113.

Wang J, Shih TT, Yen RF. Multiparametric evaluation of treatment response to neoadjuvant chemotherapy in breast cancer using integrated PET/MR. Clin Nucl Med. 2017;42:506–13.

Watanabe H, Kanematsu M, Kondo H, et al. Preoperative detection of prostate cancer: a comparison with 11C-choline PET, 18Ffluorodeoxyglucose PET and MR imaging. J Magn Reson Imaging. 2011;31:1151–6.

Werner RA, Bluemel C, Lassmann M, et al. SPECT-and PET-based patient-tailored treatment in neuroendocrine tumors: a comprehensive multidisciplinary team approach. Clin Nucl Med. 2015;40:e271–7. https://doi.org/10.1097/RLU.0000000000000729.

Werner RA, Weich A, Higuchi T, et al. Imaging of chemokine receptor 4 expression in neuroendocrine tumors – a triple tracer comparative approach. Theranostics. 2017;7:1489–98.

Wetter A, Lipponer C, Nensa F, Heusch P, Ruebben H, Schlosser TW, et al. Evaluation of the PET component of simultaneous [(18)F]choline PET/MRI in prostate cancer: comparison with [(18)F]choline PET/CT. Eur J Nucl Med Mol Imaging. 2014;41:79–88.

Wiedenmann NE, Bucher S, Hentschel M et al. Serial [18F]-fluoromisonidazole PET during radiochemotherapy for locally advanced head and neck cancer and its correlation with outcome. Radiother Oncol 2015;117:113–7.

Technical Improvements

2

Harald H. Quick

2.1 Introduction

Hybrid imaging with combined positron emission tomography/magnetic resonance (PET/MR) imaging is the most recent hybrid imaging modality (Drzezga et al. 2012; Quick et al. 2013). It combines excellent soft tissue contrast and high spatial image resolution of MR imaging with metabolic information provided by PET, as integrated PET/MR systems acquire PET and MR data simultaneously (Delso et al. 2011; Quick 2014; Grant et al. 2016). Beyond exact coregistration of PET and MR data, this can be applied for MR-based motion correction of PET data.

The integration of PET detectors within MR imaging systems has been a challenging task that has been solved by different vendors introducing three different PET/MR systems in the years 2010–2014 (Delso et al. 2011; Quick 2014; Grant et al. 2016; Zaidi et al. 2011). When compared to hybrid PET/computed tomography (CT), PET/MR has demonstrated comparable PET image quality and PET quantification in numerous clini-

cal comparison studies (Drzezga et al. 2012; Quick et al. 2013; Wiesmüller et al. 2013). However, due to the missing CT component, attenuation correction in PET/MR has to be based on MR images and subsequent image segmentation. This turned out to be challenging and a wealth of methodological developments have been described in the recent literature.

Ultimately, the aim of all current technical and methodological developments in PET/MR is to further improve workflow, image quality, PET quantification, and to broaden the application spectrum of PET/MR in research and clinical applications. This chapter on technical developments highlights current developments in PET/MR attenuation correction and motion correction, introduces new hardware developments, and discusses current research efforts on artifact correction and dose reduction in PET/MR hybrid imaging.

2.2 Attenuation Correction in PET/MR

PET is a quantitative imaging technique that facilitates the determination of the amount of radioactive tracer accumulation in a tumour, lesion or organ within the human body. In this context, attenuation correction (AC) describes a physical method to account for the self-absorption of the emitted annihilation photons in tissue and

H.H. Quick, Ph.D.
Erwin L. Hahn Institute for MR Imaging, University of Duisburg-Essen, Essen, Germany

High Field and Hybrid MR Imaging, University Hospital Essen, Essen, Germany
e-mail: harald.quick@uni-due.de

© Springer International Publishing AG 2018
L. Umutlu, K. Herrmann (eds.), *PET/MR Imaging: Current and Emerging Applications*,
https://doi.org/10.1007/978-3-319-69641-6_2

in hardware components. Attenuation correction, thus, is a pre-requisite for accurate quantification of the PET data (Kinahan et al. 1998). More specifically, the photons that originate from a positron annihilation within the body are attenuated by the surrounding tissues and by ancillary hardware components such as the patient table before they reach the PET detectors.

In combined PET/CT systems, the attenuation properties of tissue can be derived from the complementary CT images after a fast and straightforward conversion of the photon energy levels of CT-derived Hounsfield units (HU) to linear attenuation coefficients (LAC) for PET (Kinahan et al. 1998; Carney et al. 2006). In PET/MR, however, attenuation correction is methodologically challenging (Wagenknecht et al. 2013) as MR imaging measures magnetization densities and relaxation times of hydrogen nuclei in tissue. The MR signal, thus, depends on the amount of protons and their local chemical environment in tissues. As there is no direct physical dependency of proton density and proton spin relaxation times with local electron density, which causes the photon attenuation, it is not possible to derive PET attenuation properties of tissues directly from MR imaging measurements (Wagenknecht et al. 2013). To address this issue, different concepts for attenuation correction in PET/MR have been developed (Wagenknecht et al. 2013). The most widely used method for MR-based attenuation correction relies on the segmentation of MR images into different tissue classes, based on their image-based grey scales. Following segmentation, the individual tissue compartments (e.g., background air, fat, soft tissue, lung tissue) are then assigned a predefined LAC for the corresponding tissue (Martinez-Moller et al. 2009; Schulz et al. 2011). To this day, dedicated fast MR imaging sequences, such as Dixon VIBE (Martinez-Moller et al. 2009) or a fast 3D T1-weighted gradient-echo MR sequence, are applied to obtain images of tissue distribution and subsequent segmentation (Beyer et al. 2016). This general method of tissue segmentation from MR images is widely used in all currently available PET/MR systems (Beyer et al. 2016) (Fig. 2.1).

Although the MR-based segmentation techniques for AC in general provide reproducible and straightforward results in most clinical applications, multiple initial studies directly comparing PET quantification in PET/MR with PET/CT have indicated a small but systematic underestimation of PET quantification in PET/MR studies using these MR-based AC methods (Drzezga et al. 2012; Quick et al. 2013; Wiesmüller et al. 2013; Boellaard and Quick 2015). The observed underestimation of PET quantification in PET/MR can be attributed to three methodological challenges of MR-based AC: First, MR-based AC lacks information about the attenuating properties of bone. Second, MR-imaging based AC often shows signal truncations along the patient arms, that are then not considered in MR-based AC. Third, the use of ancillary hardware components, such as RF coils in the field-of-view (FOV) of the PET-detector during simultaneous PET and MR data acquisition cause additional attenuation of photons (Boellaard and Quick 2015).

2.3 Attenuation Correction of Bone

Cortical bone is not considered in the standard MR-based AC approaches. Bone here is classified as soft tissue, consequently, the exact magnitude of PET signal attenuation of bone might be systematically underestimated (Samarin et al. 2012; Akbarzadeh et al. 2013). Samarin et al. (Samarin et al. 2012) evaluated and quantified the amount of underestimation when bone is assigned the linear attenuation coefficient of soft tissue. It was shown, that for most soft-tissue lesions in whole-body examinations, PET quantification would be biased by a few %-points only. In brain PET/MR and when imaging individual bone lesions, however, the classification of bone as soft-tissue causes a significant and regionally variable bias of 20–30% (Samarin et al. 2012). As potential solutions for AC of bone, the use of MR sequences with ultrashort echo times (UTE) (Keereman et al. 2010; Johansson et al. 2011; Navalpakkam et al. 2013; Berker et al. 2012; Grodzki et al. 2012) or zero echo time (ZTE) have been

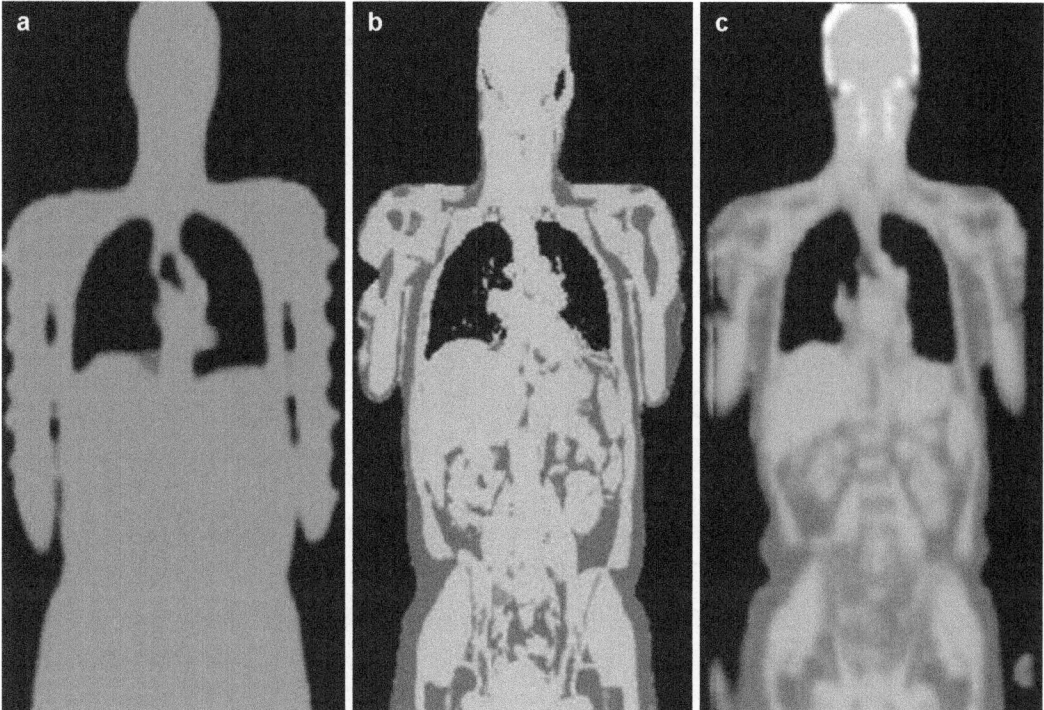

Fig. 2.1 Whole-body MR-based attenuation correction maps in coronal orientation. The AC maps were acquired by scanning one volunteer on all three current PET/MR systems, the Philips Ingenuity TF PET/MR (**a**), the Siemens Biograph mMR (**b**), and the GE Signa PET/MR (**c**). Note that MR-based AC in (**a**) provides three attenuation classes (background, soft tissue and lung), while MR-based AC in (**b** and **c**) provides four classes (background, fat, soft tissue, lung). At the time of this study (2014), system (**c**) additionally provided bone in the head station based on ultrashort echo time sequences. All three AC maps are limited by field-of-view truncations along the arms. Another general limitation in AC is the substitution of major bones by the attenuation coefficients of soft tissue. The figure reflects the state of MR-based AC in the year of measurement, i.e. 2014 (Beyer et al. 2016). To date (2017) further improvements such as bone detection and MR-based truncation correction have been implemented into new product software versions of the PET/MRI systems. (Modified from Beyer et al. 2016)

proposed (Wiesinger et al. 2016; Delso et al. 2015). While studies have shown that UTE-based AC provide accurate PET quantification results when imaging the brain (Johansson et al. 2011; Navalpakkam et al. 2013), their use in body imaging applications is limited (Aasheim 2015). Here, the fact that UTE and ZTE sequences tend to increase image artifacts in large FOV applications such as in body imaging (Navalpakkam et al. 2013) is a practical limitation.

A fast and practical solution for bone AC in whole-body PET/MR has recently been suggested and evaluated (Paulus et al. 2015). This method applies a CT-based 3-dimensional bone-model of the major bones (skull, spine, pelvic bones, upper femora) to the actual MR-based AC

data of the patient under examination and, thus, adds another compartment for the AC of bone in whole-body PET/MR exams (Fig. 2.2) (Paulus et al. 2015). This method has recently been validated in whole-body and brain PET/MR exams with promising results towards improved MR-based AC (Paulus et al. 2015; Koesters et al. 2016; Rausch et al. 2017; Oehmigen et al. 2017).

2.4 Truncation Correction

Another limitation of MR-based AC is the fact that the transaxial FOV in MR imaging is limited to about 50 cm in diameter. Beyond these dimensions, MR images show geometric distortions and

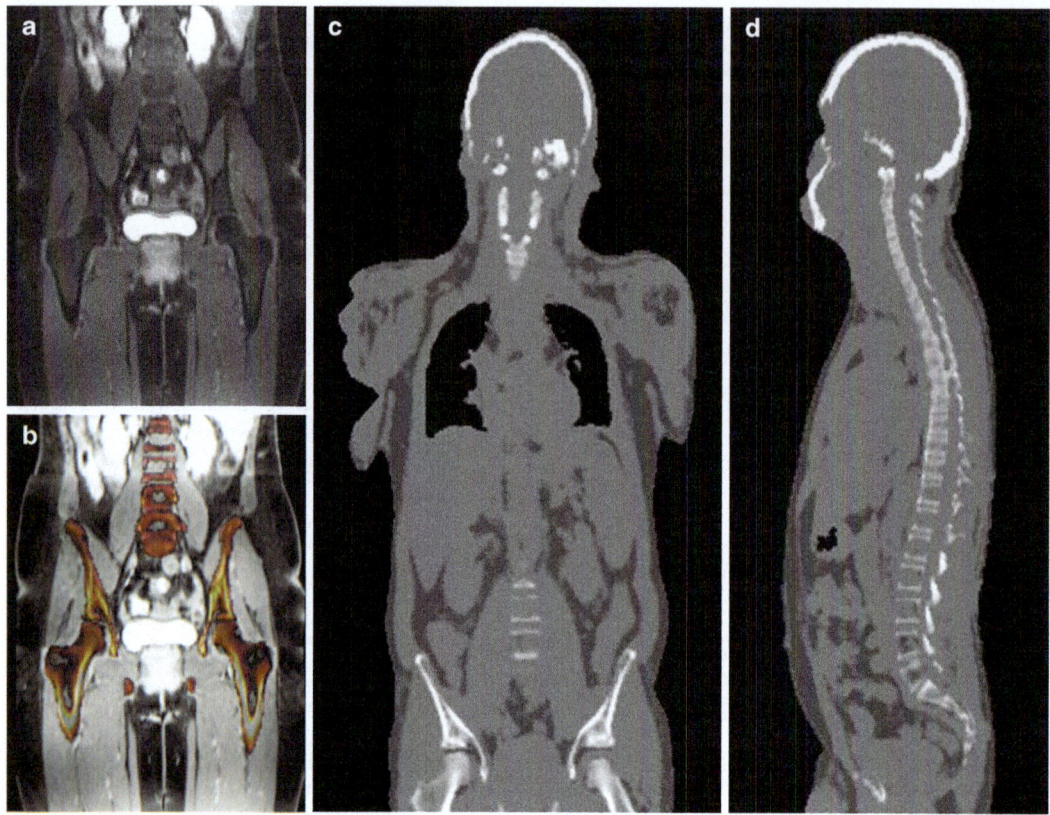

Fig. 2.2 Example for model-based addition of major bones to patient-individual MR data as shown for the pelvic region (**a**, **b**). The bone model consists of a set of MR image and bone mask pairs that are registered to subject's Dixon-sequence images for each major bone individually. Panels (**c** and **d**) show the result of adding bone as additional attenuation class to a whole-body MR-based attenuation map in coronal and sagittal orientation, respectively. (Modified from Paulus et al. 2015)

significant signal voids (Keller et al. 2013; Brendle et al. 2015a). This frequently results in truncation artifacts along the patient arms in MR-based AC, as has been shown for all three currently available PET/MR system designs (Beyer et al. 2016). Therefore, the patient body is not completely and correctly assessed in its overall dimensions and current shape. Thus, the human tissue AC based on truncated MR images does not consider the exact amount and position of tissues that contribute to PET signal attenuation, resulting in inaccurate values for PET quantification (Delso et al. 2010a; Schramm et al. 2013). Accurate PET quantification in PET/MR, thus, requires appropriate methods for truncation correction as part of the attenuation correction strategy.

An appropriate method for truncation correction that is used on all three currently available PET/MR systems is the so-called MLAA (maximum likelihood estimation of attenuation and activity) algorithm (Nuyts et al. 1999, 2013). This PET-based technique derives the outer patient contours from non-AC PET data. This information is then used to complement missing attenuation information from MR imaging data that is truncated due to the limited transaxial FOV of MR imaging (Nuyts et al. 2013). However, MLAA-based contour detection is mostly limited to radiotracers that show a considerable unspecific accumulation in the human body and blood pool, thus enabling the detection of the outer patient contour from PET signals.

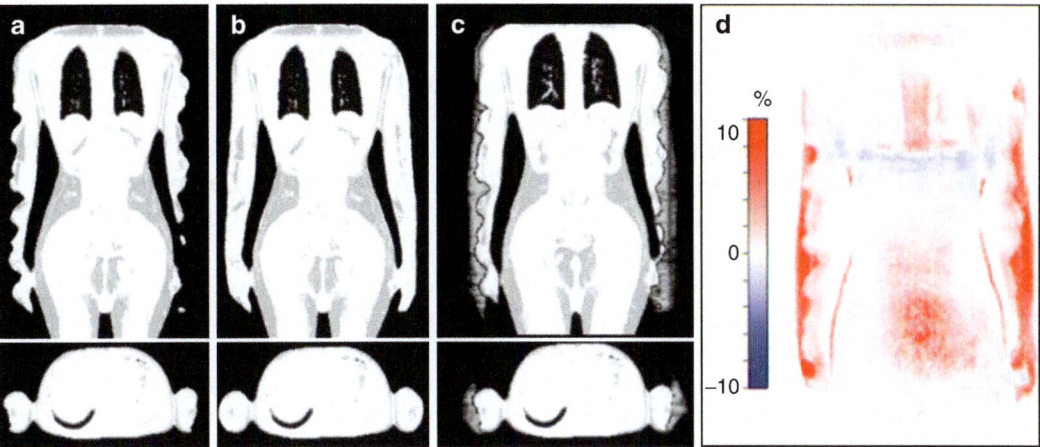

Fig. 2.3 Example for a MR-based attenuation map showing the typical lateral signal truncations along the subjects arms in coronal and transaxial orientation (**a**). Truncations result from the limited field-of-view in MR imaging. Image (**b**) was acquired by applying an optimized readout gradient field provided with the HUGE-method (Blumhagen et al. 2012, 2014). This results in a field-of-view extension and enables truncation correction of the MR-based attenuation correction maps (**b**). Truncation correction of the arms in (**c**) was achieved by applying the widely established MLAA method that derives truncated regions from PET data. The difference map in (**d**) visualizes the quantification bias (in %) between images (**a**) and (**b**), i.e. the quantitative gain by applying HUGE truncation correction. Note that truncation correction applied along the arms has also quantitative impact on the entire body volume (red and blue areas in (**d**)). (Modified from Lindemann et al. 2017)

Another method for truncation correction based on MR data was developed by Blumhagen et al. (Blumhagen et al. 2012). The method is referred to as HUGE ((B_0 homogenization using gradient enhancement) and enlarges the field-of-view in MR imaging beyond the conventional 50 cm diameter (Blumhagen et al. 2012). Foundation of the HUGE method is the measurement of the static magnetic field (B0) and gradient field distributions in the specific PET/MR system. Then, an ideal, non-distorted gradient field is calculated that is applied during MR-based AC in the lateral regions of the MR imaging FOV (Blumhagen et al. 2012). Thus, the lateral MR-based field-of-view can be extended to 60 cm in left-right direction to fully cover the patient's arms. The HUGE method has been successfully evaluated for truncation correction in whole-body PET/MR examinations in the past (Blumhagen et al. 2014). Further technical refinements of the prototype sequence and the combination of HUGE with a moving table acquisition have now resulted in the product version of HUGE that provides seamless MR

data for truncation correction in PET/MR (Lindemann et al. 2017) (Fig. 2.3).

2.5   Motion Correction

The independent and simultaneous PET and MR data acquisition in integrated PET/MR systems inherently offers the potential for motion correction and co-registration of PET and MR data (Quick 2014). This can be considered a potential advantage over PET/CT, which is currently being further explored (Tsoumpas et al. 2010; Tsoumpas et al. 2011; Wuerslin et al. 2013; Grimm et al. 2015; Baumgartner et al. 2014; Catana 2015; Manber et al. 2015; Fürst et al. 2015; Fayad et al. 2015; Gratz et al. 2017). In PET/CT the CT data is static and is acquired only once at the beginning of a typical hybrid examination. Since CT data acquisition is very fast (seconds), CT images provides a snapshot of the body anatomy and state of motion at the time of data acquisition while whole-body PET data is acquired stepwise over several minutes. In

PET/MR, the MR data is acquired simultaneous to PET data, which usually takes several minutes, both for PET and MR data. This leads to less deviation and less gross motion between both imaging modalities when compared to PET/CT hybrid imaging (Brendle et al. 2013). Moreover, real-time MR imaging and 4D MR data of breathing motion can be used to retrospectively perform motion correction of PET data, providing improved fusion of PET and MR data sets (Tsoumpas et al. 2010; 2011; Wuerslin et al. 2013; Grimm et al. 2015; Baumgartner et al. 2014; Catana 2015; Manber et al. 2015; Fürst et al. 2015; Fayad et al. 2015; Gratz et al. 2017). Motion correction strategies in PET/MR, thus, potentially lead to improved lesion visibility in the upper abdomen and liver (Fig. 2.4). Additionally, motion correction may also result in better quantification of activity in lesions and tumours as well as in cardiovascular PET/MR studies since all moving structures are depicted with sharper contours and less smeared over a larger volume, which otherwise leads to reduced standardized uptake values (SUV) of regions subject to motion (Grimm et al. 2015) (Fig. 2.4). In a recent cardiac PET/MR feasibility study, motion correction strategies have been applied to

breathing and cardiac motion to assess atherosclerotic plaques in the coronary arteries (Robson et al. 2017).

2.6 Attenuation Correction of Hardware Components

The previous sections have discussed techniques, limitations, and recent solutions for MR-based AC of the patient body. An additional source of attenuation of the annihilation photons in PET/MR is the use of ancillary hardware components, such as the patient table and radiofrequency (RF) receiver coils that are placed around the patient body for MR signal detection. These hardware components also attenuate photons before they reach the PET detector and, therefore, may cause a bias of the PET quantification, as demonstrated in earlier studies (Delso et al. 2010b; Tellmann et al. 2011). The general concept for AC of hardware components in PET/MR is to generate CT-based attenuation maps of each hardware component that has to be corrected (Quick et al. 2013; Quick 2014), as it is the current standard method on all three current PET/MR systems. Therefore, three-dimensional (3D) CT-based

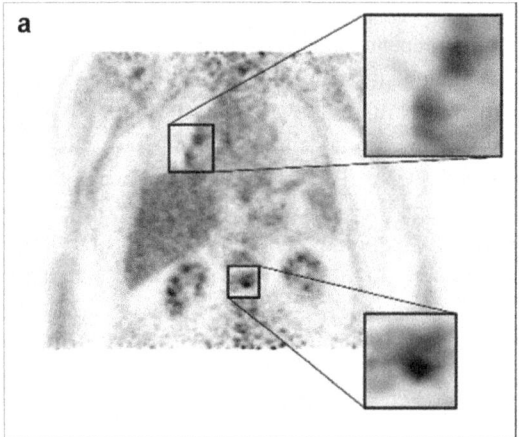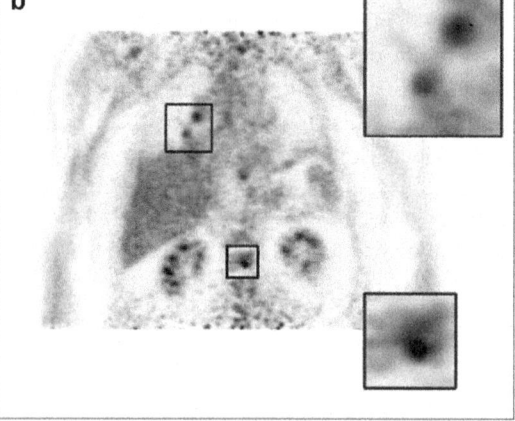

Fig. 2.4 Application of motion correction in a patient with two lesions in the lung and one lesion in the spine. A coronal PET image from a PET/MR study is shown. Image (**a**) was acquired using the standard free-breathing PET protocol with an acquisition time of several minutes. Image (**b**) was acquired by applying respiratory motion correction. For motion correction the MR data was used to derive 3-dimensional motion fields over time that were then used for non-rigid registration of the PET data to one static, motion corrected 3D image. The motion corrected data in (**b**) provides sharper visualization and higher contrast of the two lesions in the lung, while the non-moving lesion in the spine shows identical image features (Modified from Gratz et al. 2017)

attenuation templates for rigid and stationary RF coils such as the head/neck RF coil are added to the overall patient attenuation map prior to the PET data reconstruction (Quick 2014). By automatically linking the current patient table position during a patient examination to the known position of the individual RF coil on the system's patient table, CT-template-based AC can be performed during the PET data reconstruction process (Delso et al. 2010b). This AC method provides fast and accurate results for most of the RF coils that are delivered with the current PET/MR systems. However, the 3D attenuation templates used during reconstruction can be misaligned with the actual RF coil position or not represent the actual attenuation of the RF coils used (Paulus et al. 2012). This is an inherent limitation for flexible (non-rigid) RF surface coils, which are frequently used in whole-body imaging applications to provide excellent MRI signal from the anterior body parts. Flexible RF coils are currently not routinely considered in CT-template-based AC since their position and/or geometry during a PET/MR examination is not known and may differ from a pre-acquired 3D AC template (Paulus et al. 2012). It has been shown in previous studies, that the flexible standard multi-channel RF surface body coils attenuate the PET signal by only few %-points (Paulus et al. 2012, 2013; Wollenweber et al. 2014; Paulus and Quick 2016). Thus, the average attenuation due to flexible RF coils in routine applications of PET/MR seems negligible. However, PET quantification may be locally biased by up to 10–20% due to increased attenuation of PET signal in the immediate vicinity of single hardware components of the RF coils (Paulus et al. 2012, 2013; Paulus and Quick 2016). As an improvement to also consider flexible RF coils in AC, it has been suggested to detect the actual position of flexible RF coils in MR images by using MR visible markers (Kartmann et al. 2013; Eldib et al. 2014) or by using residual MR signal from the RF coil housing when applying UTE sequences (Paulus et al. 2012; Eldib et al. 2015). This spatial information could then be used to align a pre-defined 3D AC template of the respective RF coil with its actual position during a PET/MR examination as derived from MR images. The general concept for CT-based AC of hardware components in PET/MR is implemented in all currently available PET/MR systems for the range of rigid RF coils that are delivered with each PET/MR system (Quick 2014; Paulus and Quick 2016).

2.7 New Hardware Developments

The current PET/MR systems are all equipped with numerous RF coils to cover the patient from head to toe in whole-body imaging applications (Quick 2014; Beyer et al. 2016). Coverage of the entire patient body with RF surface coils is a general precondition for high quality MR imaging. In combined PET/MR, the RF coils are located in the FOV of the PET detector during simultaneous PET and MRI data acquisition. Thus, an additional design requirement for RF coil in PET/MR is, that the RF coils need to be as PET transparent as possible in order to reduce unwanted PET signal attenuation. Nevertheless, although designed PET transparent, all RF coils are subject to attenuation correction to provide accurate PET quantification as has been described in the previous section. A recent overview article by Paulus and Quick (2016) provides a summary of numerous RF coil developments for PET/MR applications and their individual impact on PET quantification (Paulus and Quick 2016).

To expand the portfolio of clinical applications of PET/MR and to improve dedicated examinations, new and specific RF coils were designed over the recent years for combined use in PET/MR. For example, new multi-channel RF head coils have been designed to improve neuro imaging and to increase the performance of simultaneous functional MR imaging (fMRI) with PET imaging (Sander et al. 2015). Three recent studies have described the design and implementation of bilateral breast RF coils for PET/MR breast imaging (Aklan et al. 2013; Dregely et al. 2015; Oehmigen et al. 2016). The integration of such breast RF coils requires a PET-transparent design and consideration of the ancillary RF coil

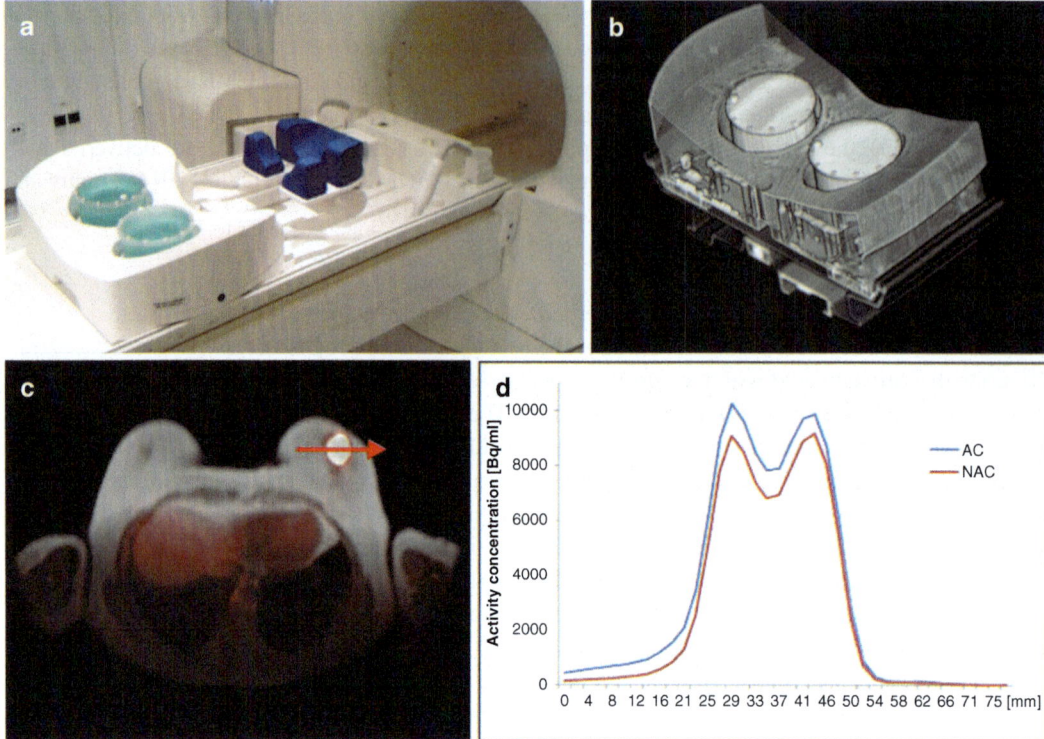

Fig. 2.5 Broadening the application spectrum of PET/MR by integration of a breast radiofrequency (RF) coil. 16-channel breast RF coil that was designed PET transparent for use in PET/MR systems (Rapid Biomedical, Germany) (**a**). (**b**) 3-Dimensional CT-based attenuation template for attenuation correction of the RF coil housing. (**c**) Example case of patient with breast carcinoma imaged on PET/MR with the RF breast coil. (**d**) Quantitative evaluation of activity concentration in the breast tumour along the red arrow (in **c**). The blue line plot shows the activity in the tumour after attenuation correction of the RF breast coil. The red line plot shows lower activity values because the RF breast coil here was not included in attenuation correction. (Modified from Oehmigen et al. 2016)

hardware in the attenuation correction (Aklan et al. 2013; Dregely et al. 2015, 2016). Figure 2.5 provides an example of a 16-channel breast RF coil that was implemented into an integrated PET/MR system with hardware attenuation correction (Oehmigen et al. 2016).

Two recent studies describe the development of equipment for radiation therapy (RT) planning for use in PET/MR. The overall aim of this endeavour is to integrate PET/MR hybrid imaging into the concept of RT planning, which would further broaden the application spectrum of PET/MR (Paulus et al. 2014, 2016). The developments encompass PET transparent hardware components such as a table platform with indexing system and RF coil holders for head/neck imaging as well as for body imaging (Paulus et al. 2014, 2016). All components have been evaluated for use in PET/MR. A systematic μmap generator ensures accurate attenuation correction of all RT equipment in the FOV of the PET detector (Paulus et al. 2014). All these recent RF coil and hardware component developments have laid the groundwork for new clinical applications of PET/MR and further developments of dedicated RF coils are ongoing. The additional efforts in hardware component AC at the same time ensure accurate PET quantification for these exciting new applications (Paulus and Quick 2016).

2.8 Artifact Correction

The implementation of new imaging modalities and / or technical systems goes hand in hand with new types of artifacts. The complexity of integrated PET/MR hybrid imaging bears the potential for an exaggeration of new artifacts, when compared to two independent systems. Beyond the potential affection of the visual impression of either PET or MR data, artifacts in PET/MR may also have a significant effect on quantification of PET data. Artifacts in integrated PET/MR may result from the technical crosstalk between the PET and the MR components (Delso et al. 2011; Quick 2014), e.g. when both imaging centers may not be co-aligned correctly (Brendle et al. 2013). Differences in the data acquisition speed between PET and MR might lead to local misalignments and motion artifacts due to patient and organ motion (Brendle et al. 2013). In MR-based AC all deviations from the real physical photon attenuation will ultimately lead to inaccurate values in PET quantification following AC (Keereman et al. 2011; Ladefoged et al. 2014; Brendle et al. 2015). Furthermore, the administration of contrast agents before the application of MR-based AC may lead to errors in MR-based tissue segmentation due to changes in tissue contrast (Ruhlmann et al. 2016). Per definition, the signal truncations as discussed above also represent MR-based artifacts that have an influence on PET quantification (Delso et al. 2010a; Blumhagen et al. 2012, 2014). A frequent source for MR-based artifacts are dental and metal implants that are found in a large and increasing group of patients (Gunzinger et al. 2014; Ladefoged et al. 2015; Schramm et al. 2014). Apart from the safety aspects of metal implants that have to be clarified for any MR examination, all metal implants might cause signal voids or local distortions in MR images and in MR-based AC, that exceed the physical implant volume. During image segmentation, such signal voids might then be assigned with the low linear attenuation coefficients of air (Gunzinger et al. 2014; Ladefoged et al. 2015; Schramm et al. 2014).

While initial publications dealt with the description of artifacts and evaluation of their impact on PET/MR, more recent studies now report about developments to correct for artifacts. A relatively simple approach to improve the MR-based µmap, is to use inpainting to fill signal voids arising from metal artifacts (Ladefoged et al. 2013). Thus, signal voids simulating regions with the low LAC of air are removed and the higher value LAC of the surrounding tissue is assigned (Ladefoged et al. 2013). Beyond the visual improvement of data, this may improve PET quantification as well. However, when larger metal and ceramic implants such as knee or hip joints are involved, PET quantification following µmap inpainting will still be biased due to the fact, that the real high LAC of these metallic implants is not accurately considered. Fuin et al. have suggested a method to complete signal voids in the MR-based attenuation correction data caused by implants by deriving the shape and AC values of metal implants from PET emission data (Fuin et al. 2017). In the context of metal artifact reduction in PET/MR, it has been shown that time-of-flight (TOF) PET detection with fast PET detectors allows for a significant visual reduction of artifacts in the µmap (Davison et al. 2015; Ter Voert et al. 2017), albeit PET quantification may still be biased. For the near future, it is expected that also the current breed of new artifact reducing MR imaging sequences (e.g. MAVRIC, VAT, WARP, etc.) (Sutter et al. 2012; Talbot and Weinberg 2016; Dillenseger et al. 2016; Jungmann et al. 2017) will find their implementation in dedicated PET/MR imaging protocols. In MR-only applications, such sequences have facilitated a significant reduction of the volume of distortions and signal voids around metallic implants (Sutter et al. 2012; Talbot and Weinberg 2016; Dillenseger et al. 2016; Jungmann et al. 2017). In the PET/MR regime, this could be used to further improve µmaps, and consequently, to improve PET quantification in PET/MR of patients with implants.

2.9   Dose Reduction

Integrated PET/MR hybrid imaging in selected clinical applications inherently reduces the overall patient radiation dose when compared with PET/CT by replacing ionizing CT imaging by non-ionizing MR imaging (Boellaard et al.

2010). Depending on the clinical indication, replacing CT by MR imaging in the context of PET hybrid imaging theoretically may save half of the overall radiation dose or an even higher fraction when compared with high-resolution diagnostic CT imaging (Boellaard et al. 2010). Further potential for radiotracer dose reduction in integrated PET/MR resides in the possibility of decreasing the applied activity deriving from the administered PET radiotracer. PET image quality in general is influenced by two key factors, acquisition time and injected activity, as both affect count statistics, image signal, and image noise. In PET/MR imaging, radiotracer dose reduction by injecting less tracer activity may be achieved by turning the comparatively prolonged data acquisition times into an advantage. In conventional PET/CT hybrid imaging, the PET data acquisition times typically amount to 2–3 min per bed position (Boellaard et al. 2010). In integrated PET/MR hybrid imaging, the MR examination time may be longer depending on the study protocol and clinical application field, respectively.

The higher sensitivity and larger volume coverage of new PET detectors in PET/MR systems compared to PET/CT (Delso et al. 2011) provides a third precondition for the potential to reduce the applied activity while maintaining high SNR and excellent PET image quality (Queiroz et al. 2015).

These potential advantages of PET/MR towards reducing the overall radiation dose compared to PET/CT is currently explored in selected studies. Based on the findings in controlled phantom studies (Oehmigen et al. 2014), or by simulating reduced amounts of applied activity by shortening the acquired PET list-mode data (Hartung-Knemeyer et al. 2013; Gatidis et al. 2016c), initial studies indicate that the reduction of radiotracer does not hamper diagnostic image quality in PET/MR examinations (Hartung-Knemeyer et al. 2013; Seith et al. 2017). These efforts can be considered particularly important in clinical settings for pediatric imaging or repetitive scans for therapy monitoring or surveillance (Gatidis et al. 2016a, b).

Conclusion

Today, many of the technical and methodological challenges of PET/MR imaging that were considered roadblocks to clinical PET/MRI during the early phase of implementation have been overcome. Numerous innovative solutions for attenuation correction, truncation correction, and motion correction have been suggested and scientifically evaluated during the past years. Of these, some of the most accurate and practical developments have found their way from research applications into the most recent product software applications of all PET/MR systems. Together with further hardware developments, this emerging hybrid imaging method is constantly improved and the clinical application spectrum of PET/MR is further increased.

References

Aasheim LB, Karlberg A, Goa PE, et al. PET/MR brain imaging: evaluation of clinical UTE-based attenuation correction. Eur J Nucl Med Mol Imaging. 2015;42(2015):1439–46.

Akbarzadeh A, Ay MR, Ahmadian A, Alam NR, Zaidi H. MRI-guided attenuation correction in whole-body PET/MR: assessment of the effect of bone attenuation. Ann Nucl Med. 2013;27:152–62.

Aklan B, Paulus DH, Wenkel E, Braun H, Navalpakkam BK, Ziegler S, Geppert C, Sigmund EE, Melsaether A, Quick HH. Toward simultaneous PET/MR breast imaging: systematic evaluation and integration of a radiofrequency breast coil. Med Phys. 2013;40(2):024301.

Baumgartner CF, Kolbitsch C, Balfour DR, Marsden PK, McClelland JR, Rueckert D, King AP. High-resolution dynamic MR imaging of the thorax for respiratory motion correction of PET using groupwise manifold alignment. Med Image Anal. 2014;18:939–52.

Berker Y, Franke J, Salomon A, Palmowski M, Donker HC, Temur Y, Mottaghy FM, Kuhl C, Izquierdo-Garcia D, Fayad ZA, Kiessling F, Schulz V. MRI-based attenuation correction for hybrid PET/MRI systems: a 4-class tissue segmentation technique using a combined ultrashort-echo-time/Dixon MRI sequence. J Nucl Med. 2012;53:796–804.

Beyer T, Lassen ML, Boellaard R, Delso G, Yaqub M, Sattler B, Quick HH. Investigating the state-of-the-art in whole-body MR-based attenuation correction: an intra-individual, inter-system, inventory study on three clinical PET/MR systems. MAGMA. 2016;29:75–87.

Blumhagen JO, Braun H, Ladebeck R, Fenchel M, Faul D, Scheffler K, Quick HH. Field of view extension and truncation correction for MR-based human attenuation correction in simultaneous MR/PET imaging. Med Phys. 2014;41:022303.

Blumhagen JO, Ladebeck R, Fenchel M, Scheffler K. MR-based field-of-view extension in MR/PET: B(0) homogenization using gradient enhancement (HUGE). Magn Reson Med. 2012;70:1047–57.

Boellaard R, O'Doherty MJ, Weber WA, et al. FDG PET and PET/CT: EANM procedure guidelines for tumor PET imaging—version 1.0. Eur J Nucl Med Mol Imaging. 2010;37:181–200.

Boellaard R, Quick HH. Current image acquisition options in PET/MR. Semin Nucl Med. 2015;45:192–200. Review

Brendle C, Schmidt H, Oergel A, Bezrukov I, Mueller M, Schraml C, Pfannenberg C, la Fougère C, Nikolaou K, Schwenzer N. Segmentation-based attenuation correction in positron emission tomography/magnetic resonance: erroneous tissue identification and its impact on positron emission tomography interpretation. Investig Radiol. 2015a;50(5):339–46.

Brendle C, Schmidt H, Oergel A, Bezrukov I, Mueller M, Schraml C, Pfannenberg C, la Fougère C, Nikolaou K, Schwenzer N. Segmentation-based attenuation correction in positron emission tomography/magnetic resonance: erroneous tissue identification and its impact on positron emission tomography interpretation. Investig Radiol. 2015b;50(5):339–46.

Brendle CB, Schmidt H, Fleischer S, Braeuning UH, Pfannenberg CA, Schwenzer NF. Simultaneously acquired MR/PET images compared with sequential MR/PET and PET/CT: alignment quality. Radiology. 2013;268(1):190–9.

Carney JP, Townsend DW, Rappoport V, Bendriem B. Method for transforming CT images for attenuation correction in PET/CT imaging. Med Phys. 2006;33:976–83.

Catana C. Motion correction options in PET/MRI. Semin Nucl Med. 2015;45:212–23. Review

Davison H, ter Voert EE, de Galiza Barbosa F, Veit-Haibach P, Delso G. Incorporation of time-of-flight information reduces metal artifacts in simultaneous positron emission tomography/magnetic resonance imaging: a simulation study. Investig Radiol. 2015;50(7):423–9.

Delso G, Furst S, Jakoby B, Ladebeck R, Ganter C, Nekolla SG, et al. Performance measurements of the Siemens mMR integrated whole-body PET/MR scanner. J Nucl Med. 2011;52:1914–22.

Delso G, Martinez-Möller A, Bundschuh RA, Ladebeck R, Candidus Y, Faul D, Ziegler SI. Evaluation of the attenuation properties of MR equipment for its use in a whole-body PET/MR scanner. Phys Med Biol. 2010b;55:4361–74.

Delso G, Martinez-Möller A, Bundschuh RA, Nekolla SG, Ziegler SI. The effect of limited MR field of view in MR/PET attenuation correction. Med Phys. 2010a;37:2804–12.

Delso G, Wiesinger F, Sacolick LI, Kaushik SS, Shanbhag DD, Hüllner M, Veit-Haibach P. Clinical evaluation of zero-echo-time MR imaging for the segmentation of the skull. J Nucl Med. 2015;56(3):417–22.

Dillenseger JP, Molière S, Choquet P, Goetz C, Ehlinger M, Bierry G. An illustrative review to understand and manage metal-induced artifacts in musculoskeletal MRI: a primer and updates. Skelet Radiol. 2016;45(5):677–88. https://doi.org/10.1007/s00256-016-2338-2. Epub 2016 Feb 2. Review.

Dregely I, Lanz T, Metz S, Mueller MF, Kuschan M, Nimbalkar M, Bundschuh RA, Ziegler SI, Haase A, Nekolla SG, Schwaiger M. A 16-channel MR coil for simultaneous PET/MR imaging in breast cancer. Eur Radiol. 2015;25(4):1154–61.

Drzezga A, Souvatzoglou M, Eiber M, Beer AJ, Fürst S, Martinez-Möller A, Nekolla SG, Ziegler S, Ganter C, Rummeny EJ, Schwaiger M. First clinical experience with integrated whole-body PET/MR: comparison to PET/CT in patients with oncologic diagnoses. J Nucl Med. 2012;53:845–55.

Eldib M, Bini J, Calcagno C, Robson PM, Mani V, Fayad ZA. Attenuation correction for flexible magnetic resonance coils in combined magnetic resonance/positron emission tomography imaging. Investig Radiol. 2014;49:63–9.

Eldib M, Bini J, Robson PM, Calcagno C, Faul DD, Tsoumpas C, Fayad ZA. Markerless attenuation correction for carotid MRI surface receiver coils in combined PET/MR imaging. Phys Med Biol. 2015;60:4705–17.

Fayad H, Schmidt H, Wuerslin C, Visvikis D. Reconstruction-incorporated respiratory motion correction in clinical simultaneous PET/MR imaging for oncology applications. J Nucl Med. 2015;56:884–9.

Fuin N, Pedemonte S, Catalano OA, Izquierdo-Garcia D, Soricelli A, Salvatore M, Heberlein K, Hooker JM, Van Leemput K, Catana C. PET/MRI in the presence of metal implants: completion of the attenuation map from PET emission data. J Nucl Med. 2017;58(5):840–5.

Fürst S, Grimm R, Hong I, Souvatzoglou M, Casey ME, Schwaiger M, Nekolla SG, Ziegler SI. Motion correction strategies for integrated PET/MR. J Nucl Med. 2015;56:261–9.

Gatidis S, Schmidt H, Gücke B, Bezrukov I, Seitz G, Ebinger M, Reimold M, Pfannenberg CA, Nikolaou K, Schwenzer NF, Schäfer JF. Comprehensive oncologic imaging in infants and preschool children with substantially reduced radiation exposure using combined simultaneous ^{18}F-fluorodeoxyglucose positron emission tomography/magnetic resonance imaging: a direct comparison to ^{18}F-fluorodeoxyglucose positron emission tomography/computed tomography. Investig Radiol. 2016b;51(1):7–14.

Gatidis S, Schmidt H, la Fougère C, Nikolaou K, Schwenzer NF, Schäfer JF. Defining optimal tracer activities in pediatric oncologic whole-body ^{18}F-FDG-PET/MRI. Eur J Nucl Med Mol Imaging. 2016a;43(13):2283–9.

Gatidis S, Würslin C, Seith F, Schäfer JF, la Fougère C, Nikolaou K, Schwenzer NF, Schmidt H. Towards tracer dose reduction in PET studies: Simulation of dose reduction by retrospective randomized undersampling of list-mode data. Hell J Nucl Med. 2016c;19(1):15–8. https://doi.org/10.1967/s002449910333. Epub 2016 Mar 1

Grant AM, Deller TW, Khalighi MM, Maramraju SH, Delso G, Levin CS. NEMA NU 2-2012 performance studies for the SiPM-based ToF-PET component of the GE SIGNA PET/MR system. Med Phys. 2016;43:2334.

Gratz M, Ruhlmann V, Umutlu L, Fenchel M, Quick HH. Impact of MR-based motion correction on clinical PET/MR data of patients with thoracic pathologies. In Proc. ISMRM 2017, Apr 21–27; Honolulu, HI, USA. 2017 p. 3899.

Grimm R, Fürst S, Souvatzoglou M, Forman C, Hutter J, Dregely I, Ziegler SI, Kiefer B, Hornegger J, Block KT, Nekolla SG. Self-gated MRI motion modeling for respiratory motion compensation in integrated PET/MRI. Med Image Anal. 2015;19:110–20.

Grodzki DM, Jakob PM, Heismann B. Ultrashort echo time imaging using pointwise encoding time reduction with radial acquisition (PETRA). Magn Reson Med. 2012;67:510–8.

Gunzinger JM, Delso G, Boss A, Porto M, Davison H, von Schulthess GK, Huellner M, Stolzmann P, Veit-Haibach P, Burger IA. Metal artifact reduction in patients with dental implants using multispectral three-dimensional data acquisition for hybrid PET/MRI. EJNMMI Phys. 2014;1(1):102.

Hartung-Knemeyer V, Beiderwellen KJ, Buchbender C, Kuehl H, Lauenstein TC, Bockisch A, Poeppel TD. Optimizing positron emission tomography image acquisition protocols in integrated positron emission tomography/magnetic resonance imaging. Investig Radiol. 2013;48(5):290–4.

Johansson A, Karlsson M, Nyholm T. CT substitute derived from MRI sequences with ultrashort echo time. Med Phys. 2011;38:2708–14.

Jungmann PM, Agten CA, Pfirrmann CW, Sutter R. Advances in MRI around metal. J Magn Reson Imaging 2017. doi: https://doi.org/10.1002/jmri.25708. [Epub ahead of print] Review.

Kartmann R, Paulus DH, Braun H, Aklan B, Ziegler S, Navalpakkam BK, Lentschig M, Quick HH. Integrated PET/MR imaging: automatic attenuation correction of flexible RF coils. Med Phys. 2013;40:082301.

Keereman V, Fierens Y, Broux T, De Deene Y, Lonneux M, Vandenberghe S. MRI-based attenuation correction for PET/MRI using ultrashort echo time sequences. J Nucl Med. 2010;51:812–8.

Keereman V, Holen RV, Mollet P, Vandenberghe S. The effect of errors in segmented attenuation maps on PET quantification. Med Phys. 2011;38:6010–9.

Keller SH, Holm S, Hansen AE, Sattler B, Andersen F, Klausen TL, Højgaard L, Kjær A, Beyer T. Image artifacts from MR-based attenuation correction in clinical, whole-body PET/MRI. MAGMA. 2013;26(1):173–81.

Kinahan PE, Townsend DW, Beyer T, Sashin D. Attenuation correction for a combined 3D PET/CT scanner. Med Phys. 1998;25:2046–53.

Koesters T, Friedman KP, Fenchel M, Zhan Y, Hermosillo G, Babb J, Jelescu IO, Faul D, Boada FE, Shepherd TM. Dixon sequence with superimposed model-based bone compartment provides highly accurate PET/MR attenuation correction of the brain. J Nucl Med. 2016;57(6):918–24.

Ladefoged CN, Andersen FL, Keller SH, Löfgren J, Hansen AE, Holm S, Højgaard L, Beyer T. PET/MR imaging of the pelvis in the presence of endoprostheses: reducing image artifacts and increasing accuracy through inpainting. Eur J Nucl Med Mol Imaging. 2013;40(4):594–601.

Ladefoged CN, Hansen AE, Keller SH, Fischer BM, Rasmussen JH, Law I, Kjær A, Højgaard L, Lauze F, Beyer T, Andersen FL. Dental artifacts in the head and neck region: implications for Dixon-based attenuation correction in PET/MR. EJNMMI Phys. 2015;2(1):8. https://doi.org/10.1186/s40658-015-0112-5.

Ladefoged CN, Hansen AE, Keller SH, Holm S, Law I, Beyer T, Højgaard L, Kjær A, Andersen FL. Impact of incorrect tissue classification in Dixon-based MR-AC: fat-water tissue inversion. EJNMMI Phys. 2014;1(1):101. https://doi.org/10.1186/s40658-014-0101-0. Epub 2014 Dec 14

Lindemann ME, Oehmigen M, Blumhagen JO, Gratz M, Quick HH. MR-based truncation and attenuation correction in integrated PET/MR hybrid imaging using HUGE with continuous table motion. Med Phys. 2017;44(9):4559–72.

Manber R, Thielemans K, Hutton BF, Barnes A, Ourselin S, Arridge S, O'Meara C, Wan S, Atkinson D. Practical PET respiratory motion correction in clinical PET/MR. J Nucl Med. 2015;56:890–6.

Martinez-Moller A, Souvatzoglou M, Delso G, Bundschuh RA, Chefd'hotel C, Ziegler SI, Navab N, Schwaiger M, Nekolla SG. Tissue classification as a potential approach for attenuation correction in whole-body PET/MRI: evaluation with PET/CT data. J Nucl Med. 2009;50:520–6.

Navalpakkam BK, Braun H, Kuwert T, Quick HH. Magnetic resonance-based attenuation correction for PET/MR hybrid imaging using continuous valued attenuation maps. Investig Radiol. 2013;48:323–32.

Nuyts J, Bal G, Kehren F, Fenchel M, Michel C, Watson C. Completion of a truncated attenuation image from the attenuated PET emission data. IEEE Trans Med Imaging. 2013;32:237–46.

Nuyts J, Dupont P, Stroobants S, Benninck R, Mortelmans L, Suetens P. Simultaneous maximum a posteriori reconstruction of attenuation and activity distributions from emission sinograms. IEEE Trans Med Imaging. 1999;18:393–403.

Oehmigen M, Lindemann ME, Gratz M, Kirchner J, Ruhlmann V, Umutlu L, Blumhagen JO, Fenchel M, Quick HH. Impact of improved attenuation correction featuring a bone atlas and truncation correction on PET quantification in whole-body PET/MR. Eur J Nucl Med Mol Imaging. 2017 Nov 9. doi:10.1007/s00259-017-3864-4. [Epub ahead of print]

Oehmigen M, Lindemann ME, Lanz T, Kinner S, Quick HH. Integrated PET/MR breast cancer imaging: Attenuation correction and implementation of a 16-channel RF coil. Med Phys. 2016;43(8):4808.

Oehmigen M, Ziegler S, Jakoby BW, Georgi JC, Paulus DH, Quick HH. Radiotracer dose reduction in integrated PET/MR: implications from national electrical manufacturers association phantom studies. J Nucl Med. 2014;55(8):1361–7.

Paulus D, Braun H, Aklan B, Quick HH, Simultaneous PET. MR imaging: MR-based attenuation correction of local radiofrequency surface coils. Med Phys. 2012;39:4306–15.

Paulus DH, Oehmigen M, Grüneisen J, Umutlu L, Quick HH. Whole-body hybrid imaging concept for the integration of PET/MR into radiation therapy treatment planning. Phys Med Biol. 2016;61(9):3504–20.

Paulus DH, Quick HH. Hybrid positron emission tomography/magnetic resonance imaging: challenges, methods, and state of the art of hardware component attenuation correction. Investig Radiol. 2016;51:624–34.

Paulus DH, Quick HH, Geppert C, Fenchel M, Zhan Y, Hermosillo G, Faul D, Boada F, Friedman KP, Koesters T. Whole-body PET/MR imaging: quantitative evaluation of a novel model-based MR attenuation correction method including bone. J Nucl Med. 2015;56:1061–6.

Paulus DH, Tellmann L, Quick HH. Towards improved hardware component attenuation correction in PET/MR hybrid imaging. Phys Med Biol. 2013;58: 8021–40.

Paulus DH, Thorwath D, Schmidt H, Quick HH. Towards integration of PET/MR hybrid imaging into radiation therapy treatment planning. Med Phys. 2014;41(7):072505.

Queiroz MA, Delso G, Wollenweber S, Deller T, Zeimpekis K, Huellner M, de Galiza Barbosa F, von Schulthess G, Veit-Haibach P. Dose Optimization in TOF-PET/MR Compared to TOF-PET/CT. PLoS One. 2015;10(7):e0128842.

Quick HH. Integrated PET/MR. J Magn Reson Imaging. 2014;39:243–58.

Quick HH, von Gall C, Zeilinger M, Wiesmüller M, Braun H, Ziegler S, Kuwert T, Uder M, Dörfler A, Kalender WA, Lell M. Integrated whole-body PET/MR hybrid imaging: clinical experience. Investig Radiol. 2013;48:280–9.

Rausch I, Quick HH, Cal-Gonzalez J, Sattler B, Boellaard R, Beyer T. Technical and instrumentational foundations of PET/MRI. Eur J Radiol. 2017;94:A3-A13. doi: 10.1016/j.ejrad.2017.04.004. Epub 2017 Apr 8. Review

Robson PM, Dweck MR, Trivieri MG, Abgral R, Karakatsanis NA, Contreras J, Gidwani U, Narula JP, Fuster V, Kovacic JC, Fayad ZA. Coronary Artery PET/MR imaging: feasibility, limitations, and solutions. JACC Cardiovasc Imaging. 2017. https://doi.org/10.1016/j.jcmg.2016.09.029. [Epub ahead of print]

Ruhlmann V, Heusch P, Kühl H, Beiderwellen K, Antoch G, Forsting M, Bockisch A, Buchbender C, Quick HH. Potential influence of Gadolinium contrast on image segmentation in MR-based attenuation correction with Dixon sequences in whole-body 18F-FDG PET/MR. MAGMA. 2016;29(2):301–8.

Samarin A, Burger C, Wollenweber SD, Crook DW, Burger IA, Schmid DT, von Schulthess GK, Kuhn FP. PET/MR imaging of bone lesions - implications for PET quantification from imperfect attenuation correction. Eur J Nucl Med Mol Imaging. 2012;39:1154–60.

Sander CY, Keil B, Chonde DB, Rosen BR, Catana C, Wald LL. A 31-channel MR brain array coil compatible with positron emission tomography. Magn Reson Med. 2015;73(6):2363–75.

Schramm G, Langner J, Hofheinz F, Petr J, Lougovski A, Beuthien-Baumann B, Platzek I, van den Hoff J. Influence and compensation of truncation artifacts in MR-based attenuation correction in PET/MR. IEEE Trans Med Imaging. 2013;32:2056–63.

Schramm G, Maus J, Hofheinz F, Petr J, Lougovski A, Beuthien-Baumann B, Platzek I, van den Hoff J. Evaluation and automatic correction of metal-implant-induced artifacts in MR-based attenuation correction in whole-body PET/MR imaging. Phys Med Biol. 2014;59(11):2713–26.

Schulz V, Torres-Espallardo I, Renisch S, Hu Z, Ojha N, Börnert P, Perkuhn M, Niendorf T, Schäfer WM, Brockmann H, Krohn T, Buhl A, Günther RW, Mottaghy FM, Krombach GA. Automatic, three-segment, MR-based attenuation correction for whole-body PET/MR data. Eur J Nucl Med Mol Imaging. 2011;38:138–52.

Seith F, Schmidt H, Kunz J, Kuestner T, Gatidis S, Nikolaou K, la Fougère C, Schwenzer NF. Simulation of tracer dose reduction in ^{18}F-FDG-Positron emission tomography / magnetic resonance imaging (PET/MRI): Effects on oncologic reading, image quality and artifacts. J Nucl Med. 2017. https://doi.org/10.2967/jnumed.116.184440. pii: jnumed.116.184440. [Epub ahead of print]

Sutter R, Ulbrich EJ, Jellus V, Nittka M, Pfirrmann CW. Reduction of metal artifacts in patients with total hip arthroplasty with slice-encoding metal artifact correction and view-angle tilting MR imaging. Radiology. 2012;265(1):204–14.

Talbot BS, Weinberg EP. MR Imaging with metal-suppression sequences for evaluation of total joint arthroplasty. Radiographics. 2016;36(1):209–25. https://doi.org/10.1148/rg.2016150075. Epub 2015 Nov 20. Review

Tellmann L, Quick HH, Bockisch A, Herzog H, Beyer T. The effect of MR surface coils on PET quantification in whole-body PET/MR: results from a pseudo-PET/MR phantom study. Med Phys. 2011;38(5):2795–805.

Ter Voert EE, Veit-Haibach P, Ahn S, Wiesinger F, Khalighi MM, Levin CS, Iagaru AH, Zaharchuk G, Huellner M, Delso G. Clinical evaluation of TOF versus non-TOF on PET artifacts in simultaneous PET/MR: a dual centre experience. Eur J Nucl Med Mol

Imaging. 2017. https://doi.org/10.1007/s00259-017-3619-2. [Epub ahead of print].

Tsoumpas C, Buerger C, King AP, Mollet P, Keereman V, Vandenberghe S, Schulz V, Schleyer P, Schaeffter T, Marsden PK. Fast generation of 4D PET-MR data from real dynamic MR acquisitions. Phys Med Biol. 2011;56:6597–613.

Tsoumpas C, Mackewn JE, Halsted P, King AP, Buerger C, Totman JJ, Schaeffter T, Marsden PK. Simultaneous PET-MR acquisition and MR-derived motion fields for correction of non-rigid motion in PET. Ann Nucl Med. 2010;24:745–50.

Wagenknecht G, Kaiser H-JJ, Mottaghy FM, Herzog H. MRI for attenuation correction in PET: Methods and challenges. Magn Reson Mater Phys Biol Med. 2013;26:99–113.

Wiesinger F, Sacolick LI, Menini A, Kaushik SS, Ahn S, Veit-Haibach P, Delso G, Shanbhag DD. Zero TE MR bone imaging in the head. Magn Reson Med. 2016;75:107–14.

Wiesmüller M, Quick HH, Navalpakkam B, Lell MM, Uder M, Ritt P, Schmidt D, Beck M, Kuwert T, von Gall CC. Comparison of lesion detection and quantitation of tracer uptake between PET from a simultaneously acquiring whole-body PET/MR hybrid scanner and PET from PET/CT. Eur J Nucl Med Mol Imaging. 2013;40(1):12–21.

Wollenweber SD, Delso G, Deller T, Goldhaber D, Hüllner M, Veit-Haibach P. Characterization of the impact to PET quantification and image quality of an anterior array surface coil for PET/MR imaging. MAGMA. 2014;27:149–59. Review

Wuerslin C, Schmidt H, Martirosian P, Brendle C, Boss A, Schwenzer NF, Stegger L. Respiratory motion correction in oncologic PET using T1-weighted MR imaging on a simultaneous whole-body PET/MR system. J Nucl Med. 2013;54:464–71.

Zaidi H, Ojha N, Morich M, Griesmer J, Hu Z, Maniawski P, Ratib O, Izquierdo-Garcia D, Fayad ZA, Shao L. Design and performance evaluation of a whole-body Ingenuity TF PET-MRI system. Phys Med Biol. 2011;56(10):3091–106.

Oncology

3

Benedikt M. Schaarschmidt, Lino M. Sawicki,
Gerald Antoch, and Philipp Heusch

3.1 Introduction

^{18}F-FDG PET/CT imaging has become an integral part in oncological imaging. Albeit an unspecific tracer for glucose metabolism, the increased uptake of ^{18}F-FDG in tumor cells due to their increased glucose metabolism, known as the "warburg effect", makes ^{18}F-FDG a highly useful tracer for the detection of metastatic disease in many cancer types (Warburg 1924; Lewis et al. 1994). However, the true potential of this imaging method can only be unleashed if a precise anatomic allocation of a focus exhibiting an increased glucose metabolism can be achieved. Hence, only the combination of PET and CT imaging in one single modality, PET/CT, has led to the widespread use of ^{18}F-FDG PET imaging in clinical practice and the introduction into several guidelines, most notably in lung and head and neck cancer (Grégoire et al. 2010; Goeckenjan et al. 2010; National Collaborating Centre for Cancer (UK) 2011; Wolff et al. 2012).

Despite its advantages, the low soft tissue contrast of CT makes the evaluation of several body regions difficult. In local tumor assessment, especially the precise prediction of local tumor infiltration can be problematic, most notably in head and neck cancer or soft tissue sarcoma (Antoch and Bockisch 2009; Pichler et al. 2010). In the evaluation of distant metastases, especially small metastases can be difficult to detect on PET images in tissues with a high background uptake such as the liver or the brain (Posther et al. 2006; Kong et al. 2008). Unfortunately, even contrast enhanced CT imaging does not increase the diagnostic accuracy in this regard.

Therefore, the idea of combining PET and MRI in one single scanner was applauded by radiologists and nuclear medicine physicians alike and the introduction of integrated PET/MRI scanners into clinical practice was accompanied by a tremendous hype (Catalano et al. 2013). The most recent publications show, however, that the differences between the two hybrid modalities are smaller than initially expected (Tian et al. 2014; Huellner et al. 2014; Heusch et al. 2014; Spick et al. 2016). This is most likely caused by the high sensitivity and specificity of PET for detection of distant metastases. To unleash the full potential of PET/MRI, it is therefore necessary to combine a fast whole-body protocol comprising only few selected sequences with high resolution MR imaging of selected regions to assess local tumor extent and to detect metastases in frequently affected regions such as the brain in lung cancer or the liver in colorectal cancer, to

B.M. Schaarschmidt (✉) • L.M. Sawicki
G. Antoch • P. Heusch
Department of Diagnostic and Interventional
Radiology, University Dusseldorf, Medical Faculty,
Dusseldorf, Germany
e-mail: benedikt.schaarschmidt@med.uni-
duesseldorf.de

© Springer International Publishing AG 2018
L. Umutlu, K. Herrmann (eds.), *PET/MR Imaging: Current and Emerging Applications*,
https://doi.org/10.1007/978-3-319-69641-6_3

perform true "one stop shop" examinations (Martinez-Möller et al. 2012; Schulthess and Veit-Haibach 2014). Another advantage of PET/MRI is the simultaneous acquisition of functional MRI and PET data, allowing true multiparametric tumor evaluation (Gatidis et al. 2013). Especially diffusion weighted imaging (DWI) as a marker of cellular density and perfusion imaging are promising techniques.

Therefore, the advantages, disadvantages and potential pitfalls in oncological 18F-FDG PET/MRI imaging concerning local tumor evaluation, lymph node and distant metastasis staging as well as restaging and therapy response assessment will be discussed and differences in comparison to 18F-FDG PET/CT will be highlighted.

3.2 Head and Neck

3.2.1 Squamous Cell Carcinoma

In the head and neck, squamous cell carcinoma amounts to up to 90% of all histological subtypes. Its association with the use of alcohol and tobacco leads to an increased incidence in male patients, but the number of female patients has been shown to rise over the last years (Wolff et al. 2012; Robert Koch-Institut und Gesellschaft der epidemiologischen Krebsregister in Deutschland e.V. 2015). As patient survival is highly dependent on complete surgical tumor removal, surgery is considered the therapy of choice (Howaldt et al. 2000). However, the complicated anatomy of the head and neck area and the need to preserve complex motoric functions to ensure a high postoperative quality of life make a complete tumor removal difficult. Hence, high resolution preoperative imaging is crucial for appropriate patient selection and preoperative planning. Additionally, reliable follow-up examinations are mandatory in these patients as tumor recurrence or secondary tumors are frequent and are important independent risk factors for survival (Ogden 1991; Schwartz et al. 1994).

Therefore, the combination of high resolution MRI and 18F-FDG PET imaging in one single

modality offers new possibilities in head and neck tumor imaging, which will be discussed in this chapter.

Local Tumor Evaluation

In squamous cell carcinoma of the head and neck, surgery is the treatment modality of choice (Howaldt et al. 2000; Grégoire et al. 2010; Wolff et al. 2012). However, surgical removal of a tumor located in an unfavorable anatomical region can lead to a severe functional impairment of the patient, thus considerably decreasing the postoperative quality of life. Hence, cross sectional imaging has to be considered a cornerstone in the preoperative assessment which is supplemented by a clinical examination, endoscopy and ultrasound evaluation of the head and neck (Grégoire et al. 2010; Wolff et al. 2012). In preoperative tumor staging of the head and neck, MRI offers a significantly higher soft tissue contrast compared to contrast enhanced CT imaging (Sigal et al. 1996; Leslie et al. 1999). However, CT is still a potential alternative that is considered as sufficient by the latest guidelines (Grégoire et al. 2010; Wolff et al. 2012). Local tumor staging is mainly based on morphological changes, as studies have shown that the addition of metabolic information by 18F-FDG PET does not increase the diagnostic accuracy in local tumor evaluation in comparison to CT or MRI if the location of the primary is known (Laubenbacher et al. 1995; Hafidh et al. 2006). While initial studies on hybrid imaging failed to demonstrate significant differences among conventional and hybrid imaging for T and N staging in patients with squamous cell carcinoma of the head and neck, the results indicated the superiority of integrated PET/MRI over PET/CT and MRI, revealing higher diagnostic accuracy rates of 75% in PET/MRI over 59% in PET/CT and 50% in MRI, respectively (Rodrigues et al. 2009; Schaarschmidt et al. 2015d).

Furthermore, additional 18F-FDG PET or 18F-FDG PET/CT might be helpful in the identification of the primary tumor site in patients with squamous cell carcinoma of unknown primary (Fig. 3.1) (Wong and Saunders 2003; Paul et al. 2007; Wong et al. 2012). A recent publication by Ruhlmann et al.

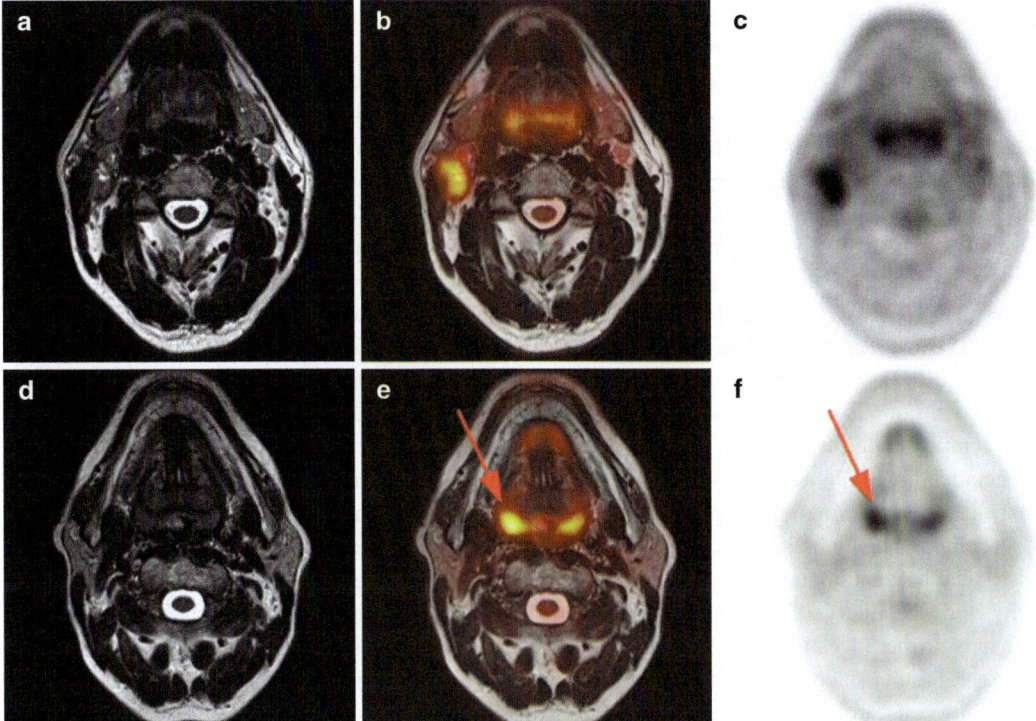

Fig. 3.1 59 year old patient with newly diagnosed lymphadenopathy of the right neck undergoing integrated ^{18}F-FDG PET/MRI for tumor localization. Two representative slices are displayed in morphological MRI (**a**, **d**), fused (**b**, **f**) and ^{18}F-FDG PET images (**c**, **f**) While the metastatic lymph node can be depicted by morphological MRI and indicates a comparable diagnostic accuracy of ^{18}F-FDG PET (**a–c**), no primary was found in morphological imaging (**d**). However, a discrepant tracer uptake can be found in the tonsils (**e**, **f**, right tonsil: SUVmax 9.79; left tonsil: SUVmax 6.14). This finding is indicative of a malignancy in the right tonsil. By endoscopic sampling, a tonsillar carcinoma of the right tonsil was confirmed

indicates a comparable diagnostic accuracy of ^{18}F-FDG PET/CT and ^{18}F-FDG PET/MRI (Ruhlmann et al. 2016). However, due to the low specificity of ^{18}F-FDG for squamous cell carcinoma, frequently observed incidental tracer uptake still poses a significant problem in the identification of tumorous tissue that cannot be overcome by the increased soft tissue contrast of the MRI component in PET/MRI examinations (Schaarschmidt et al. 2017a).

Lymph Node and Distant Metastasis Staging

The value of ^{18}F-FDG PET and ^{18}F-FDG PET/CT in preoperative lymph node assessment is controversially discussed. ^{18}F-FDG PET/CT is known to increase the sensitivity and specificity in the detection of metastatic lymph nodes when compared to sole morphological CT or MR imaging (Grégoire et al. 2010; Wolff et al. 2012). However,

especially patients without clinically identifiable nodal metastatic spread are problematic. In this specific cohort, N-staging accuracy of ^{18}F-FDG PET/CT is too low to guide surgical lymph node removal or to identify patients that do no profit from additional neck dissection (Schöder et al. 2006; Hafidh et al. 2006; Nahmias et al. 2007; Schroeder et al. 2008; Sohn et al. 2016). Similar problems were encountered in preliminary ^{18}F-FDG PET/MRI studies using retrospectively fused PET- and MRI data sets (Nakamoto et al. 2009; Kanda et al. 2013; Heusch et al. 2014c). In studies on small cohorts using integrated PET/MRI scanners, no significant differences between ^{18}F-FDG PET/CT and integrated ^{18}F-FDG PET/MRI could be detected concerning N-staging (Partovi et al. 2014a; Schaarschmidt et al. 2015d).

Although the superior co-registration of the PET and the MR data set in integrated PET/MRI could reduce misinterpretations caused by co-registration errors that are frequently encountered in retrospectively fused data sets due to patient movement, it cannot overcome the fact that ^{18}F-FDG is an unspecific tracer with a low sensitivity for micrometastases. Furthermore, the low spatial resolution of PET leads to considerate partial volume effects in small metastatic lesions, further impairing the detection of micrometastases in ^{18}F-FDG PET/CT and ^{18}F-FDG PET/MRI imaging (Buchbender et al. 2012a).

Despite these sobering preliminary data, the definite role of ^{18}F-FDG PET/MRI in preoperative lymph node evaluation is still unclear. Especially the combined analysis of simultaneously acquired information on glucose uptake by PET, cellular density by improved DWI and morphological MR parameters might excel the sensitivity and specificity of ^{18}F-FDG PET/CT and demands further investigation.

In early tumor stages of patients suffering from squamous cell carcinoma of the head and neck, distant metastases are rare. In these cases, whole-body cross sectional imaging is not generally recommended and methods such as chest x-ray or abdominal ultrasound are considered as sufficient (Grégoire et al. 2010; Wolff et al. 2012).

In advanced local tumor stages, metastatic disease is frequent. Here, lung and bone metastases are most commonly observed, making chest CT the modality of choice for the detection of distant metastases (de Bree et al. 2000; Wolff et al. 2012). While most mucosal tumors can be diagnosed by endoscopy alone, precise whole body staging by ^{18}F-FDG PET/CT can be of considerate help in these patients in detecting cancers of the lung and the esophagus (Strobel et al. 2009; Haerle et al. 2011). Nevertheless, while ^{18}F-FDG PET/MRI might be beneficial in the detection of bone metastases in comparison to ^{18}F-FDG PET/CT (see 3.7.2), the lower sensitivity for lung nodules might be problematic (see Sect. Local Tumor Evaluation). As no comparative studies between ^{18}F-FDG PET/CT and ^{18}F-FDG PET/MRI are available at the current time point, the clinical impact of these potential differences should be the focus of future studies.

Restaging and Response to Therapy

In contrast to other oncological diseases, tumor recurrence or secondary malignancies are frequent after the successful treatment of squamous cell carcinoma in the head and neck area and lead to a significant decrease in patient survival (Liu et al. 2007; Mücke et al. 2009). As these malignancies are most frequently observed over a period of five years after successful tumor treatment and frequently do not cause distinctive clinical symptoms, regular patient follow up and restaging is necessary (Ogden 1991; Boysen et al. 1990; Schwartz et al. 1994; Rogers et al. 2009). Here, morphological imaging plays a major role in tumor detection and regular cross sectional examinations, therefore either CT or MRI is recommended (Loeffelbein et al. 2015). However, recent studies indicate that ^{18}F-FDG PET imaging is highly sensitive and specific in the identification of small lymph node metastases and unknown primary tumors in follow up examinations alike (Lonneux et al. 2000; Abgral et al. 2009; Rodrigues et al. 2009). Still, the use of ^{18}F-FDG PET/CT in postoperative patients is challenging as scar tissue may frequently display a marked glucose uptake and can be mistaken for tumor recurrence. Due to the high soft tissue contrast of MRI, the differentiation between malignant and benign glucose uptake might be superior in ^{18}F-FDG PET/MRI in comparison to ^{18}F-FDG PET/CT (Engelbrecht et al. 1995; Lell et al. 2000). Hence, it is not surprising that the combined analysis of ^{18}F-FDG PET and MRI datasets in patients undergoing MRI and subsequent ^{18}F-FDG PET/CT is superior to the interpretation of either modality alone (Comoretto et al. 2008; Queiroz et al. 2014). Nevertheless, based on preliminary data, a superior detection for malignant lesions in integrated ^{18}F-FDG PET/MRI has not been demonstrated in follow-up examinations until now, although the superior soft tissue contrast is helpful to identify patients that are eligible for surgery (Fig. 3.2) (Schaarschmidt et al. 2015d).

Within the last few years, therapy response assessment became a focus of research in head and neck imaging. Recently published results

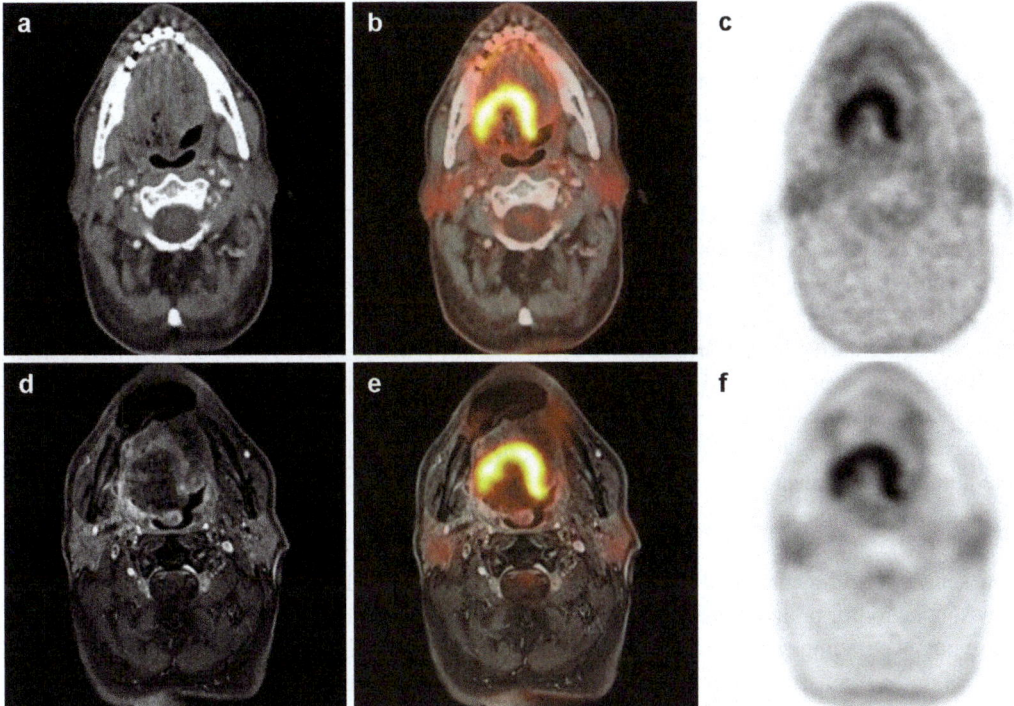

Fig. 3.2 61 year old patient after tongue tumor resection undergoing hybrid imaging because of suspected tumor recurrence. Morphological, fused and ^{18}F-FDG PET images are displayed for ^{18}F-FDG PET/CT (**a–c**) and ^{18}F-FDG PET/MRI (**d–f**). While the tumor can be detected in ^{18}F-FDG PET/CT and ^{18}F-FDG PET/MRI, contrast enhanced, high resolution MR images (**d**) provide additional data concerning local tumor invasion in comparison to contrast enhanced CT (**a**).

indicate that ^{18}F-FDG PET/CT imaging is sufficient to select patients that do not profit from neck dissection after the completion of radiochemotherapy (Mehanna et al. 2016). However, early therapy response assessment is desirable to identify non-responders and potentially change the treatment regimen. Here, changes in glucose metabolism detected by ^{18}F-FDG PET can be observed in patients responding to therapy, while in contrast to positive response in PET, at the same time a considerate increase of the apparent diffusion coefficient (ADC) derived from DWI can be observed (Vandecaveye et al. 2010; Wong et al. 2016). Hence, further research is needed to investigate whether the combined analysis of glucose metabolism and functional MRI parameters can be used to precisely identify patients that do not profit from radiochemotherapy.

3.3 Thorax

3.3.1 Lung Cancer

Lung cancer is responsible for the highest amount of cancer related deaths in the western world (Siegel et al. 2014; Robert Koch-Institut und Gesellschaft der epidemiologischen Krebsregister in Deutschland e.V. 2015). Since its commercial introduction at the beginning of the twenty-first century, ^{18}F-FDG PET/CT has become the modality of choice for assessing the tumor extent in patients suffering from lung cancer. The combination of high quality morphological imaging by CT and metabolic imaging of increased, tumor associated glucose metabolism by ^{18}F-FDG PET has led to an unprecedented high sensitivity and specificity in the evaluation of lymph node and distant metastases, especially in non-small cell lung cancer (NSCLC) (Lardinois et al. 2003; Antoch et al. 2003). Therefore, ^{18}F-FDG PET/CT has now become firmly incorporated in the latest guidelines for initial tumor staging (Goeckenjan et al. 2010; National Collaborating Centre for Cancer (UK) 2011). Additionally, recent literature shows that a decrease of ^{18}F-FDG uptake in patients undergoing chemo- or radiochemotherapy is an independent predictor of survival (Pöttgen et al. 2016; Shang et al. 2016). Hence, further ^{18}F-FDG PET/CT imaging during treatment might be used for early response evaluation and treatment planning in the near future. Nevertheless, despite its many advantages, ^{18}F-FDG PET/CT bears a few shortcomings that demand the introduction of new imaging techniques:

- low sensitivity for mediastinal infiltration.
- low sensitivity for brain metastases.
- false positive findings in adrenal lesions.
- lack of multiparametric tumor evaluation.

^{18}F-FDG PET/MRI is a potential alternative to ^{18}F-FDG PET/CT for lung cancer staging. Due to the higher soft tissue contrast and the possibility to acquire functional PET and MRI data (e.g. diffusion weighted imaging, perfusion imaging etc.), it may offer a new platform for improved assessment of tumor biology. Nevertheless, the lower sensitivity for detection of lung nodules might lead to a decrease in staging accuracy in comparison to ^{18}F-FDG PET/CT (Sawicki et al. 2016a). Hence, thoracic imaging in lung cancer in ^{18}F-FDG PET/MRI and potential advantages and pitfalls of ^{18}F-FDG PET/MRI will be discussed in the upcoming paragraphs.

Local Tumor Evaluation

Although CT is still favored by most radiologists, recent literature shows that ^{18}F-FDG PET/CT and ^{18}F-FDG PET/MRI provide similar local staging results in NSCLC patients (Schwenzer et al. 2012; Heusch et al. 2014a). However, these results highly depend on the correct choice of pulse sequences. After the commercial introduction of integrated PET/MRI scanners, various researchers proposed PET/MRI protocols solely depending on the two-point 3D-Dixon VIBE sequence for morphological imaging to decrease scan time (Eiber et al. 2011; Stolzmann et al. 2013). However, recent literature shows, that particularly T2 sequences in PROPELLER technique and contrast enhanced 3D gradient echo sequences provide the most accurate local tumor evaluation and should therefore be incorporated in dedicated lung cancer ^{18}F-FDG PET/MRI protocols (Fig. 3.3) (Hintze et al. 2006; Biederer et al. 2012; Schaarschmidt et al. 2015a). Based on elaborate sequence selection, recent studies demonstrated the possibility to perform whole-body ^{18}F-FDG PET/MRI examinations including dedicated sequences for thoracic imaging in an acquisition time that is comparable to ^{18}F-FDG PET/CT (Huellner 2016).

MRI has always been considered to be superior to CT for the assessment of mediastinal or chest wall infiltration (Landwehr et al. 1999). Therefore, ^{18}F-FDG PET/MRI has been considered to be superior to ^{18}F-FDG PET/CT for staging of locally advanced lung cancer. However, no significant differences have been found in local tumor evaluation between ^{18}F-FDG PET/CT and PET/MRI in several studies and the impact on patient management seems to be low (Heusch et al. 2014a; Fraioli et al. 2014; Schaarschmidt et al. 2017b). Hence, the use of ^{18}F-FDG PET/MRI in the evaluation of locally advanced lung cancer lies at the discretion of the examiner.

According to the latest TNM classification system, pulmonary metastases have a strong impact on the T-stage of lung cancers, upstaging patients to a T3 stage if found in the same lobe or to a T4 stage if found in the ipsilateral lung (Sobin et al. 2011). Therefore, the detection of additional pulmonary metastases is crucial for local tumor evaluation, rendering the detection of even small pulmonary nodules a necessity. The latest publications demonstrate that ^{18}F-FDG PET/MRI is inferior to ^{18}F-FDG PET/CT in the detection of pulmonary nodules, especially in subcentimeter lesions (Fig. 3.4) (Chandarana et al. 2013; Sawicki et al. 2016a). However, the clinical impact of missed pulmonary nodules is still unknown. Although missed pulmonary metastases might lead to a downstaging if primary ^{18}F-FDG PET/MRI was performed, a recent study by Schaarschmidt et al. found no changes in clinical management in lung cancer patients due to missed pulmonary nodules (Sawicki et al. 2016b; Schaarschmidt et al. 2017b). Additionally, new

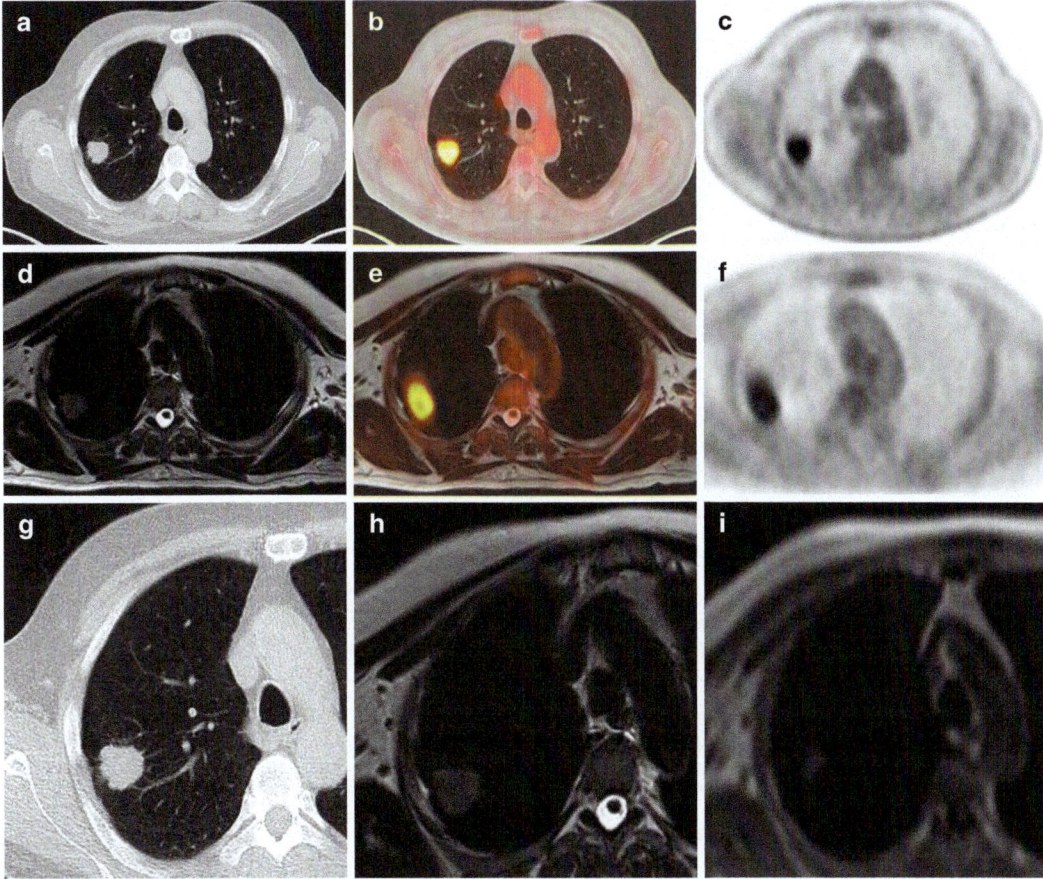

Fig. 3.3 66 year old male patient suffering from an adenocarcinoma of the right upper lobe (G1). Morphological, fused and PET images are displayed for ^{18}F-FDG PET/CT (**a–c**) and ^{18}F-FDG PET/MRI (**d–f**). Additionally, enlarged CT (**g**), T2 BLADE (**h**) and two-point 3D-Dixon VIBE images (**i**) are shown. While local staging results are concordant in ^{18}F-FDG PET/CT and high quality ^{18}F-FDG PET/MRI using a T2 BLADE sequence (T1b due to a tumor size of 2.5 cm in both hybrid imaging modalities), sole evaluation of the tumor size in the two-point 3D-Dixon VIBE sequence (tumor size: 1.4 cm) would have led to a downstaging of local tumor extent to T1a.

MRI sequences, like ultra short echo time (UTE) or zero echo time (ZTE) sequences, might improve the sensitivity of ^{18}F-FDG PET/MRI for pulmonary nodules even further (Burris et al. 2016).

Lymph Node and Distant Metastasis Staging

Especially in non-small cell lung cancer, the extent of metastatic lymph node spread is the most important prognostic factor for survival (Leyn et al. 2007). Therefore, the precise assessment of the N-Stage is of utmost importance to decide on the most appropriate treatment regimen. Due to the high specificity and sensitivity of ^{18}F-FDG PET for lymph node metastases and the potential

to precisely locate the increased tracer uptake in the co-registered data set in PET/CT, ^{18}F-FDG PET/CT has occupied a central role in the pretherapeutic assessment of patients suffering from non-small cell lung cancer (Lardinois et al. 2003; Antoch et al. 2003; Goeckenjan et al. 2010; National Collaborating Centre for Cancer (UK) 2011). As differences in attenuation correction and detector technology do not seem to influence the detection rate of tumorous lesions, it is expected that ^{18}F-FDG PET images acquired in PET/CT and PET/MRI provide the same diagnostic reliability (Hartung-Knemeyer et al. 2013). Nevertheless, recent data revealed differences in the diagnostic accuracy of [18]FDG-PET/MRI and ^{18}F-FDG PET/

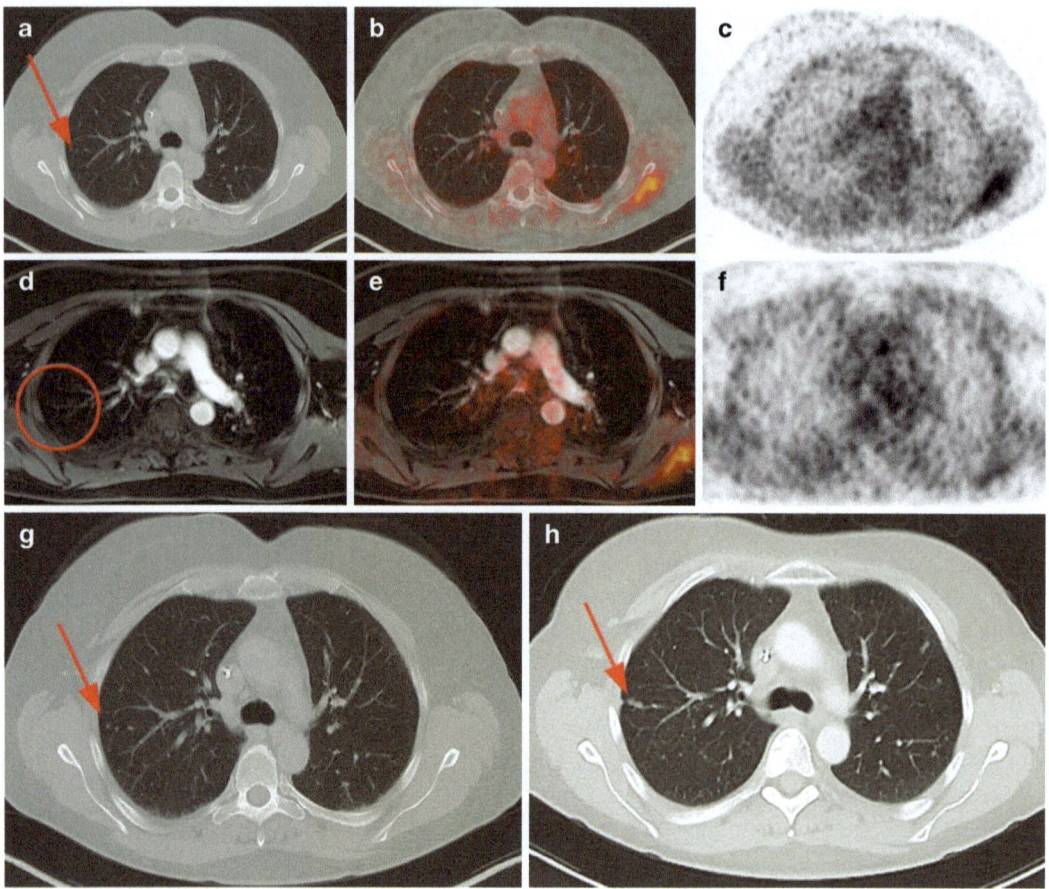

Fig. 3.4 52 year old female patient suffering from metastatic breast cancer. Morphological, fused and PET images are displayed for ¹⁸F-FDG PET/CT (**a–c**) and ¹⁸F-FDG PET/MRI (**d–f**). Additionally, CT images of the initial ¹⁸F-FDG PET/CT scan (**g**) and of the follow-up examination (**h**) are shown. While clearly visible in ¹⁸F-FDG PET/CT (**a**), a small, non ¹⁸F-FDG-avid pulmonary nodule in the right upper lobe was missed on high quality 3D gradient echo sequence images in the ¹⁸F-FDG PET/MRI examination (D) which turned out to be a pulmonary metastasis in follow-up after one year (**g, h**)

CT for lymph node staging (Heusch et al. 2014a; Schaarschmidt et al. 2017b). However, as ¹⁸F-FDG PET/CT and ¹⁸F-FDG PET/MRI examinations were performed subsequently in the majority of the comparison studies in non-small cell lung cancer patients, the observed differences were rather caused by the different acquisition time points due to the study design than by differences in scanner technology (Hahn et al. 2012).

In the last years, DWI has been investigated for lymph node staging in lung cancer and has been advocated as a potential alternative to PET (Nomori et al. 2008). First studies indicate an inverse correlation between the apparent diffusion coefficient derived from DWI and the standardized uptake value derived from PET in the primary tumor and in lymph node metastases (Regier et al. 2012; Heusch et al. 2013; Schaarschmidt et al. 2015b). But although these two imaging biomarkers seem to be intertwined, they depict different pathophysiological processes (Schaarschmidt et al. 2015b). Therefore, the potential of simultaneous assessment of PET and DWI data provides new possibilities in lymph node characterization, which should be further explored in the future.

¹⁸F-FDG PET/CT is a highly sensitive imaging modality for distant metastases in non-small cell lung cancer patients. Nevertheless, the detection of brain and adrenal metastases in ¹⁸F-FDG PET/CT remains problematic, leaving room for potential improvement based on MRI. Due to the low soft tissue contrast of CT and the low sensitivity

and specificity of PET for brain metastases, MRI is considered to be superior to ^{18}F-FDG PET/CT for the detection of brain metastases and therefore incorporated in the latest guidelines (Posther et al. 2006; Goeckenjan et al. 2010). Integrated PET/MRI scanners allow the additional acquisition of dedicated high resolution images of the brain during a whole body examination. By performing a real "one stop shop" examination, a subsequent brain MRI scan is redundant leading to a much more streamlined diagnostic process, reducing the time span for the overall diagnostic workup and thus increasing patient satisfaction while only moderately increasing the acquisition time of the whole-body scan (Martinez-Möller et al. 2012; Schulthess and Veit-Haibach 2014).

The diagnosis of adrenal metastases can be challenging in ^{18}F-FDG PET/CT. Increased ^{18}F-FDG uptake is a strong predictor for malignancy, but still, some case reports indicate that also benign adrenal lesions such as adrenocortical adenoma can exhibit a markedly increased glucose metabolism (Yun et al. 2001; Shimizu et al. 2003; Basu and Nair 2005). Although adrenocortical adenomas can be safely identified by additional unenhanced CT scans or an additional delayed contrast enhanced CT scan after 15 minutes, these techniques demand additional radiation exposure and are difficult to incorporate in the clinical workflow (Park et al. 2007). Chemical shift imaging, however, is a reliable technique to characterize adrenal lesions and can be helpful in these equivocal cases (Fig. 3.5).

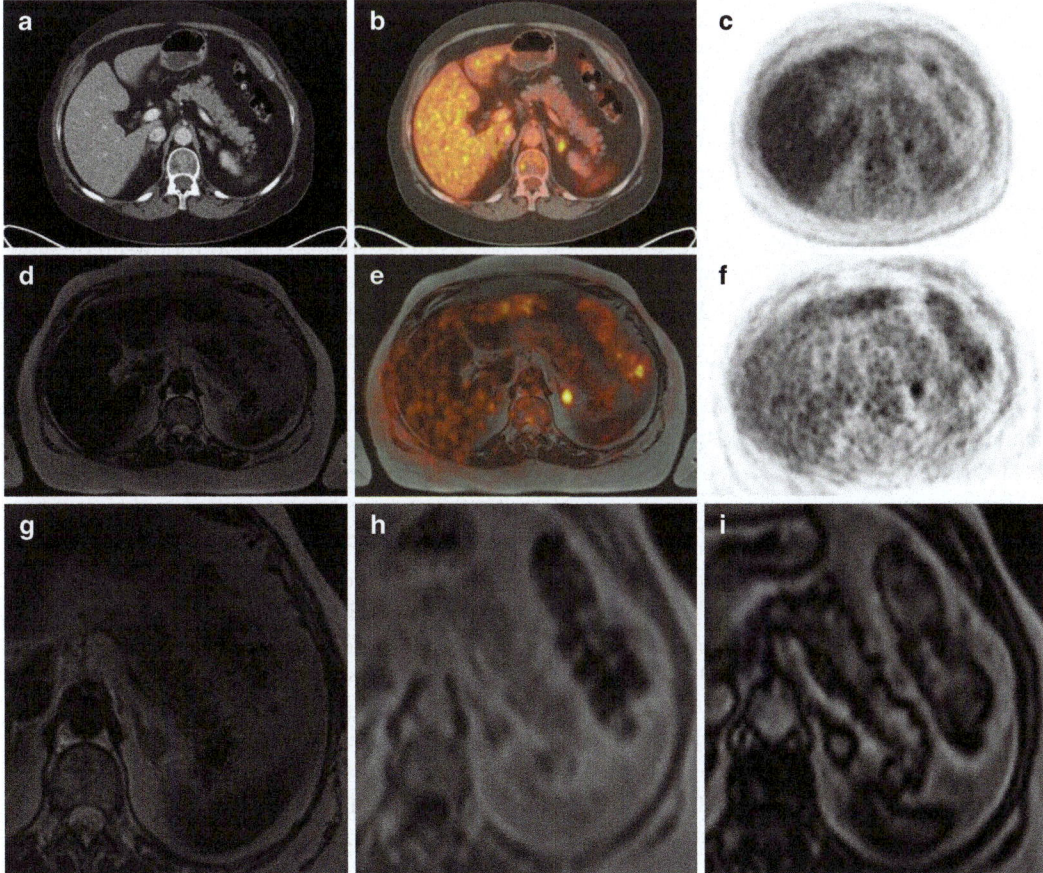

Fig. 3.5 59 year old female patient suffering from Stage IV non-small cell lung cancer (adenocarcinoma). Morphological, fused and PET images are displayed for ^{18}F-FDG PET/CT (**a–c**) and ^{18}F-FDG PET/MRI (**d–f**). Additionally, T1 FLASH (**g**) as well as in- (**h**) and opposed phase (**i**) T1 images are shown. Increased tracer uptake of a mass in the left adrenal gland is suspicious for malignancy (**c, f**), but due to the low uptake (SUVmax 4.53) similar to the liver parenchyma, a benign lesion (e.g. adrenal adenoma) cannot be safely excluded. In PET/MRI, the lack of signal loss in the in- and opposed phase images (**h, i**) is indicative for an adrenal metastasis, which was confirmed by follow-up after 6 months

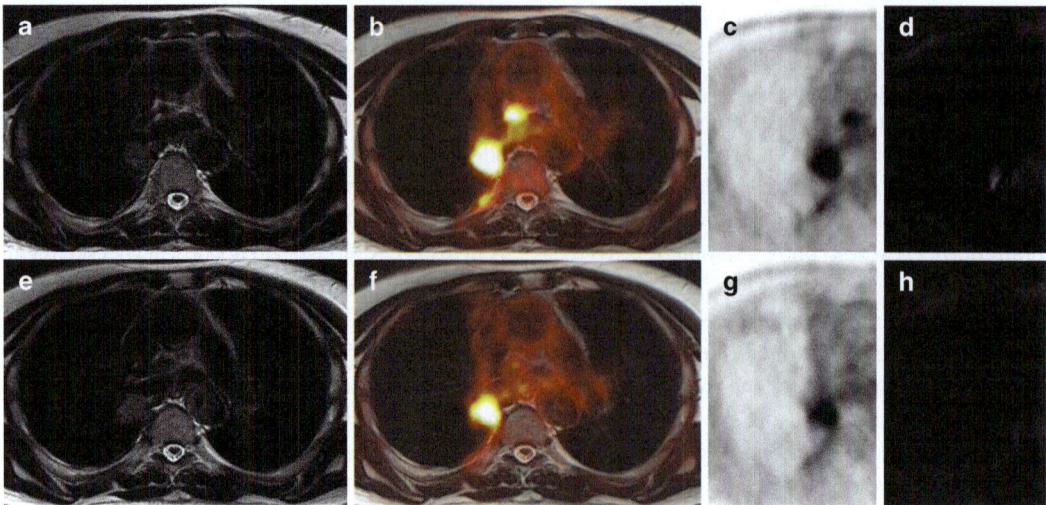

Fig. 3.6 71 year old male patient suffering from Stage IV non-small cell lung cancer (adenocarcinoma, G2). Morphological, fused and PET images as well as DWI are displayed for ^{18}F-FDG PET/MRI before (**a–d**) and during treatment (**e–h**). After two cycles of chemotherapy, no obvious morphological changes can be observed (**a, f**), but a marked decrease in glucose metabolism in the primary tumor in the right lower lobe (before treatment: SUVmean 10,03, **b, c**; after treatment: SUVmean 7,65, **f, g**) and in the mediastinal lymph nodes can be found. Additionally, early changes can be noted in DWI (**d, h**)

As chemical shift imaging is incorporated in the MR-based attenuation correction of ^{18}F-FDG PET/MRI, these pre-existing data may be used for further differentiation of adrenal lesions and have been shown to significantly improve the diagnostic certainty of correct assessment of suspicious adrenal lesions in ^{18}F-FDG PET/MRI when compared to ^{18}F-FDG PET/CT without prolonging the examination time (Haider et al. 2004; Schaarschmidt et al. 2015c).

Restaging and Response to Therapy

Recent therapeutic advances in lung cancer treatment, most notably multimodal treatment regimes, have drastically increased lung cancer survival. Therefore, restaging and response assessment of lung cancer patients has become a focus of interest in clinical research. To avoid adverse side effects, it is important to assess the effectiveness of radio- or chemotherapy as quickly as possible after the start of treatment.

Latest publications indicate that changes in glucose metabolism detected by ^{18}F-FDG PET/CT are not only capable to predict survival after combined radiochemotherapy, but are also more accurate than morphological CT in the detection of early therapeutic response to chemotherapy (Pöttgen et al. 2016; Shang et al. 2016). Albeit promising, this one dimensional approach will not be sufficient in the future. Especially in stage IV lung cancer, cytotoxic chemotherapy is only of limited use and despite multiple innovations in the twentieth century, the overall increase in survival is sobering (Breathnach et al. 2001). Therefore, research has shifted to the identification of tumor specific mutations which can be targeted by novel therapeutic agents. However, changes induced by these new drugs can be difficult to detect by one imaging biomarker alone, especially in equivocal cases (Nishino et al. 2014). Here, the simultaneous acquisition of multiple imaging biomarkers such as glucose metabolism depicted by ^{18}F-FDG PET, tissue cellularity depicted by DWI, tissue vascularization by dynamic contrast enhanced imaging (DCE) and further molecular imaging biomarkers acquired in one single ^{18}F-FDG PET/MRI scan may be particularly helpful (Fig. 3.6) (Ohno et al. 2012; Nensa et al. 2014a, b).

3.3.2 Malignant Pleural Mesothelioma

Malignant pleural mesothelioma is a rare tumor entity mainly caused by asbestos exposition. Although asbestos has been banned in most countries of the western world since the beginning of the twenty-first century, it is expected that the peak of mesothelioma associated mortality has not been reached (Peto et al. 1999). As personalized, multimodal treatment combining surgery, chemotherapy and radiation therapy is heavily relying on the tumor stage, highly accurate imaging is necessary to choose the most appropriate treatment regimen and assess treatment response (Neumann et al. 2013; Opitz 2014).

At the moment, CT is still considered as the modality of choice for the initial diagnosis, staging and assessment of therapy (Armato et al. 2013). However, the low soft tissue contrast, even of contrast enhanced CT, is problematic in the diagnosis of local tumor invasion (Heelan et al. 1999). Furthermore, the differentiation between asbestos related benign pleural disease and early malignant pleural mesothelioma is extraordinarily difficult.

Therefore, the use of other imaging modalities like MRI or ^{18}F-FDG PET/CT for detection and staging of malignant pleural mesothelioma is discussed in recent literature (Armato et al. 2013; Nickell et al. 2014). ^{18}F-FDG PET/CT offers unprecedented accuracy in the detection of malignant pleural lesions as well as lymph node and distant metastases (Plathow et al. 2008; Wilcox et al. 2009; Yildirim et al. 2009). Additionally, changes in glucose metabolism could be used for therapy response assessment (Veit-Haibach et al. 2010). In local tumor evaluation, ^{18}F-FDG PET/CT is not superior to MRI, as MRI is considered to be more sensitive for the detection of chest wall and diaphragmatic infiltration (Heelan et al. 1999; Wilcox et al. 2009). Additionally, DWI has been found to be highly sensitive for the detection of malignant pleural lesions (Coolen et al. 2014). Hence, ^{18}F-FDG PET/MRI may be a potential alternative to ^{18}F-FDG PET/CT in malignant pleural mesothelioma imaging, as comparable staging results have been reported in small cohorts between both hybrid imaging modalities (Fig. 3.7) (Martini et al. 2016; Schaarschmidt et al. 2016).

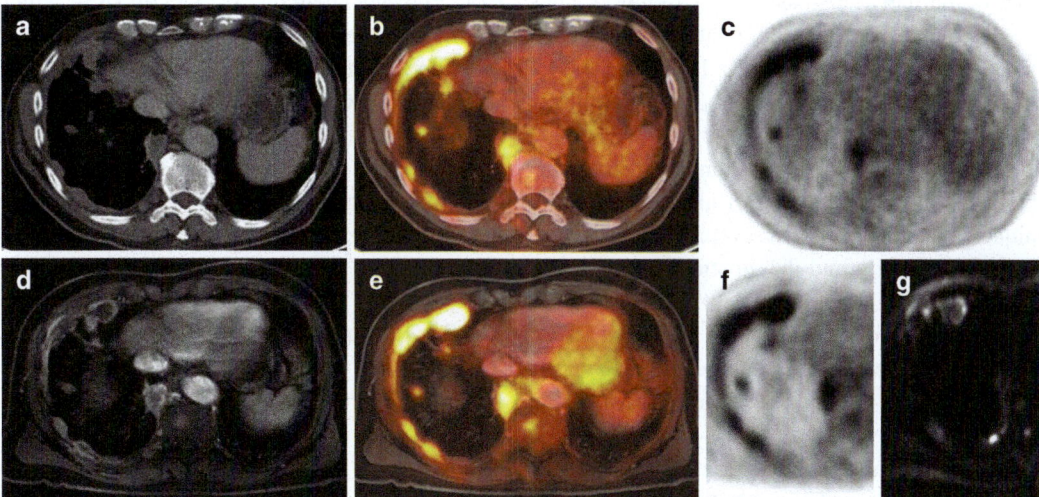

Fig. 3.7 73 year old male patient suffering from advanced malignant pleural mesothelioma (cT4 cN0 cM1) with diffuse left-sided pleural tumor spread with additional mediastinal and chest wall infiltration. Morphological, fused and PET images are displayed for ^{18}F-FDG PET/CT (A-C) and ^{18}F-FDG PET/MRI including DWI (D-G). Contrast enhanced T1-weighted imaging and DWI incorporated in the PET/MRI protocol are more conspicuous for chest wall infiltration and the additional bone metastasis in the vertebral body than CT- or PET-imaging

3.4 Upper Abdomen and Upper Gastrointestinal Tract

3.4.1 Liver Metastases

The liver is the most frequent site of hematogenous metastases and liver metastases are far more common than primary hepatic neoplasms. Typical primary tumors that are associated with the development of liver metastases are colorectal cancer, lung cancer, breast cancer and neuroendocrine tumors. Since the presence and extent of distant metastatic spread is the most important factor for patient prognosis, detection of liver metastases as well as their discrimination from benign lesions such as follicular nodular hyperplasia (FNH), adenoma or hemangioma is critical for selecting the ideal treatment and estimation of prognosis. According to current NCCN guidelines, CT is suggested as the first-line imaging modality for liver metastases (NCCN 2016). However, the sensitivity of CT for liver metastases is limited due to the inherently low soft-tissue contrast, and thus, more accurate imaging modalities are necessary when exact assessment of the hepatic spread is inevitable, such as when a decision regarding curative vs. palliative management is required. Due to the increased glucose metabolism of most liver metastases, ^{18}F-FDG PET/CT is able to improve the sensitivity for their detection to 76–97% (D'souza et al. 2009; Donati et al. 2010). MRI, on the other hand, offering the highest soft-tissue contrast of all imaging techniques, has been shown to provide an even higher sensitivity and diagnostic accuracy than ^{18}F-FDG PET/CT (Seo et al. 2011). MRI offers an unparalleled detectability of small liver lesions, and specific patterns of enhancement on dynamic T1w imaging in combination with DWI, in/opposed phase, and T2-weighted imaging enable advanced characterization of hepatic lesions, rendering MRI a promising alternative to CT in hybrid imaging. Moreover, the soft-tissue contrast of MRI compensates for inherent limitations of the PET component, such as the comparatively high background ^{18}F-FDG uptake

of the liver parenchyma which may mask lesions with liver-equivalent uptake. The diagnostic accuracy of MRI can be further enhanced by applying liver-specific contrast agents (Goodwin et al. 2011). The combination of the advantageous features of MRI and PET in a hybrid imaging modality was expected to constitute a new gold standard of liver imaging. Early studies using retrospectively fused PET and MRI datasets already indicated high synergistic potential of PET/MRI for liver imaging (Donati et al. 2010). However, the quality of retrospective fusion PET/MRI is inferior to that of simultaneous PET/MRI as differences due to different patient positioning and breath-hold imaging in PET/CT and MRI lead to a distorted coregistration. Since simultaneous PET/MRI is still a new imaging technique, current evidence concerning its diagnostic capability in liver imaging is limited. Nevertheless, two comparative studies by Beiderwellen et al. showed an incremental value of ^{18}F-FDG PET/MRI over ^{18}F-FDG PET/CT and MRI in the detection of liver metastases, providing superior sensitivity, specificity, and diagnostic confidence (Fig. 3.8) (Beiderwellen et al. 2013a, 2015). More patients with liver metastases were identified by ^{18}F-FDG PET/MRI than by ^{18}F-FDG PET/CT, which adumbrates the potential clinical impact of PET/MRI on a patient basis. Based on current evidence, ^{18}F-FDG PET/MRI may play an important role in whole-body staging of cancers with high potential for liver metastases that would usually be staged with ^{18}F-FDG PET/CT but do not require high-resolution pulmonary imaging.

3.4.2 Hepatocellular Carcinoma

Hepatocellular carcinoma (HCC) has an increasing incidence in patients with chronic hepatic disease and is associated with a high mortality rate (Mittal and El-Serag 2013). The ^{18}F-FDG uptake of HCC is variable due to considerable differences in glucose-6-phosphatase activity and cell surface glucose transporters in HCC. The preoperative SUVmax has been found to be a

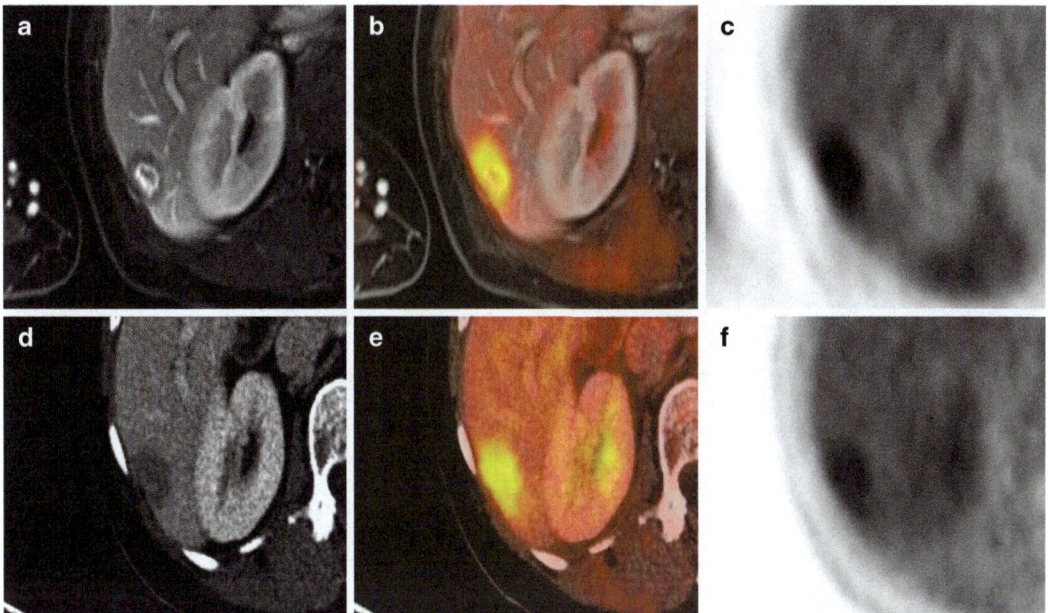

Fig. 3.8 Patient with hepatic recurrence of breast cancer. The metastasis is detectable on post-contrast fat-saturated T1w MRI (**a**), ¹⁸F-FDG PET/MRI (**b**), PET from PET/MRI (**c**), CT (**d**), ¹⁸F-FDG PET/CT (**e**), and PET from PET/CT (**f**) due to contrast enhancement on MRI, ill-defined hypodense appearance on CT and increased ¹⁸F-FDG FDG uptake

surrogate for survival and correlates with the degree of differentiation of HCC (Torizuka et al. 1995; Lee et al. 2011). Herein, high-grade HCC show significantly higher ¹⁸F-FDG uptake than low-grade HCC. Therefore, ¹⁸F-FDG PET tends to better detect high-grade HCC while the sensitivity for lower grade HCC is limited due to their lower ¹⁸F-FDG uptake against the physiologically high background uptake of normal hepatic parenchyma. As a result, the overall detectability of HCC in FDG-imaging is impaired, with a reported sensitivity of only 55–68%, and thus, ¹⁸F-FDG PET/CT is considered to have limited value in assessing primary HCC (Khan et al. 2000; Talbot et al. 2010). Although to date there is no dedicated study on the diagnostic accuracy of ¹⁸F-FDG PET/MRI in HCC, an increased accuracy in comparison to ¹⁸F-FDG PET/CT can be expected based on the superior soft-tissue contrast of MRI, as MRIalone has a sensitivity and specificity of 81% and 85% for the detection of HCC, respectively (Colli et al. 2006). The possibility of obtaining simultaneous functional

tumor information from dedicated MRI sequences and PET is another advantage of PET/MRI (Fig. 3.9). For instance, DWI has been shown to improve the detectability of subcentimeter satellite HCC metastases (Xu et al. 2010; Park et al. 2012). In contrary to primary HCC, ¹⁸F-FDG PET/CT has a high diagnostic potential in detecting recurrent HCC. Studies that evaluated ¹⁸F-FDG PET/CT in case of disease recurrence reported a 90% sensitivity and >80% specificity (Sun et al. 2009). ¹⁸F-FDG PET/MRI is expected to further exceed the diagnostic performance of PET/CT in recurrent HCC. ¹⁸F-FDG PET/MRI may be particularly appealing as disease recurrence tends to be isolocal and MRI, by means of dynamic contrast T1w imaging and DWI, provides a better capability to differentiate local recurrence from post-therapeutic changes than CT. Two recent studies evaluated the role of ¹⁸F-FDG PET/MRI in interventional treatment for HCC. Fowler et al. investigated a potential link between dose deposition from Y-90 microspheres radio-embolization measured on PET/

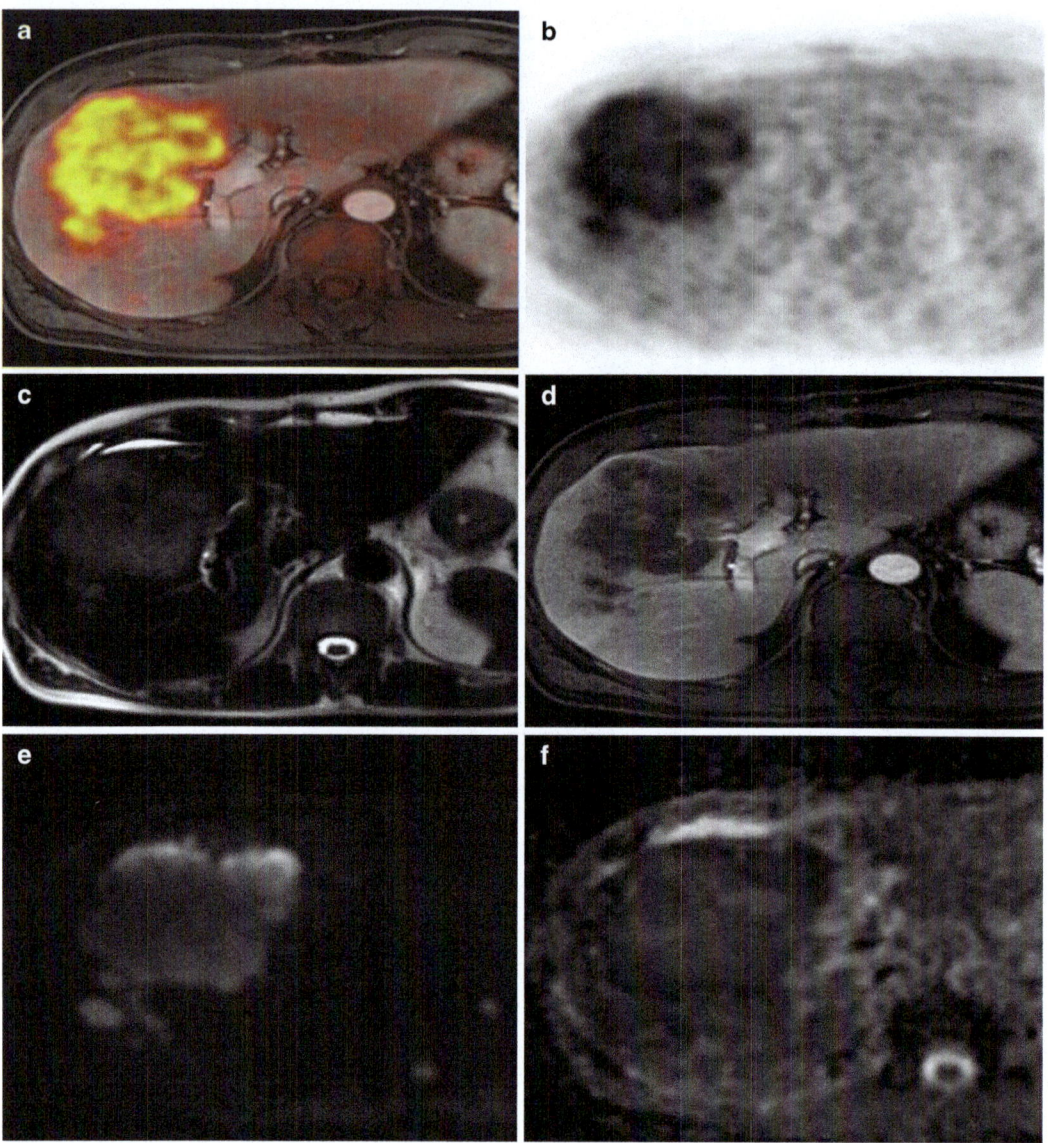

Fig. 3.9 Patient with a large HCC in the right liver lobe. ^{18}F-FDG PET/MRI (**a**), PET (**b**), PET from PET/MRI (**c**), Post-contrast fat-saturated T1w MRI (**d**), *b*-1000 DWI (**e**), ADC map (**f**). The HCC shows strong ^{18}F-FDG uptake (SUVmax: 14.7) and also restricted diffusion

MRI and individual lesion response. Their results showed that the average dose deposition measured on PET/MRI might serve as an independent predictor of local treatment response (Fowler et al. 2016). Another study by Ramalho et al. found that ^{18}F-FDG PET/MRI is useful to detect residual tumor following thermoablation therapy (Ramalho et al. 2015). Metastases to the lungs, abdominal lymph nodes, and bone are the most frequent sites of extrahepatic metastatic HCC (Katyal et al. 2000). According to a meta-analysis by Lin et al., ^{18}F-FDG PET/CT is beneficial in detecting extrahepatic disease with pooled estimates of sensitivity and specificity of 77% and 98%, respectively (Lin et al. 2012). In the light of current knowledge, whole-body staging of HCC using ^{18}F-FDG PET/MRI should provide equal detectability of lymph node metastases, identify less lung metastases but improve the depiction of soft-tissue and osseous metastases (Beiderwellen et al. 2014; Sawicki et al. 2016b, a). However, it is for future studies to investigate the actual role of ^{18}F-FDG PET/MRI in whole-body staging of HCC.

3.4.3 Neuroendocrine Tumors

Neuroendocrine tumors (NETs) originate from endocrine and neural cells dispersed throughout the body. As a heterogeneous group of tumors there is a large variety of histopathological patterns, endocrine potential, and degree of aggressiveness (Klimstra et al. 2015). Pancreas, rectum, small bowel, appendix and the lung are considered among the most frequent primary tumor sites of NETs, despite their rare incidence. However, most probably due to the continuous improvement of imaging techniques their detection rate has multiplied up to fivefold over the last decades (1970's: 1.09/100.000, 2004: 5.25/100.000) (Yao et al. 2008). Metastases are found in up to 50% of NET patients at initial diagnosis, with the liver being the most common site of metastatic spread (Oberg and Eriksson 2005). In fact, about 80% of NET patients develop liver metastases during the course of the disease. Therefore, assessment of local tumor burden and metastatic spread is highly important both for choosing the appropriate treatment (surgery vs. chemotherapy) and estimation of prognosis. Pathologic expression of cell-surface somatostatin receptors (SSTR) - especially SSTR type 2—is a unique feature of NETs that has been used as a target structure for radiolabeled somatostatin analogues in nuclear medical imaging (Kulaksiz et al. 2002; Kaemmerer et al. 2011). SSTR targeting ^{111}In-labeled octreotide scintigraphy and single photon emission tomography (SPECT) have been widely used for NET imaging. However, the low anatomic and spatial resolution of scintigraphy and SPECT often lead to false negative scans. With the introduction of PET/CT and more SSTR avid tetraazacyclododecane-tetraacetic acid (DOTA) peptides, accurate localization and depiction of even subcentimeter NET lesions has become possible. According to recent meta-analyses ^{68}Ga-DOTA peptide-based PET/CT has a pooled sensitivity of 93% and specificity of 96% and is considered the diagnostic gold standard in NET imaging, especially for differentiated NETs that typically show high SSTR cell surface expression (Treglia et al. 2012; Hofman et al. 2015). Hybrid PET/MRI enables the simultaneous acquisition of ^{68}Ga-DOTA peptide-based PET imaging along with high soft-tissue contrast and functional MRI (Fig. 3.3). With regard to NET staging, ^{68}Ga-DOTA peptide-based PET/MRI might offer several potential benefits over PET/CT. As liver metastases are a frequent occurrence in NET patients, assessment of the presence and the extent of liver metastases is of particular clinical relevance. The superior soft-tissue contrast of MRI as well as diffusion-weighted imaging facilitate an improved detectability of small lesions that—due to their small size and/ or low radiotracer avidity—remained undetected on ^{68}Ga-DOTA peptide-based PET/CT (Fig. 3.10) (Sawicki et al. 2017). This is relevant since NET metastases partly exhibit low SSTR expression, although originating from a well-differentiated tumor. Furthermore, characterization of sites with physiologically high radiotracer uptake remains a problem in ^{68}Ga-DOTA peptide-based PET/CT. For instance, normal ^{68}Ga-DOTA-peptide uptake of the uncinate process of the pancreas often mimics malignancy on PET/CT (Jacobsson et al. 2012). By means of the inherently higher soft-tissue contrast of MRI, ^{68}Ga-DOTA peptide-based PET/MRI rather than PET/CT could differentiate physiologic uptake of the uncinate process from an actual NET manifestation. Current literature endorses the use of ^{68}Ga-DOTA peptide-based PET/MRI as an alternative to ^{68}Ga-DOTA peptide-based PET/CT in whole-body staging of NET (Jacobsson et al. 2012; Sawicki et al. 2017). The SUVs from ^{68}Ga-DOTATOC PET/MRI and PET/CT show strong correlations. In relation to extrahepatic disease, both modalities provide a similarly high diagnostic performance both in morphologic and ^{68}Ga-DOTA peptide-based PET imaging,

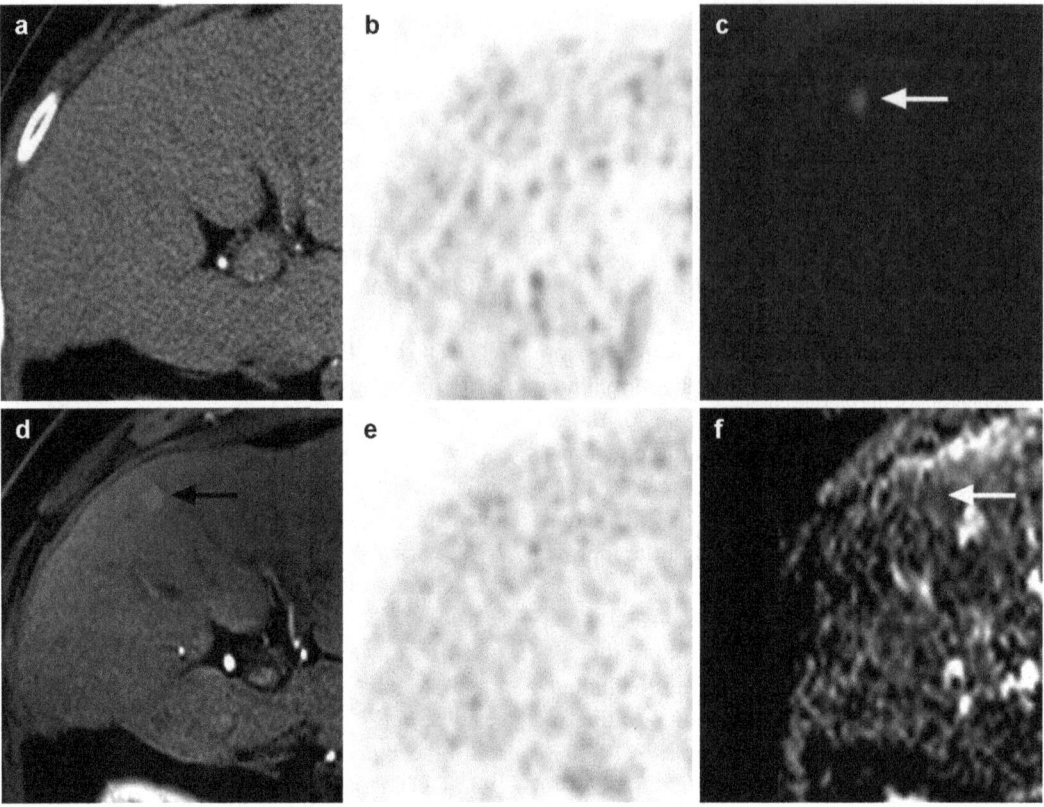

Fig. 3.10 Patient with NET metastasis in segment 5 of the liver. The metastasis does not exhibit pathologic SSTR expression on PET images from ^{68}Ga-DOTATOC PET/CT (**b**) or PET images from ^{68}Ga-DOTATOC PET/MRI (**e**). Since there was no morphologic correlate on CT (**a**), the metastasis is missed on ^{68}Ga-DOTATOC PET/CT. The metastasis is identified by ^{68}Ga-DOTATOC PET/MRI as a small hypervascularized lesion on contrast-enhanced arterial phase fat-saturated T1w images (arrow in **d**) with restricted diffusion as shown by high signal intensity on b-1000 DWI (arrow in **c**) and low ADC values (arrow in **f**)

although ^{68}Ga-DOTA peptide-based PET/MRI revealed minor disadvantages inherent to MRI regarding lung nodules and sclerotic bone lesions. In relation to liver metastases, studies unanimously show a clear superiority of PET/MRI based on the ability to detect small liver lesions and the higher lesion-to-background contrast on MRI (Schreiter et al. 2012; Beiderwellen et al. 2013b; Hope et al. 2015; Sawicki et al. 2017). Whether this translates to a change in therapy or survival is yet to be evaluated.

3.4.4 Esophageal Carcinoma

Esophageal cancer is the ninth most frequent cancer worldwide and represents about 4–10%

of gastrointestinal malignancies. The two main histological subtypes are squamous cell carcinoma and adenocarcinoma. While squamous cell carcinomas are more common in developing countries, adenocarcinomas are the predominant esophageal cancer type in the western world. Adenocarcinomas are located in the lower third of the esophagus, where they originate from metaplastic glandular cells. Risk factors include alcohol, tobacco, gastro-esophageal reflux, and obesity. In patients with early-stage disease, curative esophagectomy is the treatment of choice and post-surgical patients have a 5-year survival rate of 41%. However, the majority of patients present with locally advanced cancer at initial referral, and up to 30% already suffer from distant metastases, which dramatically decreases the chances of 5-year survival to 4% (Institute NC 2017a). In addition to biopsy, pre-surgical endoscopic ultrasound (EUS), CT, and ^{18}F-FDG PET/CT are frequently applied for judgment of operability and evaluation of the local tumor extent, lymph node status and distant metastases. EUS is relevant for the evaluation of tumor size and local invasiveness and recommended as imaging of choice for T-staging by current guidelines (Varghese et al. 2013). CT is the most widely used imaging technique for thoracoabdominal staging of esophagus carcinoma. For N-Staging and M-Staging, CT has a reported sensitivity of 84% and 81% and a specificity of 67% and 82%, respectively (Lowe et al. 2005). The low specificity in N-Staging is without a doubt attributable to the size criterion applied by CT for characterization of lymph node metastasis (> 1 cm). Since most esophageal cancers are ^{18}F-FDG-avid, the role of ^{18}F-FDG PET/CT for staging has also been evaluated. ^{18}F-FDG PET-based detectability of the primary tumor is possible in >95% of all cases. However false-positive reports can occur due to functional ^{18}F-FDG uptake or esophagitis. ^{18}F-FDG PET/CT is inferior to EUS in the evaluation of local tumor invasiveness (Lowe et al. 2005). There are conflicting results for ^{18}F-FDG PET/CT regarding locoregional nodal assessment. Increased glucose metabolism of mediastinal lymph nodes close to the primary tumor can be hard to discriminate from esophageal uptake due to the limited spatial resolution of PET and flawed co-registration from peristalsis. False-negatives are possible in micro-metastatic lymph nodes, and false-positives can occur in esophagitis, sarcoidosis, or tuberculosis. A meta-analysis that evaluated the diagnostic accuracy of preoperative ^{18}F-FDG PET/CT reported a sensitivity of 51% and specificity of 84% for locoregional lymph node involvement (van Westreenen et al. 2004). The integration of ^{18}F-FDG PET/CT into the conventional work-up was found to improve staging and potentially avoid unnecessary surgery based on the excellent ability to detect distant metastases (Flamen et al. 2000; Liberale et al. 2004; van Westreenen

et al. 2005). According to current guidelines MRI is not intended as a first-line modality but has a role in determining indistinctive liver or adrenal lesions. Evidence for ^{18}F-FDG PET/MRI is based on a recent pilot study of 19 patients that compared EUS, CT, ^{18}F-FDG PET/CT and ^{18}F-FDG PET/MRI in pre-surgical local and locoregional esophageal cancer staging. ^{18}F-FDG PET/MRI provided high accuracy for T staging, and better accuracy than EUS, CT, and ^{18}F-FDG PET/CT in locoregional lymph nodes (Lee et al. 2014). Concerning M-staging, ^{18}F-FDG PET/MRI is expected to be superior in parenchymatous organs such as the liver and inferior in low-proton density organs such as the lung. The role of ^{18}F-FDG PET/MRI in recurrent esophageal cancer is yet to be explored. Based on the combined high soft-tissue contrast and its potential for functional imaging, PET/MRI might be beneficial to discriminate local recurrence from scar tissue, monitor treatment response, and guide irradiation planning.

3.5 Lower Gastrointestinal Tract

3.5.1 Colorectal Cancer

Colorectal cancer is the third most common cancer in the western world and the fourth most common cause of cancer-related death. It accounts for about 95% of gastrointestinal malignancies. There has been a rising incidence of colorectal cancer worldwide over the last three decades, although in recent years, numbers are gradually declining in well-developed countries (Haggar and Boushey 2009). The vast majority of colorectal cancers are adenocarcinomas (~95%). Endoscopic biopsy is performed to determine colorectal cancer. Contrast-enhanced CT of the chest and abdomen is recommended as first-line imaging to estimate the stage of disease and also for re-staging (NCCN 2016). In patients with rectal cancer MRI of the pelvis should be applied in order to assess T- and N-staging and the risk of local recurrence, as determined by the presumed resection margin (Nougaret et al.

2013). While MRI provides accurate T-staging and evaluation of resection margin, N-staging is hampered both in MRI and CT due to possible reactive enlargement of perirectal lymph nodes or small, morphologically unsuspicious lymph node metastases (Vag et al. 2014). Hybrid imaging with ^{18}F-FDG PET/CT has been found to improve the specificity of N-staging in colorectal cancer (85%). Nevertheless, in clinical routine, whole-body ^{18}F-FDG PET/CT is reserved for staging of patients expected to be curable by resection, clarification of equivocal findings, or suspected cancer recurrence. Because of its excellent M-staging capabilities, ^{18}F-FDG PET/CT has a significant clinical impact, leading to up- or down-staging of up to 31% of patients (Kochhar et al. 2010). Moreover, the use of ^{18}F-FDG PET/CT instead of conventional imaging changes treatment plans from curative to palliative or vice versa in about 30% of the cases (Petersen et al. 2014). ^{18}F-FDG uptake correlates with prognosis and is predictive of mortality in liver metastasis from colorectal cancer (Riedl et al. 2007). ^{18}F-FDG PET/MRI may be a potential alternative to ^{18}F-FDG PET/CT in colorectal cancer staging, particularly in primary rectal cancer. Based on its higher soft tissue contrast and the benefits of DWI, ^{18}F-FDG PET/MRI is expected to provide more exact T-staging and at least equivalent accuracy in N- and M-staging compared to ^{18}F-FDG PET/CT. Furthermore, ^{18}F-FDG PET/MRI has been shown to be superior in evaluating hepatic lesions, which is particularly relevant because of the high rate of liver metastases in colorectal cancer (Beiderwellen et al. 2013a, 2015). Recently, the accuracy of ^{18}F-FDG PET/MRI has been compared with that of contrast-enhanced CT in 51 patients with colorectal cancer (Kang et al. 2016). ^{18}F-FDG PET/MRI showed an incremental diagnostic value over CT in 28% of patients, providing improved characterization and additional detection of distant metastases, although it missed a few pulmonary lesions. Initial studies on UTE sequences indicated a high potential for reliably depicting subcentimeter lung lesions and may improve the detection rate of MRI in the future,

but this requires additional investigation (Burris et al. 2016). According to the authors, the information from ^{18}F-FDG PET/MRI led to an alternative treatment strategy in one fifth of the patients. Notwithstanding these promising data, current evidence is limited and there are many open questions concerning ^{18}F-FDG PET/MRI in colorectal cancer, such as its role in disease recurrence or evaluation of treatment response.

3.6   Lymphatic System

3.6.1   Lymphoma

In 2016 about 72,000 new cases of non-Hodgkin lymphoma (NHL) and 8500 new cases of Hodgkin's lymphoma were expected in the USA (Institute NC 2017b, c). Current lymphoma classifications recognize >50 subtypes of lymphoma based on differences in histopathology, cytogenetics, and immunohistochemistry. In clinical routine, a limited number of subtypes account for the majority of cases, including Hodgkin's lymphoma (10% of lymphoma), diffuse large B-cell lymphoma (33% of NHL), follicular lymphoma (20% of NHL), marginal zone lymphoma (10% of NHL), chronic lymphatic leukemia (7% of NHL), and mantle cell lymphoma (7% of NHL). The Ann Arbor classification, introduced in 1971 and revised in 1989, is used to stage both Hodgkin lymphoma and non-Hodgkin lymphoma based on the extent of nodal group involvement, extranodal lymphoma manifestation and presence of B-symptoms. On a metabolic level, lymphoma can be categorized according to ^{18}F-FDG avidity, based on expression of cell surface glucose transporter proteins such as GLUT-1. CT is used for whole-body staging in non ^{18}F-FDG-avid lymphoma (Cheson et al. 2014). ^{18}F-FDG PET/CT is the modality of choice for staging of all ^{18}F-FDG - avid lymphoma, such as Hodgkin lymphoma and diffuse large B-cell lymphoma (Weiler-Sagie et al. 2010; Cheson et al. 2014). However, as certain subtypes of lymphoma vary in their ^{18}F-FDG - avidity, ^{18}F-FDG PET/CT initial staging should entail high quality morphological CT imaging to enable best possible staging for lymphoma of any kind. Studies have shown that ^{18}F-FDG PET/CT provides more exact staging than CT and ^{18}F-FDG PET alone with a reported sensitivity, specificity, PPV and NPV of 96%, 99%, 96%, and 99% (Freudenberg et al. 2004). The 2014 Lugano guidelines recommend ^{18}F-FDG PET/CT for the following indications: (a) initial staging, (b) re-staging, and (c) evaluation of therapy response (Cheson et al. 2014). Compared to conventional imaging, ^{18}F-FDG PET/CT changes staging results of up to 20% of patients at initial staging and induces change of treatment in about 15% of patients. The combined information on lymphoma extent and vitality offers the basis for a sophisticated evaluation of treatment response through changes in lesion size and glucose metabolism. Today, ^{18}F-FDG PET/CT is an integral part of most large-scale lymphoma trials and has a key role for initial and re-staging during and after completion of chemotherapy. The particular charm of ^{18}F-FDG PET/CT lies in its ability to discriminate vital from non-vital residual masses, which is crucial for treatment planning. The Deauville criteria propagate an ^{18}F-FDG PET/CT-based response evaluation using a 5-point scale: (1) No uptake, (2) slight uptake, below mediastinal blood pool, (3) uptake above mediastinal blood pool, but below or equal to uptake of liver, (4) uptake moderately higher than uptake of liver, and (5) uptake markedly higher than uptake of liver (Meignan et al. 2009). ^{18}F-FDG PET-negativity after completion of therapy indicates a low chance for disease recurrence, and data from the HD15 study showed that ^{18}F-FDG PET/CT performed after chemotherapy can guide the need for additional radiotherapy (Engert et al. 2012). ^{18}F-FDG PET/MRI may be an alternative to ^{18}F-FDG PET/CT for whole-body imaging of lymphoma, entailing the following potential advantages:

– Lower radiation exposition.
– Superior assessment of extra-nodal involvement.

– More differentiated (re-)staging due to simultaneous acquisition of (multiparametric) MRI and ^{18}F-FDG PET.

Several groups have evaluated the role of ^{18}F-FDG PET/MRI in staging of lymphoma (Heacock et al. 2015; Herrmann et al. 2015; Sher et al. 2016; Grueneisen et al. 2016; Atkinson et al. 2016; Ponisio et al. 2016; Afaq et al. 2017; Kirchner et al. 2017a, b). Existing evidence indicate a diagnostic accuracy in lymphoma staging equivalent to ^{18}F-FDG PET/CT at 39–64% less radiation dose (Fig. 3.11). Considering the young age of many patients, ^{18}F-FDG PET/MRI might aid to reduce the risk of radiation-induced secondary neoplasms. Grueneisen et al. investigated a fast ^{18}F-FDG PET/MRI protocol (whole-body T1w VIBE, T2w HASTE, DWI) and were able to reduce the scan duration of whole-body PET/MRI to under 30 min without compromising the diagnostic performance (Grueneisen et al. 2016). Lesion detection and Ann Arbor staging were shown equivalent in ^{18}F-FDG PET/MRI and ^{18}F-FDG PET/CT and SUVmax values strongly correlated. Introducing an even shorter study protocol, Kirchner et al. investigated the diagnostic performance of a so-called ultra-fast PET/MRI protocol, demonstrating its high diagnostic potential while reducing the examination time to an equally short examination time as in PET/CT (Kirchner et al. 2017a, b). In a recent study that compared different ^{18}F-FDG PET/MRI protocols, the additional application of contrast-enhanced and diffusion-weighted imaging resulted in higher diagnostic accuracy on a per lesion- and per patient basis (Kirchner et al. 2017a, b). Whole-body DWI has been shown to be inferior to PET/CT on a per-lesion basis but could be useful in low-grade lymphomas and surveillance (Herrmann et al. 2015). As they depict different pathophysiological processes, the potential of acquiring ^{18}F-FDG PET and DWI simultaneously enables the exploration of their complementary value for staging and response evaluation, which should be further investigated in future trials (Schaarschmidt et al. 2015b).

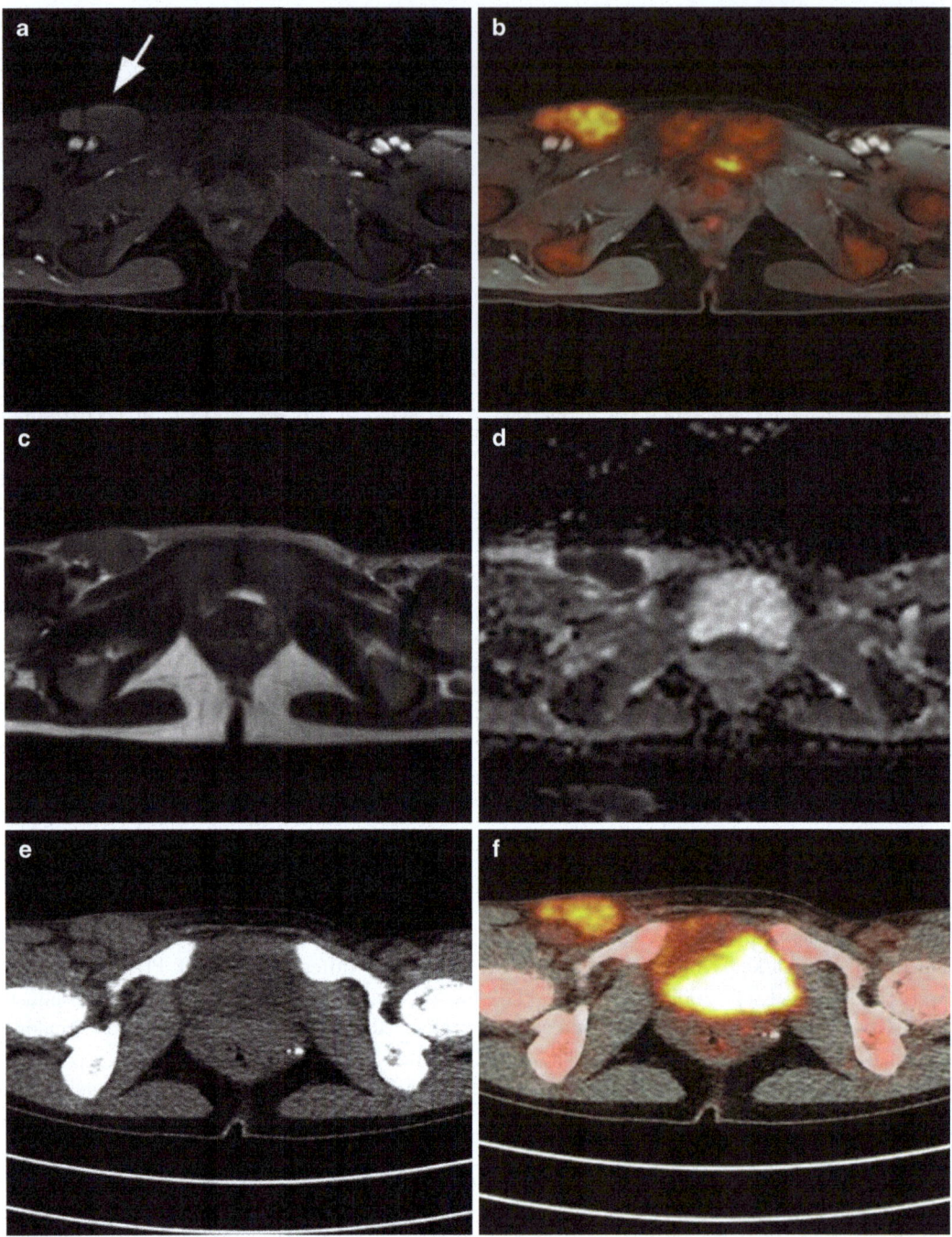

Fig. 3.11 A 20-year-old female NHL patient with two pathologic lymph nodes in the right inguinal region Shown in post-contrast fat-saturated T1w MRI (**a**), [18]F- FDG PET/MRI (**b**), T2w imaging (**c**), ADC map (**d**), CT (**e**), ^{18}F-FDG PET/CT (**f**)

3.7 Musulosceletal System

3.7.1 Malignant Primary Bone Tumors and Soft Tissue Sarcomas

Malignant primary bone tumors and soft tissue sarcomas are exceedingly rare (Siegel et al. 2014). Due to the multitude of histological subtypes, precise pretherapeautical imaging is essential for optimized patient and therapy management. While MRI excels in local tumor imaging due to its high soft tissue contrast, imaging of glucose metabolism by ^{18}F-FDG PET is of considerable value in the evaluation of lymph nodes and the detection of distant metastases (Tateishi et al. 2007). Therefore, the idea of performing high resolution MR imaging to assess local tumor extent and acquire whole-body MR and PET images for distant metastasis staging in a single examination is promising and has been discussed as a potential major advantage for integrated PET/MRI imaging in several reviews (Fig. 3.12) (Antoch and Bockisch 2009; Buchbender et al. 2012b; Andersen et al. 2016). Although several case reports indicate the

advantages of a combined acquisition of functional PET data, morphological MR imaging and functional MR imaging techniques, studies evaluating the additional value of integrated ^{18}F-FDG PET/MRI in comparison to ^{18}F-FDG PET/CT and subsequent MRI in initial tumor staging and tumor recurrence diagnostics are rare (Fig. 3.13) (Schuler et al. 2013; Partovi et al. 2014b; Zhang et al. 2016). A study published by Schuler et al. in 2015 indicates that ^{18}F-FDG PET/MRI offers a comparable staging accuracy as conventional staging in sarcoma patients (Schuler et al. 2015). Furthermore, therapy response assessment seems to be possible in ^{18}F-FDG PET/MRI (Platzek et al. 2017). However, further prospective studies are necessary to evaluate if ^{18}F-FDG PET/MRI is superior to the sequential acquisition of ^{18}F-FDG PET/CT and subsequent MRI in tumor staging and response assessment. In pediatric patients, however, integrated ^{18}F-FDG PET/MRI offers an easier clinical workflow by allowing true "one stop shop" examinations that do not only increase patient comfort but also lead to a considerable dose reduction by the omission of a whole-body CT scan (Schäfer et al. 2014).

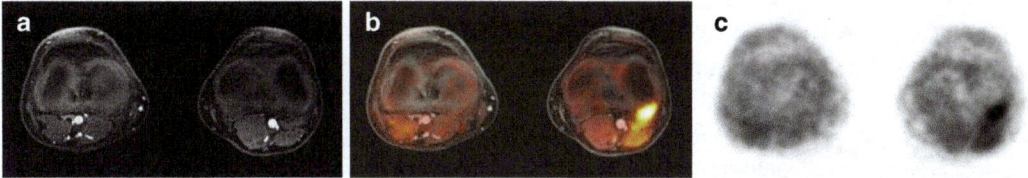

Fig. 3.12 59 year old male patient suffering from chondrosarcoma left knee undergoing PET/MRI for initial staging. Morphological, fused and PET images are displayed for ^{18}F-FDG PET/MRI (**a**–**c**). While the suspicious tissue can be easily missed even on contrast enhanced MRI (**a**), PET/MRI images are highly conspicuous for malignancy

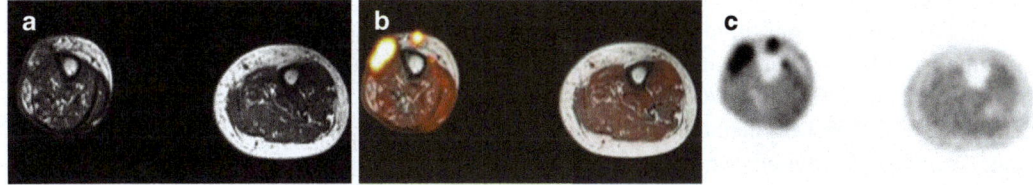

Fig. 3.13 61 year old female patient undergoing PET/MRI for tumor recurrence diagnostics after resection of a soft tissue sarcoma. Morphological, fused and PET images are displayed for ^{18}F-FDG PET/MRI (**a**–**c**)

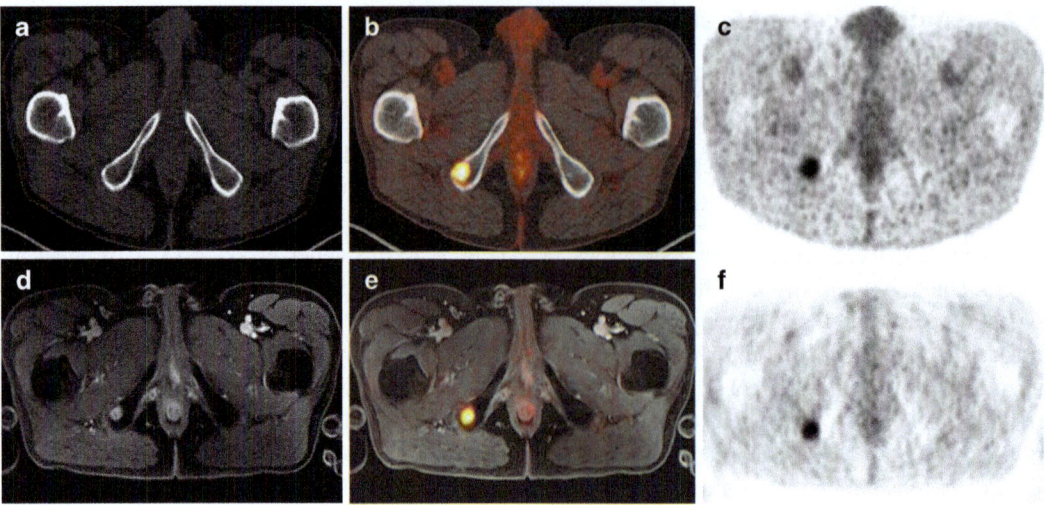

Fig. 3.14 64 year old male patient suffering from advanced non-small cell lung cancer (adenocarcinoma). Morphological, fused and PET images are displayed for ¹⁸F-FDG PET/CT (**a–c**) and ¹⁸F-FDG PET/MRI (**d–f**). While no morphological correlate can be detected for the highly suspicious tracer uptake in the right ischial tuberosity in CT (**a**), a clear morphological correlate can be detected in contrast enhanced MRI (**d**), confirming an osseous metastasis

3.7.2 Osseous Metastases

Bone metastases occur frequently in numerous cancer types and are not only associated with a considerate mortality but also a high morbidity causing frequent hospitalization due to bone pain and pathological fractures (Rubens 1998). Therefore, the detection and correct characterization of bone lesions is pivotal. While bone scintigraphy and CT imaging are still used as basic imaging tools, ¹⁸F-FDG PET/CT and MRI seem to provide a higher sensitivity and specificity in the detection of bone metastases (Even-Sapir 2005). Integrated ¹⁸F-FDG PET/MRI combines the advantages of both imaging modalities and initial studies report a superior conspicuity and diagnostic confidence for osseous metastases (Beiderwellen et al. 2014; Samarin et al. 2015). Furthermore, preliminary data suggest that ¹⁸F-FDG PET/MRI offers a sensitivity of 96.3% and a specificity of 98.8%, surpassing both whole-body MRI and ¹⁸F-FDG PET/CT (Fig. 3.14) (Catalano et al. 2015). Despite these encouraging results, caution is advised when transferring these results to clinical practice as the analyzed patient cohorts are small and the underlying oncological diseases are diverse, thus necessitating further research.

References

Abgral R, Querellou S, Potard G, et al. Does 18F-FDG PET/CT improve the detection of posttreatment recurrence of head and neck squamous cell carcinoma in patients negative for disease on clinical follow-up? J Nucl Med. 2009;50:24–9. https://doi.org/10.2967/jnumed.108.055806.

Afaq A, Fraioli F, Sidhu H, et al. Comparison of PET/MRI With PET/CT in the evaluation of disease status in lymphoma. Clin Nucl Med. 2017;42:1–7. https://doi.org/10.1097/RLU.0000000000001344.

Andersen KF, Jensen KE, Loft A. PET/MRI imaging in musculoskeletal disorders. PET Clin. 2016;11:453–63. https://doi.org/10.1016/j.cpet.2016.05.007.

Antoch G, Bockisch A. Combined PET/MRI: a new dimension in whole-body oncology imaging? Eur J Nucl Med Mol Imaging. 2009;36:113–20. https://doi.org/10.1007/s00259-008-0951-6.

Antoch G, Stattaus J, Nemat AT, et al. Non–small cell lung cancer: dual-modality PET/CT in preoperative staging. Radiology. 2003;229:526–33. https://doi.org/10.1148/radiol.2292021598.

Armato SG III, Labby ZE, Coolen J, et al. Imaging in pleural mesothelioma: a review of the 11th International Conference of the International Mesothelioma Interest Group. Lung Cancer. 2013;82:190–6. https://doi.org/10.1016/j.lungcan.2013.08.005.

Atkinson W, Catana C, Abramson JS, et al. Hybrid FDG-PET/MRI compared to FDG-PET/CT in adult lymphoma patients. Abdom Radiol NY. 2016;41:1338–48. https://doi.org/10.1007/s00261-016-0638-6.

Basu S, Nair N. 18F-FDG uptake in bilateral adrenal hyperplasia causing Cushing's syndrome. Eur J

Nucl Med Mol Imaging. 2005;32:384. https://doi.org/10.1007/s00259-004-1629-3.

Beiderwellen K, Geraldo L, Ruhlmann V, et al. Accuracy of [18F]FDG PET/MRI for the detection of liver metastases. PLoS One. 2015;10:e0137285. https://doi.org/10.1371/journal.pone.0137285.

Beiderwellen K, Gomez B, Buchbender C, et al. Depiction and characterization of liver lesions in whole body [18F]-FDG PET/MRI. Eur J Radiol. 2013a;82:e669–75. https://doi.org/10.1016/j.ejrad.2013.07.027.

Beiderwellen K, Huebner M, Heusch P, et al. Whole-body [18F]FDG PET/MRI vs. PET/CT in the assessment of bone lesions in oncological patients: initial results. Eur Radiol. 2014;24:2023–30. https://doi.org/10.1007/s00330-014-3229-3.

Beiderwellen KJ, Poeppel TD, Hartung-Knemeyer V, et al. Simultaneous 68Ga-DOTATOC PET/MRI in patients with gastroenteropancreatic neuroendocrine tumors: initial results. Investig Radiol. 2013b;48:273–9. https://doi.org/10.1097/RLI.0b013e3182871a7f.

Biederer J, Beer M, Hirsch W, et al. MRI of the lung (2/3). Why … when … how? Insights Imaging. 2012;3:355–71. https://doi.org/10.1007/s13244-011-0146-8.

Boysen M, Lövdal O, Tausjö J. Winther F (1992) The value of follow-up in patients treated for squamous cell carcinoma of the head and neck. Eur J Cancer Oxf Engl. 1990;28:426–30.

Breathnach OS, Freidlin B, Conley B, et al. Twenty-two years of phase III trials for patients with advanced non–small-cell lung cancer: sobering results. J Clin Oncol. 2001;19:1734–42.

Buchbender C, Heusner TA, Lauenstein TC, et al. Oncologic PET/MRI, part 1: tumors of the brain, head and neck, chest, abdomen, and pelvis. J Nucl Med. 2012a;53:928–38. https://doi.org/10.2967/jnumed.112.105338.

Buchbender C, Heusner TA, Lauenstein TC, et al. Oncologic PET/MRI, part 2: bone tumors, soft-tissue tumors, melanoma, and lymphoma. J Nucl Med. 2012b;53:1244–52. https://doi.org/10.2967/jnumed.112.109306.

Burris NS, Johnson KM, Larson PEZ, et al. Detection of small pulmonary nodules with ultrashort echo time sequences in oncology patients by using a PET/MRI system. Radiology. 2016;278:239–46. https://doi.org/10.1148/radiol.2015150489.

Catalano OA, Nicolai E, Rosen BR, et al. Comparison of CE-FDG-PET/CT with CE-FDG-PET/MRI in the evaluation of osseous metastases in breast cancer patients. Br J Cancer. 2015;112:1452–60. https://doi.org/10.1038/bjc.2015.112.

Catalano OA, Rosen BR, Sahani DV, et al. Clinical impact of PET/MRI imaging in patients with cancer undergoing same-day PET/CT: initial experience in 134 patients—a hypothesis-generating exploratory study. Radiology. 2013;269:857–69. https://doi.org/10.1148/radiol.13131306.

Chandarana H, Heacock L, Rakheja R, et al. Pulmonary nodules in patients with primary malignancy: comparison of hybrid PET/MRI and PET/CT imaging.

Radiology. 2013;268:874–81. https://doi.org/10.1148/radiol.13130620.

Cheson BD, Fisher RI, Barrington SF, et al. Recommendations for initial evaluation, staging, and response assessment of Hodgkin and non-Hodgkin lymphoma: The Lugano classification. J Clin Oncol. 2014;32:3059–67. https://doi.org/10.1200/JCO.2013.54.8800.

Colli A, Fraquelli M, Casazza G, et al. Accuracy of ultrasonography, spiral CT, magnetic resonance, and alpha-fetoprotein in diagnosing hepatocellular carcinoma: a systematic review. Am J Gastroenterol. 2006;101:513–23. https://doi.org/10.1111/j.1572-0241.2006.00467.x.

Comoretto M, Balestreri L, Borsatti E, et al. Detection and restaging of residual and/or recurrent nasopharyngeal carcinoma after chemotherapy and radiation therapy: comparison of MR imaging and FDG PET/CT. Radiology. 2008;249:203–11. https://doi.org/10.1148/radiol.2491071753.

Coolen J, De Keyzer F, Nafteux P, et al. Malignant pleural mesothelioma: visual assessment by using pleural pointillism at diffusion-weighted MR imaging. Radiology. 2014;274:576–84. https://doi.org/10.1148/radiol.14132111.

de Bree R, Deurloo EE, Snow GB, Leemans CR. Screening for distant metastases in patients with head and neck cancer. Laryngoscope. 2000;110:397–401. https://doi.org/10.1097/00005537-200003000-00012.

Donati OF, Hany TF, Reiner CS, et al. Value of retrospective fusion of PET and MR images in detection of hepatic metastases: comparison with 18F-FDG PET/CT and Gd-EOB-DTPA-enhanced MRI. J Nucl Med Off Publ Soc Nucl Med. 2010;51:692–9. https://doi.org/10.2967/jnumed.109.068510.

D'souza MM, Sharma R, Mondal A, et al. Prospective evaluation of CECT and 18F-FDG-PET/CT in detection of hepatic metastases. Nucl Med Commun. 2009;30:117–25. https://doi.org/10.1097/MNM.0b013e32831ec57b.

Eiber M, Martinez-Möller A, Souvatzoglou M, et al. Value of a Dixon-based MR/PET attenuation correction sequence for the localization and evaluation of PET-positive lesions. Eur J Nucl Med Mol Imaging. 2011;38:1691–701. https://doi.org/10.1007/s00259-011-1842-9.

Engelbrecht V, Pisar E, Fürst G, Mödder U. Verlaufskontrolle und Rezidivdiagnostik maligner Kopf- und Halstumoren nach Radiochemotherapie. RöFo - Fortschritte Auf Dem Geb Röntgenstrahlen Bildgeb Verfahr. 1995;162:304–10. https://doi.org/10.1055/s-2007-1015887.

Engert A, Haverkamp H, Kobe C, et al. Reduced-intensity chemotherapy and PET-guided radiotherapy in patients with advanced stage Hodgkin's lymphoma (HD15 trial): a randomised, open-label, phase 3 non-inferiority trial. Lancet. 2012;379:1791–9. https://doi.org/10.1016/S0140-6736(11)61940-5.

Even-Sapir E. Imaging of malignant bone involvement by morphologic, scintigraphic, and hybrid modalities. J Nucl Med. 2005;46:1356–67.

Flamen P, Lerut A, Van Cutsem E, et al. Utility of positron emission tomography for the staging of patients with potentially operable esophageal carcinoma. J Clin Oncol Off J Am Soc Clin Oncol. 2000;18:3202–10. https://doi.org/10.1200/JCO.2000.18.18.3202.

Fowler KJ, Maughan NM, Laforest R, et al. PET/MRI of hepatic 90Y microsphere deposition determines individual tumor response. Cardiovasc Intervent Radiol. 2016;39:855–64. https://doi.org/10.1007/s00270-015-1285-y.

Fraioli F, Screaton NJ, Janes SM, et al. Non-small-cell lung cancer resectability: diagnostic value of PET/MRI. Eur J Nucl Med Mol Imaging. 2014;42:49–55. https://doi.org/10.1007/s00259-014-2873-9.

Freudenberg LS, Antoch G, Schütt P, et al. FDG-PET/CT in re-staging of patients with lymphoma. Eur J Nucl Med Mol Imaging. 2004;31:325–9. https://doi.org/10.1007/s00259-003-1375-y.

Gatidis S, Schmidt H, Claussen CD, Schwenzer NF. Multiparametrische Bildgebung mittels simultaner MR/PET. Radiology. 2013;53:669–75. https://doi.org/10.1007/s00117-013-2496-3.

Goeckenjan G, Sitter H, Thomas M, et al. Prevention, diagnosis, therapy, and follow-up of lung cancer. Pneumologie. 2010;65:39–59. https://doi.org/10.1055/s-0030-1255961.

Goodwin MD, Dobson JE, Sirlin CB, et al. Diagnostic challenges and pitfalls in MR imaging with hepatocyte-specific contrast agents. Radiographics. 2011;31:1547–68. https://doi.org/10.1148/rg.316115528.

Grégoire V, Lefebvre J-L, Licitra L, Felip E. Squamous cell carcinoma of the head and neck: EHNS–ESMO–ESTRO Clinical Practice Guidelines for diagnosis, treatment and follow-up. Ann Oncol. 2010;21:v184–6. https://doi.org/10.1093/annonc/mdq185.

Grueneisen J, Sawicki LM, Schaarschmidt BM, et al. Evaluation of a fast protocol for staging lymphoma patients with integrated PET/MRI. PLoS One. 2016;11:e0157880. https://doi.org/10.1371/journal.pone.0157880.

Haerle SK, Schmid DT, Ahmad N, et al. The value of (18)F-FDG PET/CT for the detection of distant metastases in high-risk patients with head and neck squamous cell carcinoma. Oral Oncol. 2011;47:653–9. https://doi.org/10.1016/j.oraloncology.2011.05.011.

Hafidh MA, Lacy PD, Hughes JP, et al. Evaluation of the impact of addition of PET to CT and MR scanning in the staging of patients with head and neck carcinomas. Eur Arch Oto-Rhino-Laryngol Head Neck. 2006;263:853–9. https://doi.org/10.1007/s00405-006-0067-1.

Haggar FA, Boushey RP. Colorectal cancer epidemiology: incidence, mortality, survival, and risk factors. Clin Colon Rectal Surg. 2009;22:191–7. https://doi.org/10.1055/s-0029-1242458.

Hahn S, Hecktor J, Grabellus F, et al. Diagnostic accuracy of dual-time-point 18F-FDG PET/CT for the detection of axillary lymph node metastases in breast cancer patients. Acta Radiol. 2012;53:518–23. https://doi.org/10.1258/ar.2012.110420.

Haider MA, Ghai S, Jhaveri K, Lockwood G. Chemical Shift MR imaging of hyperattenuating (>10 HU) adrenal masses: does it still have a role? Radiology. 2004;231:711–6. https://doi.org/10.1148/radiol.2313030676.

Hartung-Knemeyer V, Beiderwellen KJ, Buchbender C, et al. Optimizing positron emission tomography image acquisition protocols in integrated positron emission tomography/magnetic resonance imaging. Investig Radiol. 2013;48:290–4. https://doi.org/10.1097/RLI.0b013e3182823695.

Heacock L, Weissbrot J, Raad R, et al. PET/MRI for the evaluation of patients with lymphoma: initial observations. AJR Am J Roentgenol. 2015;204:842–8. https://doi.org/10.2214/AJR.14.13181.

Heelan RT, Rusch VW, Begg CB, et al. Staging of malignant pleural mesothelioma: comparison of CT and MR imaging. Am J Roentgenol. 1999;172:1039–47. https://doi.org/10.2214/ajr.172.4.10587144.

Herrmann K, Queiroz M, Huellner MW, et al. Diagnostic performance of FDG-PET/MRI and WB-DW-MRI in the evaluation of lymphoma: a prospective comparison to standard FDG-PET/CT. BMC Cancer. 2015;15:1002. https://doi.org/10.1186/s12885-015-2009-z.

Heusch P, Buchbender C, Köhler J, et al. Correlation of the Apparent Diffusion Coefficient (ADC) with the Standardized Uptake Value (SUV) in hybrid 18F-FDG PET/MRI in Non-Small Cell Lung Cancer (NSCLC) lesions: initial results. RöFo - Fortschritte Auf Dem Geb Röntgenstrahlen Bildgeb Verfahr. 2013;185:1056–62. https://doi.org/10.1055/s-0033-1350110.

Heusch P, Buchbender C, Köhler J, et al. Thoracic staging in lung cancer: prospective comparison of 18F-FDG PET/MRI imaging and 18F-FDG PET/CT. J Nucl Med. 2014a;55:373–8. https://doi.org/10.2967/jnumed.113.129825.

Heusch P, Nensa F, Schaarschmidt B, et al. Diagnostic accuracy of whole-body PET/MRI and whole-body PET/CT for TNM staging in oncology. Eur J Nucl Med Mol Imaging. 2014b;42:42–8. https://doi.org/10.1007/s00259-014-2885-5.

Heusch P, Sproll C, Buchbender C, et al. Diagnostic accuracy of ultrasound, 18F-FDG-PET/CT, and fused 18F-FDG-PET-MR images with DWI for the detection of cervical lymph node metastases of HNSCC. Clin Oral Investig. 2014c;18:969–78. https://doi.org/10.1007/s00784-013-1050-z.

Hintze C, Biederer J, Wenz HW, et al. MRI in staging of lung cancer. Radiology. 2006;46:251–254., 256–259. https://doi.org/10.1007/s00117-005-1334-7.

Hofman MS, Lau WFE, Hicks RJ. Somatostatin receptor imaging with 68Ga DOTATATE PET/CT: clinical utility, normal patterns, pearls, and pitfalls in interpretation. Radiographics. 2015;35:500–16. https://doi.org/10.1148/rg.352140164.

Hope TA, Pampaloni MH, Nakakura E, et al. Simultaneous (68)Ga-DOTA-TOC PET/MRI with gadoxetate disodium in patients with neuroendocrine tumor. Abdom

Imaging. 2015;40:1432–40. https://doi.org/10.1007/s00261-015-0409-9.

Howaldt HP, Vorast H, Blecher JC, et al. Results of the DOSAK tumor register. Mund- Kiefer-Gesichtschirurgie MKG. 2000;4(Suppl 1):S216–25.

Huellner MW, Appenzeller P, Kuhn FP, et al. Whole-body nonenhanced PET/MRI versus PET/CT in the staging and restaging of cancers: preliminary observations. Radiology. 2014;273:859–69. https://doi.org/10.1148/radiol.14140090.

Huellner MW, Barbosa F de G, Husmann L, et al (2016) TNM staging of non–small cell lung cancer: comparison of PET/MRI and PET/CT. J Nucl Med 57:21–26. doi: https://doi.org/10.2967/jnumed.115.162040.

Institute NC (2017a). Cancer stat facts: esophageal cancer. 2017.

Institute NC (2017b). Cancer stat facts: non-hodgkin lymphoma. 2017.

Institute NC (2017c). Cancer stat facts: hodgkin lymphoma. 2017.

Jacobsson H, Larsson P, Jonsson C, et al. Normal uptake of 68Ga-DOTA-TOC by the pancreas uncinate process mimicking malignancy at somatostatin receptor PET. Clin Nucl Med. 2012;37:362–5. https://doi.org/10.1097/RLU.0b013e3182485110.

Kaemmerer D, Peter L, Lupp A, et al. Molecular imaging with ^{68}Ga-SSTR PET/CT and correlation to immunohistochemistry of somatostatin receptors in neuroendocrine tumours. Eur J Nucl Med Mol Imaging. 2011;38:1659–68. https://doi.org/10.1007/s00259-011-1846-5.

Kanda T, Kitajima K, Suenaga Y, et al. Value of retrospective image fusion of 18F-FDG PET and MRI for preoperative staging of head and neck cancer: Comparison with PET/CT and contrast-enhanced neck MRI. Eur J Radiol. 2013;82:2005–10. https://doi.org/10.1016/j.ejrad.2013.06.025.

Kang B, Lee JM, Song YS, et al. Added value of integrated whole-body PET/MRI for evaluation of colorectal cancer: comparison with contrast-enhanced MDCT. AJR Am J Roentgenol. 2016;206:10–20. https://doi.org/10.2214/AJR.14.13818.

Katyal S, Oliver JH, Peterson MS, et al. Extrahepatic metastases of hepatocellular carcinoma. Radiology. 2000;216:698–703. https://doi.org/10.1148/radiology.216.3.r00se24698.

Khan MA, Combs CS, Brunt EM, et al. Positron emission tomography scanning in the evaluation of hepatocellular carcinoma. J Hepatol. 2000;32:792–7.

Kirchner J, Deuschl C, Grueneisen J, et al. $^{(18)}$F-FDG PET/MRI in patients suffering from lymphoma: how much MRI information is really needed? Eur J Nucl Med Mol Imaging. 2017a. https://doi.org/10.1007/s00259-017-3635-2.

Kirchner J, Sawicki LM, Suntharalingam S, Grueneisen J, Ruhlmann V, Aktas B, Deuschl C, Herrmann K, Antoch G, Forsting M, Umutlu L. Whole-body staging of female patients with recurrent pelvic malignancies: Ultra-fast 18F-FDG PET/MRI compared to 18F-FDG PET/CT and CT. PLoS One. 2017b;12(2):e0172553. https://doi.org/10.1371/journal.pone.0172553. eCollection 2017.

Klimstra DS, Beltran H, Lilenbaum R, Bergsland E. The spectrum of neuroendocrine tumors: histologic classification, unique features and areas of overlap. Am Soc Clin Oncol Educ Book Am Soc Clin Oncol Meet. 2015:92–103. 10.14694/EdBook_AM.2015.35.92.

Kochhar R, Liong S, Manoharan P. The role of FDG PET/CT in patients with colorectal cancer metastases. Cancer Biomark Sect Dis Markers. 2010;7:235–48. https://doi.org/10.3233/CBM-2010-0201.

Kong G, Jackson C, Koh DM, et al. The use of 18F-FDG PET/CT in colorectal liver metastases—comparison with CT and liver MRI. Eur J Nucl Med Mol Imaging. 2008;35:1323–9. https://doi.org/10.1007/s00259-008-0743-z.

Kulaksiz H, Eissele R, Rössler D, et al. Identification of somatostatin receptor subtypes 1, 2A, 3, and 5 in neuroendocrine tumours with subtype specific antibodies. Gut. 2002;50:52–60.

Landwehr P, Schulte O, Lackner K. MR imaging of the chest: mediastinum and chest wall. Eur Radiol. 1999;9:1737–44. https://doi.org/10.1007/s003300050917

Lardinois D, Weder W, Hany TF, et al. Staging of non–small-cell lung cancer with integrated positron-emission tomography and computed tomography. N Engl J Med. 2003;348:2500–7. https://doi.org/10.1056/NEJMoa022136.

Laubenbacher C, Saumweber D, Wagner-Manslau C, et al. Comparison of fluorine-18-fluorodeoxyglucose pet, mri and endoscopy for staging head and neck squamous-cell carcinomas. J Nucl Med. 1995;36:1747–57.

Lee G, H I, Kim S-J, et al. Clinical implication of PET/MRI imaging in preoperative esophageal cancer staging: comparison with PET/CT, endoscopic ultrasonography, and CT. J Nucl Med. 2014;55:1242–7. https://doi.org/10.2967/jnumed.114.138974.

Lee JH, Park JY, Kim DY, et al. Prognostic value of 18F-FDG PET for hepatocellular carcinoma patients treated with sorafenib. Liver. 2011;31:1144–9. https://doi.org/10.1111/j.1478-3231.2011.02541.x.

Lell M, Baum U, Greess H, et al. Head and neck tumors: imaging recurrent tumor and post-therapeutic changes with CT and MRI. Eur J Radiol. 2000;33:239–47. https://doi.org/10.1016/S0720-048X(99)00120-5.

Leslie A, Fyfe E, Guest P, et al. Staging of squamous cell carcinoma of the oral cavity and oropharynx: a comparison of MRI and CT in T- and N-staging. [miscellaneous article]. J Comput Assist Tomogr. 1999;23:43–9.

Lewis P, Marsden P, Gee T, et al. 18F-fluorodeoxyglucose positron emission tomography in preoperative evaluation of lung cancer. Lancet. 1994;344:1265–6. https://doi.org/10.1016/S0140-6736(94)90753-6.

Leyn PD, Lardinois D, Schil PEV, et al. ESTS guidelines for preoperative lymph node staging for non-small cell lung cancer. Eur J Cardiothorac Surg. 2007;32:1–8. https://doi.org/10.1016/j.ejcts.2007.01.075.

Liberale G, Van Laethem JL, Gay F, et al. The role of PET scan in the preoperative management of oesophageal cancer. Eur J Surg Oncol. 2004;30:942–7. https://doi.org/10.1016/j.ejso.2004.07.020.

Lin C-Y, Chen J-H, Liang J-A, et al. 18F-FDG PET or PET/CT for detecting extrahepatic metastases or recurrent hepatocellular carcinoma: a systematic review and meta-analysis. Eur J Radiol. 2012;81:2417–22. https://doi.org/10.1016/j.ejrad.2011.08.004.

Liu S-A, Wong Y-K, Lin J-C, et al. Impact of recurrence interval on survival of oral cavity squamous cell carcinoma patients after local relapse. Otolaryngol Head Neck Surg. 2007;136:112–8. https://doi.org/10.1016/j.otohns.2006.07.002.

Loeffelbein DJ, Eiber M, Mayr P, et al. Loco-regional recurrence after surgical treatment of oral squamous cell carcinoma: Proposals for follow-up imaging based on literature, national guidelines and institutional experience. J Cranio-Maxillofac Surg. 2015;43:1546–52. https://doi.org/10.1016/j.jcms.2015.06.020.

Lonneux M, Lawson G, Ide C, et al. Positron emission tomography with fluorodeoxyglucose for suspected head and neck tumor recurrence in the symptomatic patient. Laryngoscope. 2000;110:1493–7. https://doi.org/10.1097/00005537-200009000-00016.

Lowe VJ, Booya F, Fletcher JG, et al. Comparison of positron emission tomography, computed tomography, and endoscopic ultrasound in the initial staging of patients with esophageal cancer. Mol Imaging Biol. 2005;7:422–30. https://doi.org/10.1007/s11307-005-0017-0.

Martinez-Möller A, Eiber M, Nekolla SG, et al. Workflow and scan protocol considerations for integrated whole-body PET/MRI in oncology. J Nucl Med. 2012;53:1415–26. https://doi.org/10.2967/jnumed.112.109348.

Martini K, Meier A, Opitz I, et al. Diagnostic accuracy of sequential co-registered PET+MR in comparison to PET/CT in local thoracic staging of malignant pleural mesothelioma. Lung Cancer. 2016;94:40–5. https://doi.org/10.1016/j.lungcan.2016.01.017.

Mehanna H, Wong W-L, McConkey CC, et al. PET-CT surveillance versus neck dissection in advanced head and neck cancer. N Engl J Med. 2016;374:1444–54. https://doi.org/10.1056/NEJMoa1514493.

Meignan M, Gallamini A, Meignan M, et al. Report on the First International Workshop on interim-PET scan in lymphoma. Leuk Lymphoma. 2009;50:1257–60. https://doi.org/10.1080/10428190903040048.

Mittal S, El-Serag HB. Epidemiology of hepatocellular carcinoma: consider the population. J Clin Gastroenterol. 2013;47(Suppl):S2–6. https://doi.org/10.1097/MCG.0b013e3182872f29.

Mücke T, Wagenpfeil S, Kesting MR, et al. Recurrence interval affects survival after local relapse of oral cancer. Oral Oncol. 2009;45:687–91. https://doi.org/10.1016/j.oraloncology.2008.10.011.

Nahmias C, Carlson ER, Duncan LD, et al. Positron Emission Tomography/Computerized Tomography (PET/CT) scanning for preoperative staging of patients with oral/head and neck cancer. J Oral Maxillofac Surg. 2007;65:2524–35. https://doi.org/10.1016/j.joms.2007.03.010.

Nakamoto Y, Tamai K, Saga T, et al. Clinical value of image fusion from MR and PET in patients with head and neck cancer. Mol Imaging Biol. 2009;11:46–53. https://doi.org/10.1007/s11307-008-0168-x.

National Collaborating Centre for Cancer (UK). The diagnosis and treatment of lung cancer (update). Cardiff, UK: National Collaborating Centre for Cancer (UK); 2011.

NCCN. National Comprehensive Cancer Network Guidelines for Patients. Colon Cancer. Version 1. 2016. Accessed Apr 2017

Nensa F, Beiderwellen K, Heusch P, Wetter A. Clinical applications of PET/MRI: current status and future perspectives. Diagn Interv Radiol. 2014a;20:438–47. https://doi.org/10.5152/dir.2014.14008.

Nensa F, Stattaus J, Morgan B, et al. Dynamic contrast-enhanced MRI parameters as biomarkers for the effect of vatalanib in patients with non-small-cell lung cancer. Future Oncol. 2014b;10:823–33. https://doi.org/10.2217/fon.13.248.

Neumann V, Löseke S, Nowak D, et al. Malignant pleural mesothelioma. Dtsch Ärztebl Int. 2013;110:319–26. https://doi.org/10.3238/arztebl.2013.0319.

Nickell LT, Lichtenberger JP, Khorashadi L, et al. Multimodality imaging for characterization, classification, and staging of malignant pleural mesothelioma. Radiographics. 2014;34:1692–706. https://doi.org/10.1148/rg.346130089.

Nishino M, Hatabu H, Johnson BE, McLoud TC. State of the art: response assessment in lung cancer in the era of genomic medicine. Radiology. 2014;271:6–27. https://doi.org/10.1148/radiol.14122524.

Nomori H, Mori T, Ikeda K, et al. Diffusion-weighted magnetic resonance imaging can be used in place of positron emission tomography for N staging of non–small cell lung cancer with fewer false-positive results. J Thorac Cardiovasc Surg. 2008;135:816–22. https://doi.org/10.1016/j.jtcvs.2007.10.035.

Nougaret S, Reinhold C, Mikhael HW, et al. The use of MR imaging in treatment planning for patients with rectal carcinoma: have you checked the "DISTANCE"? Radiology. 2013;268:330–44. https://doi.org/10.1148/radiol.13121361.

Oberg K, Eriksson B. Endocrine tumours of the pancreas. Best Pract Res Clin Gastroenterol. 2005;19:753–81. https://doi.org/10.1016/j.bpg.2005.06.002.

Ogden GR. Second malignant tumours in head and neck cancer. BMJ. 1991;302:193–4.

Ohno Y, Koyama H, Yoshikawa T, et al. Diffusion-weighted MRI versus 18F-FDG PET/CT: performance as predictors of tumor treatment response and patient survival in patients with non–small cell lung cancer receiving chemoradiotherapy. Am J Roentgenol. 2012;198:75–82. https://doi.org/10.2214/AJR.11.6525.

Opitz I. Management of malignant pleural mesothelioma—The European experience. J Thorac Dis. 2014;6:S238–52. https://doi.org/10.3978/j.issn.2072-1439.2014.05.03.

Park BK, Kim CK, Kim B, Lee JH. Comparison of delayed enhanced CT and chemical shift MR for evaluating hyperattenuating incidental adrenal masses. Radiology. 2007;243:760–5. https://doi.org/10.1148/radiol.2433051978.

Park M-S, Kim S, Patel J, et al. Hepatocellular carcinoma: detection with diffusion-weighted versus contrast-enhanced magnetic resonance imaging in pretransplant patients. Hepatology. 2012;56:140–8. https://doi.org/10.1002/hep.25681.

Partovi S, Kohan A, Vercher-Conejero JL, et al. Qualitative and quantitative performance of 18F-FDG-PET/MRI versus 18F-FDG-PET/CT in patients with head and neck cancer. Am J Neuroradiol. 2014a;35:1970–5. https://doi.org/10.3174/ajnr.A3993.

Partovi S, Kohan AA, Zipp L, et al. Hybrid PET/MRI imaging in two sarcoma patients – clinical benefits and implications for future trials. Int J Clin Exp Med. 2014b;7:640–8.

Paul SAM, Stoeckli SJ, von Schulthess GK, Goerres GW. FDG PET and PET/CT for the detection of the primary tumour in patients with cervical non-squamous cell carcinoma metastasis of an unknown primary. Eur Arch Oto Rhino Laryngol. 2007;264:189–95. https://doi.org/10.1007/s00405-006-0177-9.

Petersen RK, Hess S, Alavi A, Høilund-Carlsen PF. Clinical impact of FDG-PET/CT on colorectal cancer staging and treatment strategy. Am J Nucl Med Mol Imaging. 2014;4:471–82.

Peto J, Decarli A, Vecchia CL, et al. The European mesothelioma epidemic. Br J Cancer. 1999;79:666–72. https://doi.org/10.1038/sj.bjc.6690105.

Pichler BJ, Kolb A, Nägele T, Schlemmer H-P. PET/MRI: paving the way for the next generation of clinical multimodality imaging applications. J Nucl Med. 2010;51:333–6. https://doi.org/10.2967/jnumed.109.061853.

Plathow C, Staab A, Schmaehl A, et al. Computed tomography, positron emission tomography, positron emission tomography/computed tomography, and magnetic resonance imaging for staging of limited pleural mesothelioma: initial results. Investig Radiol. 2008;43:737–44. https://doi.org/10.1097/RLI.0b013e3181817b3d.

Platzek I, Beuthien-Baumann B, Schramm G, et al. FDG PET/MRI in initial staging of sarcoma: Initial experience and comparison with conventional imaging. Clin Imaging. 2017;42:126–32. https://doi.org/10.1016/j.clinimag.2016.11.016.

Ponisio MR, McConathy J, Laforest R, Khanna G. Evaluation of diagnostic performance of whole-body simultaneous PET/MRI in pediatric lymphoma. Pediatr Radiol. 2016;46:1258–68. https://doi.org/10.1007/s00247-016-3601-3.

Posther KE, McCall LM, Harpole DH, et al. Yield of brain 18F-FDG PET in evaluating patients with potentially operable non–small cell lung cancer. J Nucl Med. 2006;47:1607–11.

Pöttgen C, Gauler T, Bellendorf A, et al. Standardized uptake decrease on [18F]-fluorodeoxyglucose positron emission tomography after neoadjuvant chemotherapy is a prognostic classifier for long-term outcome after multimodality treatment: secondary analysis of a randomized trial for resectable stage IIIA/B non–small-cell lung cancer. J Clin Oncol. 2016;34:2526–33. https://doi.org/10.1200/JCO.2015.65.5167.

Queiroz MA, Hüllner M, Kuhn F, et al. PET/MRI and PET/CT in follow-up of head and neck cancer patients. Eur J Nucl Med Mol Imaging. 2014;41:1066–75. https://doi.org/10.1007/s00259-014-2707-9.

Ramalho M, AlObaidy M, Burke LM, et al. MR-PET evaluation of 1-month post-ablation therapy for hepatocellular carcinoma: preliminary observations. Abdom Imaging. 2015;40:1405–14. https://doi.org/10.1007/s00261-015-0436-6.

Regier M, Derlin T, Schwarz D, et al. Diffusion weighted MRI and 18F-FDG PET/CT in non-small cell lung cancer (NSCLC): Does the apparent diffusion coefficient (ADC) correlate with tracer uptake (SUV)? Eur J Radiol. 2012;81:2913–8. https://doi.org/10.1016/j.ejrad.2011.11.050.

Riedl CC, Akhurst T, Larson S, et al. 18F-FDG PET scanning correlates with tissue markers of poor prognosis and predicts mortality for patients after liver resection for colorectal metastases. J Nucl Med. 2007;48:771–5. https://doi.org/10.2967/jnumed.106.037291.

Robert Koch-Institut, Gesellschaft der epidemiologischen Krebsregister in Deutschland e.V, editor. Krebs in Deutschland 2011/2012. 10th ed. Berlin: Auflage; 2015.

Rodrigues RS, Bozza FA, Christian PE, et al. Comparison of whole-body PET/CT, dedicated high-resolution head and neck PET/CT, and contrast-enhanced CT in preoperative staging of clinically M0 squamous cell carcinoma of the head and neck. J Nucl Med. 2009;50:1205–13. https://doi.org/10.2967/jnumed.109.062075.

Rogers SN, Brown JS, Woolgar JA, et al. Survival following primary surgery for oral cancer. Oral Oncol. 2009;45:201–11. https://doi.org/10.1016/j.oraloncology.2008.05.008.

Rubens RD. Bone metastases – the clinical problem. Eur J Cancer. 1998;1990(34):210–3.

Ruhlmann V, Ruhlmann M, Bellendorf A, et al. Hybrid imaging for detection of carcinoma of unknown primary: a preliminary comparison trial of whole-body PET/MRI versus PET/CT. Eur J Radiol. 2016;85:1941–7. https://doi.org/10.1016/j.ejrad.2016.08.020.

Samarin A, Hüllner M, Queiroz MA, et al. 18F-FDG-PET/MRI increases diagnostic confidence in detection of bone metastases compared with 18F-FDG-PET/CT. Nucl Med Commun. 2015;36:1165–73. https://doi.org/10.1097/MNM.0000000000000387.

Sawicki LM, Deuschl C, Beiderwellen K, et al (2017) Evaluation of 68Ga-DOTATOC PET/MRI for whole-body staging of neuroendocrine tumours in comparison with 68Ga-DOTATOC PET/CT.

Sawicki LM, Grueneisen J, Buchbender C, et al. Comparative performance of 18F-FDG PET/MRI and 18F-FDG PET/CT in detection and characterization of pulmonary lesions in 121 oncologic patients. J Nucl Med. 2016a;57:582–6. https://doi.org/10.2967/jnumed.115.167486.

Sawicki LM, Grueneisen J, Buchbender C, et al. Evaluation of the outcome of lung nodules missed on 18F-FDG PET/MRI compared with 18F-FDG PET/CT in patients with known malignancies. J Nucl Med. 2016b;57:15–20. https://doi.org/10.2967/jnumed.115.162966.

Schaarschmidt B, Buchbender C, Gomez B, et al. Thoracic staging of non-small-cell lung cancer using integrated 18F-FDG PET/MRI imaging: diagnostic value of different MR sequences. Eur J Nucl Med Mol Imaging. 2015a;42:1257–67. https://doi.org/10.1007/s00259-015-3050-5.

Schaarschmidt BM, Buchbender C, Nensa F, et al. Correlation of the Apparent Diffusion Coefficient (ADC) with the Standardized Uptake Value (SUV) in lymph node metastases of Non-Small Cell Lung Cancer (NSCLC) patients using hybrid 18F-FDG PET/MRI. PLoS One. 2015b;10:e0116277. https://doi.org/10.1371/journal.pone.0116277.

Schaarschmidt BM, Gomez B, Buchbender C, et al. Is integrated 18F-FDG PET/MRI superior to 18F-FDG PET/CT in the differentiation of incidental tracer uptake in the head and neck area? Diagn Interv Radiol. 2017a;23:127–32. https://doi.org/10.5152/dir.2016.15610.

Schaarschmidt BM, Grueneisen J, Heusch P, et al. Does 18F-FDG PET/MRI reduce the number of indeterminate abdominal incidentalomas compared with 18F-FDG PET/CT? Nucl Med Commun. 2015c;36:588–95. https://doi.org/10.1097/MNM.0000000000000298.

Schaarschmidt BM, Grueneisen J, Metzenmacher M, et al. Thoracic staging with (18)F-FDG PET/MRI in non-small cell lung cancer - does it change therapeutic decisions in comparison to (18)F-FDG PET/CT? Eur Radiol. 2017b;27:681–8. https://doi.org/10.1007/s00330-016-4397-0.

Schaarschmidt BM, Heusch P, Buchbender C, et al. Locoregional tumour evaluation of squamous cell carcinoma in the head and neck area: a comparison between MRI, PET/CT and integrated PET/MRI. Eur J Nucl Med Mol Imaging. 2015d;43:92–102. https://doi.org/10.1007/s00259-015-3145-z.

Schaarschmidt BM, Sawicki LM, Gomez B, et al. Malignant pleural mesothelioma: initial experience in integrated 18F-FDG PET/MRI imaging. Clin Imaging. 2016;40:956–60. https://doi.org/10.1016/j.clinimag.2016.05.001.

Schäfer JF, Gatidis S, Schmidt H, et al. Simultaneous whole-body PET/MRI imaging in comparison to PET/CT in pediatric oncology: initial results. Radiology. 2014;273:220–31. https://doi.org/10.1148/radiol.14131732.

Schöder H, Carlson DL, Kraus DH, et al. 18F-FDG PET/CT for detecting nodal metastases in patients with oral cancer staged N0 by clinical examination and CT/MRI. J Nucl Med. 2006;47:755–62.

Schreiter NF, Nogami M, Steffen I, et al. Evaluation of the potential of PET-MRI fusion for detection of liver metastases in patients with neuroendocrine tumours. Eur Radiol. 2012;22:458–67. https://doi.org/10.1007/s00330-011-2266-4.

Schroeder U, Dietlein M, Wittekindt C, et al. Is there a need for positron emission tomography imaging to stage the N0 neck in T1-T2 squamous cell carcinoma of the oral cavity or oropharynx? Ann Otol Rhinol Laryngol. 2008;117:854–63.

Schuler MK, Platzek I, Beuthien-Baumann B, et al. (18)F-FDG PET/MRI for therapy response assessment in sarcoma: comparison of PET and MR imaging results. Clin Imaging. 2015;39:866–70. https://doi.org/10.1016/j.clinimag.2015.05.014.

Schuler MK, Richter S, Beuthien-Baumann B, et al. PET/MRI imaging in high-risk sarcoma: first findings and solving clinical problems. Case Rep Oncol Med. 2013. https://doi.org/10.1155/2013/793927.

von Schulthess GK, Veit-Haibach P. Workflow considerations in PET/MRI imaging. J Nucl Med. 2014. https://doi.org/10.2967/jnumed.113.129239. jnumed.113.129239

Schwartz LH, Ozsahin M, Zhang GN, et al. Synchronous and metachronous head and neck carcinomas. Cancer. 1994;74:1933–8. https://doi.org/10.1002/1097-0142(19941001)74:7<1933::AID-CNCR2820740718>3.0.CO;2-X.

Schwenzer NF, Schraml C, Müller M, et al. Pulmonary lesion assessment: comparison of whole-body hybrid MR/PET and PET/CT imaging—pilot study. Radiology. 2012;264:551–8. https://doi.org/10.1148/radiol.12111942.

Seo HJ, Kim M-J, Lee JD, et al. Gadoxetate disodium-enhanced magnetic resonance imaging versus contrast-enhanced 18F-fluorodeoxyglucose positron emission tomography/computed tomography for the detection of colorectal liver metastases. Investig Radiol. 2011;46:548–55. https://doi.org/10.1097/RLI.0b013e31821a2163.

Shang J, Ling X, Zhang L, et al. Comparison of RECIST, EORTC criteria and PERCIST for evaluation of early response to chemotherapy in patients with non-small-cell lung cancer. Eur J Nucl Med Mol Imaging. 2016;43:1945–53. https://doi.org/10.1007/s00259-016-3420-7.

Sher AC, Seghers V, Paldino MJ, et al. Assessment of sequential PET/MRI in comparison with PET/CT of pediatric lymphoma: a prospective study. AJR

Am J Roentgenol. 2016;206:623–31. https://doi.org/10.2214/AJR.15.15083.

Shimizu A, Oriuchi N, Tsushima Y, et al. High [18F] 2-fluoro-2-deoxy-D-glucose (FDG) uptake of adrenocortical adenoma showing subclinical Cushing's syndrome. Ann Nucl Med. 2003;17:403–6.

Siegel R, Ma J, Zou Z, Jemal A. Cancer statistics, 2014. CA Cancer J Clin. 2014;64:9–29. https://doi.org/10.3322/caac.21208.

Sigal R, Zagdanski AM, Schwaab G, et al. CT and MR imaging of squamous cell carcinoma of the tongue and floor of the mouth. Radiographics. 1996;16:787–810. https://doi.org/10.1148/radiographics.16.4.8835972.

Sobin LH, Gospodarowicz MK, Wittekind C, editors. Lung. In: TNM classification of malignant tumours. Hoboken, NJ: John Wiley & Sons; 2011. p. 138–43.

Sohn B, Koh YW, Kang WJ, et al. Is there an additive value of 18 F-FDG PET-CT to CT/MRI for detecting nodal metastasis in oropharyngeal squamous cell carcinoma patients with palpably negative neck? Acta Radiol. 2016;57:1352–9. https://doi.org/10.1177/0284185115587544.

Spick C, Herrmann K, Czernin J. 18F-FDG PET/CT and PET/MRI perform equally well in cancer: evidence from studies on more than 2,300 patients. J Nucl Med. 2016;57:420–30. https://doi.org/10.2967/jnumed.115.158808.

Stolzmann P, Veit-Haibach P, Chuck N, et al. (2013) detection rate, location, and size of pulmonary nodules in trimodality PET/CT-MR: comparison of low-dose CT and Dixon-based MR imaging. Investig Radiol. 2013;48:241–6. https://doi.org/10.1097/RLI.0b013e31826f2de9.

Strobel K, Haerle SK, Stoeckli SJ, et al. Head and neck squamous cell carcinoma (HNSCC) – detection of synchronous primaries with (18)F-FDG-PET/CT. Eur J Nucl Med Mol Imaging. 2009;36:919–27. https://doi.org/10.1007/s00259-009-1064-6.

Sun L, Guan Y-S, Pan W-M, et al. Metabolic restaging of hepatocellular carcinoma using whole-body F-FDG PET/CT. World J Hepatol. 2009;1:90–7. https://doi.org/10.4254/wjh.v1.i1.90.

Talbot J-N, Fartoux L, Balogova S, et al. Detection of hepatocellular carcinoma with PET/CT: a prospective comparison of 18F-fluorocholine and 18F-FDG in patients with cirrhosis or chronic liver disease. J Nucl Med. 2010;51:1699–706. https://doi.org/10.2967/jnumed.110.075507.

Tateishi U, Yamaguchi U, Seki K, et al. Bone and soft-tissue sarcoma: preoperative staging with fluorine 18 fluorodeoxyglucose PET/CT and conventional imaging. Radiology. 2007;245:839–47. https://doi.org/10.1148/radiol.2453061538.

Tian J, Fu L, Yin D, et al. Does the novel integrated PET/MRI offer the same diagnostic performance as PET/CT for oncological indications? PLoS One. 2014;9:e90844. https://doi.org/10.1371/journal.pone.0090844.

Torizuka T, Tamaki N, Inokuma T, et al. In vivo assessment of glucose metabolism in hepatocellular carcinoma with FDG-PET. J Nucl Med. 1995;36:1811–7.

Treglia G, Castaldi P, Rindi G, et al. Diagnostic performance of Gallium-68 somatostatin receptor PET and PET/CT in patients with thoracic and gastroenteropancreatic neuroendocrine tumours: a meta-analysis. Endocrine. 2012;42:80–7. https://doi.org/10.1007/s12020-012-9631-1.

Vag T, Slotta-Huspenina J, Rosenberg R, et al. Computerized analysis of enhancement kinetics for preoperative lymph node staging in rectal cancer using dynamic contrast-enhanced magnetic resonance imaging. Clin Imaging. 2014;38:845–9. https://doi.org/10.1016/j.clinimag.2014.06.011.

van Westreenen HL, Heeren PAM, van Dullemen HM, et al. Positron emission tomography with F-18-fluorodeoxyglucose in a combined staging strategy of esophageal cancer prevents unnecessary surgical explorations. J Gastrointest Surg. 2005;9:54–61. https://doi.org/10.1016/j.gassur.2004.09.055.

van Westreenen HL, Westerterp M, Bossuyt PMM, et al. Systematic review of the staging performance of 18F-fluorodeoxyglucose positron emission tomography in esophageal cancer. J Clin Oncol. 2004;22:3805–12. https://doi.org/10.1200/JCO.2004.01.083.

Vandecaveye V, Dirix P, De Keyzer F, et al. Predictive value of diffusion-weighted magnetic resonance imaging during chemoradiotherapy for head and neck squamous cell carcinoma. Eur Radiol. 2010;20:1703–14. https://doi.org/10.1007/s00330-010-1734-6.

Varghese TK, Hofstetter WL, Rizk NP, et al. The society of thoracic surgeons guidelines on the diagnosis and staging of patients with esophageal cancer. Ann Thorac Surg. 2013;96:346–56. https://doi.org/10.1016/j.athoracsur.2013.02.069.

Veit-Haibach P, Schaefer NG, Steinert HC, et al. Combined FDG-PET/CT in response evaluation of malignant pleural mesothelioma. Lung Cancer. 2010;67:311–7. https://doi.org/10.1016/j.lungcan.2009.04.015.

Warburg O. Über den Stoffwechsel der Carcinomzelle. Naturwissenschaften. 1924;12:1131–7.

Weiler-Sagie M, Bushelev O, Epelbaum R, et al. (18) F-FDG avidity in lymphoma readdressed: a study of 766 patients. J Nucl Med. 2010;51:25–30. https://doi.org/10.2967/jnumed.109.067892.

Wilcox BE, Subramaniam RM, Peller PJ, et al. Utility of integrated computed tomography—positron emission tomography for selection of operable malignant pleural mesothelioma. Clin Lung Cancer. 2009;10:244–8. https://doi.org/10.3816/CLC.2009.n.033.

Wolff K-D, Follmann M, Nast A. The diagnosis and treatment of oral cavity cancer. Dtsch Ärztebl Int. 2012;109:829–35. https://doi.org/10.3238/arztebl.2012.0829.

Wong KH, Panek R, Welsh L, et al. The predictive value of early assessment after 1 cycle of induction chemotherapy with 18F-FDG PET/CT and diffusion-weighted MRI for response to radical chemoradiotherapy in head and neck squamous cell carcinoma. J Nucl Med. 2016;57:1843–50. https://doi.org/10.2967/jnumed.116.174433.

Wong WL, Saunders M. The impact of FDG PET on the management of occult primary head and neck tumours. Clin Oncol. 2003;15:461–6.

Wong WL, Sonoda LI, Gharpurhy A, et al. 18F-fluorodeoxyglucose positron emission tomography/computed tomography in the assessment of occult primary head and neck cancers--an audit and review of published studies. Clin Oncol. 2012;24:190–5. https://doi.org/10.1016/j.clon.2011.11.001.

Xu P-J, Yan F-H, Wang J-H, et al. Contribution of diffusion-weighted magnetic resonance imaging in the characterization of hepatocellular carcinomas and dysplastic nodules in cirrhotic liver. J Comput Assist Tomogr. 2010;34:506–12. https://doi.org/10.1097/RCT.0b013e3181da3671.

Yao JC, Hassan M, Phan A, et al. One hundred years after "carcinoid": epidemiology of and prognostic factors for neuroendocrine tumors in 35,825 cases in the United States. J Clin Oncol Off J Am Soc Clin Oncol. 2008;26:3063–72. https://doi.org/10.1200/JCO.2007.15.4377.

Yildirim H, Metintas M, Entok E, et al. Clinical value of fluorodeoxyglucose-positron emission tomography/computed tomography in differentiation of malignant mesothelioma from asbestos-related benign pleural disease: an observational pilot study. J Thorac Oncol. 2009;4:1480–4. https://doi.org/10.1097/JTO.0b013e3181c0a7ff.

Yun M, Kim W, Alnafisi N, et al. 18F-FDG PET in characterizing adrenal lesions detected on CT or MRI. J Nucl Med. 2001;42:1795–9.

Zhang X, Chen Y-LE, Lim R, et al. Synergistic role of simultaneous PET/MRI-MRS in soft tissue sarcoma metabolism imaging. Magn Reson Imaging. 2016;34:276–9. https://doi.org/10.1016/j.mri.2015.10.027.

Prostate Imaging

4

Axel Wetter and Matthias Eiber

4.1 Prostate Cancer: Epidemiology and Pathology

In developed countries, prostate cancer is one of the most common malignancies with an incidence of 69.5 cases per 100,000 men, and is considered to be among the five leading causes of death worldwide (Torre et al. 2015). In 95% of all malignant prostate tumors, prostate cancer arises from acinar epithelial cells and is therefore defined as an adenocarinoma. Rare entities of prostate cancer include neuroendocrine or sarcomatoid prostate cancers. Pathological and clinical staging of prostate cancer is based on the TNM classification, providing information about the primary tumor (T-stage), lymph node metastases (N-stage) and distant metastases (M-stage). T1 defines a clinically inapparent tumor (not detectable by imaging), T2 a tumor confined to the gland, T3 a tumor with extracapsular growth and T4 a tumor that infiltrates adjacent tissue (TNM classification of malignant tumors, eighth edi-

tion). Grading of prostate cancer is almost exclusively based on the Gleason grading system (Gleason grading), whereby the tumor is described by an increasing loss of differentiation, displayed in Gleason patterns from 1 to 5. As there are often several growth patterns within the prostate, the most common and second most common Gleason pattern is recorded and reported as the Gleason sum score, ranging from 2 to 10 (Gleason 1966). Staging and grading of prostate cancer are of utmost importance for further therapy decisions. From a clinical point of view, the information derived from staging, grading and other variables, such as the PSA value, are used for outcome prediction and are implemented in nomograms such as the Partin tables (Partin et al. 1993).

4.2 Prostate Cancer: MR Imaging

MR imaging of the prostate has become the leading imaging modality for tumor detection and local staging of prostate cancer. Due to its high soft tissue contrast, MRI enables detailed visualization of the zonal anatomy of the prostate, including differentiation of the central, peripheral and transition zone, anterior fibomuscular stroma, periurethral region and seminal vesicles. Morphological MR imaging of the prostate is primarily based on high-resolution strong T2-weighted fast-spin-echo images, where the healthy peripheral zone and the seminal vesicles exhibit a hyper-intense signal, whereas the transi-

A. Wetter, M.D. (✉)
Department of Diagnostic and Interventional Radiology and Neuroradiology, University Hospital Essen, Essen, Germany
e-mail: axel.wetter@uk-essen.de

M. Eiber, M.D.
Department of Nuclear Medicine,
Technical University Munich, Munich, Germany

© Springer International Publishing AG 2018
L. Umutlu, K. Herrmann (eds.), *PET/MR Imaging: Current and Emerging Applications*,
https://doi.org/10.1007/978-3-319-69641-6_4

tional zone exhibits a hypo-intense signal. Over the past years, MR imaging of prostate cancer has emerged from sole morphological imaging to a multiparametric imaging approach, combining anatomical and functional data by the implementation of diffusion-weighted imaging (DWI) and dynamic contrast-enhanced imaging (DCE) (Hricak et al. 1983, Fütterer et al. 2006, Morgan et al. 2007). DWI in prostate cancer is based on the presumption that high cellularity leads to decreased movement of water molecules which are insensitive for the so-called diffusion sensitizing gradients, hence resulting in retention of their high signal despite increasing diffusion sensitizing gradients. DCE is based on the assumption that prostate cancer lesions display a focal and early enhancement due to pathological tumor vessels. Numerous studies have shown that the combined analysis of morphological and functional MR-datasets leads to significantly improved detection of prostate cancer foci (Hamoen et al. 2015). The European Society of Urogenital Radiology (ESUR) and the American College of Radiologists (ACR) have made efforts to standardize mpMRI of the prostate and have proposed a standardized approach, the Prostate Imaging Reporting and Data System (PI-RADS) for lesion characterization (Barentz et al. 2012, Weinreb et al. 2016). In its newest version (PI-RADSv2),

PI-RADS is based on T2-weighted imaging, DWI and DCE. Suspicious prostate lesions are graded using both a score from 1 to 5 in T2-weighted images and DWI, whereby DWI is the dominant sequence for lesion detection of the peripheral zone, and T2-weighted imaging is dominant for lesion characterization of the transitional zone. DCE is assessed on the existence or absence of pathological early enhancement and may lead to an upgrade of a PI-RADS score 3-lesion in the peripheral zone to a score of 4. Minimum field strength of 1.5 T is recommended, but preference is given to 3 T scanners. According to PI-RADS v2, use of an endorectal coil is not necessary at 3 T, but might be useful in 1.5 T scanners in order to improve signal-to-noise ratio. Typical prostate cancer lesions are strongly hypointense in T2-weighted images and display a diffusion restriction with a high signal in the original diffusion-weighted images and a concomitant signal drop in the ADC maps. DCE typically demonstrates a focal and earlier enhancement than corresponding areas of non-malignant prostate tissue. Sufficient diagnostic accuracy for the detection of prostate cancer has been shown when using PI-RADS (Hamoen et al. 2015). Table 4.1 illustrates a typical MR sequence protocol for prostate, pelvic and whole-body MR imaging as part of a PET/MRI protocol.

Table 4.1 Set of MR-sequences combining the application of multi-parametric prostate MRI, pelvic MRI and whole-body MRI within a hybrid PET/MR examination

Sequence	TR (ms)	TE (ms)	FoV (mm)	Slice thickness (mm)	Matrix	B-values (s/mm²)
TIRM coronal pelvis	3110	56	380	5	273 × 448	
T2 FSE axial pelvis	4311	114	400	7	512	
T2 FSE axial prostate	4360	101	200	3	310 × 320	
T2 FSE coronal prostate	4000	101	200	3	310 × 320	
T2 FSE sagittal prostate	3740	101	200	3	310 × 320	
DWI prostate	7600	89	260	3	102 × 160	0, 1000, 1500, 2000
DWI pelvis	8100	70	420	5	90 × 160	0, 500, 1000
T1 vibe axial pre flip 2 deg. nativ prostate	4.24	1.31	300	3	114 × 192	
T1 vibe axial pre flip 15 deg. nativ prostate	4.24	1.31	300	3	114 × 192	
T1 vibe axial dyn prostate (DCE)	4.24	1.31	300	3	114 × 192	
T1 FSE axial 5 mm fs pelvis	606	10	400	5	176 × 512	
T1 vibe dixon axial contrast wholebody	4.05	1.29	380	3.5	173 × 320	

4.3 Prostate Cancer: PET and PET/CT Imaging

While MR imaging characterizes prostate lesions on the basis of morphological and functional data, PET imaging adds information on metabolism or target expression, depending on the specific tracer used. At present, two types of radiopharmaceuticals for PET imaging of prostate cancer are employed: choline derivatives or small molecules targeting the prostate-specific membrane antigen (PSMA). The employment of choline tracers is based on the observation that prostate cancer harbors an increased uptake of choline as a precursor for the synthesis of phosphorylcholine and ultimately phosphatidylcholine in tumor cells. Carbon-11-choline was originally introduced for PET imaging of brain tumors, but was later also utilized for prostate cancer imaging (Hara et al. 1998). The development of ^{18}F labeled choline derivatives such as ^{18}F fluoroethylcholine had the advantage of a markedly longer half-life period and shorter positron range (Hara et al. 2002). More recently, PSMA ligands have moved into the focus of prostate cancer imaging. PSMA is a transmembrane glycoprotein and functions as a cell surface peptidase (Sweat et al. 1998). It is highly over expressed (100–1000 fold) on almost all prostate cancer cells and most of its metastases, making it a highly valuable target for prostate cancer imaging. In this coherence, a ^{68}Ga labeled PSMA ligand (Glu-NH-CO-NH-Lys-(Ahx)-^{68}Ga-HBED-CC, ^{68}Ga PSMA-HEBD-CC or ^{68}Ga PSMA-11) was successfully introduced in 2012 and is the most commonly used PSMA ligand to date (Afshar-Oromieh et al. 2013). Most recently, ^{18}F-PSMA 1007, an ^{18}F labeled PSMA ligand has been developed, combining the high specificity of PSMA with reduced urinary clearance, hence reducing the diagnostically challenging "halo"-effect (caused by tracer accumulation in the bladder and consecutive overlapping uptake) (Giesel et al. 2017).

So far, main indications for PET and PET/CT imaging with radiolabeled choline focus on patients with biochemical recurrence after radical prostatectomy or radiation therapy and on patients with high-risk prostate cancer for initial staging. Emerging indications are stratifications into different therapeutic groups (e.g., eligibility for salvage lymphadenectomy) and prediction of the patient's prostate cancer-specific survival (Giovacchini et al. 2017). In recent years, PET/CT imaging with ^{68}Ga PSMA-11 has been extensively investigated and has shown high clinical value in prostate cancer imaging. It has proven to be superior over choline derivatives in terms of lesion detection, lesion-background contrast and tracer uptake in recurrent prostate cancer. Especially in early recurrent disease (e.g. PSA < 1 ng/ml) ^{68}Ga PSMA-11 has demonstrated the ability to successfully detect tumor lesions which are usually occult in other imaging modalities, including ^{18}F-Choline-PET/CT imaging (Afshar-Oromieh 2016).

4.4 Prostate Cancer: PET/MR Imaging

Integrated PET/MR imaging is based on the integration of a PET scanner into an MR scanner in order to enable simultaneous data acquisition with both modalities during one session. Simultaneous scanning without the necessity of moving the patient from one scanner to another enables excellent co-registration of suspicious lesions (even of lesions of smaller size), which is known to be hampered in sequentially fused hybrid imaging. Furthermore, the addition of excellent soft-tissue contrast and the possibility to combine functional information from MRI (DWI, DCE) with molecular information from PET holds promise of increasing the diagnostic capability. From a technical point of view, simultaneous PET/MR scanning is demanding, as several preconditions—from structural integration of both scanners to deployment of specific hardware such as receiver coils and novel PET detector crystals, as well as specific requirements such as different techniques for scatter and attenuation correction—have to be met in order to provide a well-performing employment in clinical routine. Since the first preclinical scan with an integrated PET/MR scanner in 2008 (Pichler et al. 2008), numerous studies have been carried out in order to investigate this new technology in the field of prostate cancer.

4.4.1 Technical Evaluation and Feasibility

Over the past few years, simultaneous PET/MRI has proven to be a robust method under clinical conditions. PET images derived from PET/MRI have been shown to provide the same image quality as PET images derived from PET/CT; however, certain differences in quantitative values (e.g. SUVs) calculated from both modalities can be observed for a variety of reasons, such as MR-based attenuation correction, novel image reconstruction algorithms as well as the timing and length of the PET acquisition (Drzezga et al. 2012, Souvatzoglou et al. 2013, Wetter et al. 2014). Therefore, quantification of PET data derived from PET/MR remains challenging, and bone lesions in particular require careful attention, as underestimation of tracer uptake is frequently observed (Seith et al. 2016). The possibility of combining multiparametric prostate MRI with the PET scan draws particular attendance to investigate primary prostate cancer with integrated PET/MRI. The feasibility of simultaneous PET/MRI in primary prostate cancer was demonstrated shortly after the launch of commercially available integrated PET/MR scanners in 2013 (Wetter et al. 2013).

As PET imaging of prostate cancer with ^{68}Ga PSMA-11 is regarded to be superior to choline derivatives, employing and evaluating this technique using hybrid PET/MR is of utmost promise. An initial report on the application of ^{68}Ga PSMA-11 PET/MRI demonstrated its technical feasibility (Afshar-Oromieh 2014). Drawbacks of ^{68}Ga PSMA-11 PET/MRI are "halo" artifacts around the urinary bladder and kidneys which are supposed to result from inaccurate scatter correction especially in regions with high tracer uptake. Apart from continuous work and improvement on reconstruction algorithms, a practical work-around for this challenge is forced diuresis, which reduces the tracer concen-

tration in the urinary bladder and consequently also reduces the halo effect. The recent introduction of ^{18}F PSMA-1007 might overcome this problem as it has only minimal urinary excretion (Giesel et al. 2017).

4.4.2 Clinical Workflow and Protocols

Initial investigations on PET/MRI put the focus on clinical workflow as well as protocols for whole-body fully integrated PET/MR imaging for different oncological tumor entities including prostate cancer (Martinez-Moeller et al. 2012, Souvatzoglou et al. 2013). These considerations were driven by the fact that compared with PET/CT, PET/MRI is a complex technique resulting in new problems and challenges, especially regarding workflow, scan protocols, and data analysis. This complexity applies in particular to examinations in oncology with partial- or whole-body coverage extending over several bed positions. Unlike diagnostic PET/CT, for which the clinical CT protocols can largely be copied from stand-alone CT, the design of a diagnostic MRI protocol for partial- or whole-body coverage is more complex and has to be adapted to the special requirements of PET/MRI to be both time-efficient and comprehensive.

4.5 Diagnostic Performance

4.5.1 Primary Prostate Cancer

Initial studies investigated the use of choline derivatives in PET/MR. Advantages compared to PET/CT arise from the potential of improved discrimination between malignant lesions and areas of benign prostatic hyperplasia which may exhibit similar choline uptake in PET but show different characteristics on MR. Recent studies using PET/MRI in primary prostate cancer described a higher diagnostic capability in terms of sensitivity and positive predictive value for tumor lesion detection compared to multiparametric MRI alone (Lee et al. 2017, Piert et al. 2016). This is regarded to result from the complimentary information of PET and functional MRI combined with exact matching of the PET data and MRI data in suspicious lesion.

Using ^{68}Ga PSMA-11 PET/MRI, preliminary results indicate that it might be at least equivalent to standalone multiparametric MRI for intraprostatic tumor localization (Eiber et al. 2015). Exploiting combined ^{68}Ga-PSMA11 PET/MRI for direct comparison in 53 intermediate/high risk patients the sensitivity of mpMRI using PI-RADS criteria amounted to 43% compared to 64% for ^{68}Ga-PSMA11 PET. Simultaneous PET/MRI, combining functional and mpMR data, further improved sensitivity to 76%. When com-pared to published data for mpMRI, ^{68}Ga PSMA-11 PET/MRI shows comparable sensitivity but notably higher specificity (Eiber et al. 2015). Important application areas of ^{68}Ga PSMA-11 PET/MRI may include precise radiation therapy planning or biopsy targeting with PET/MRI-based, ultrasound-guided or in-bore biopsy systems in order to use the improved tumor detection ability of ^{68}Ga PSMA-11 PET/MRI in patients with previously negative prostate biopsies. Figure 4.1 gives an example of a multi-

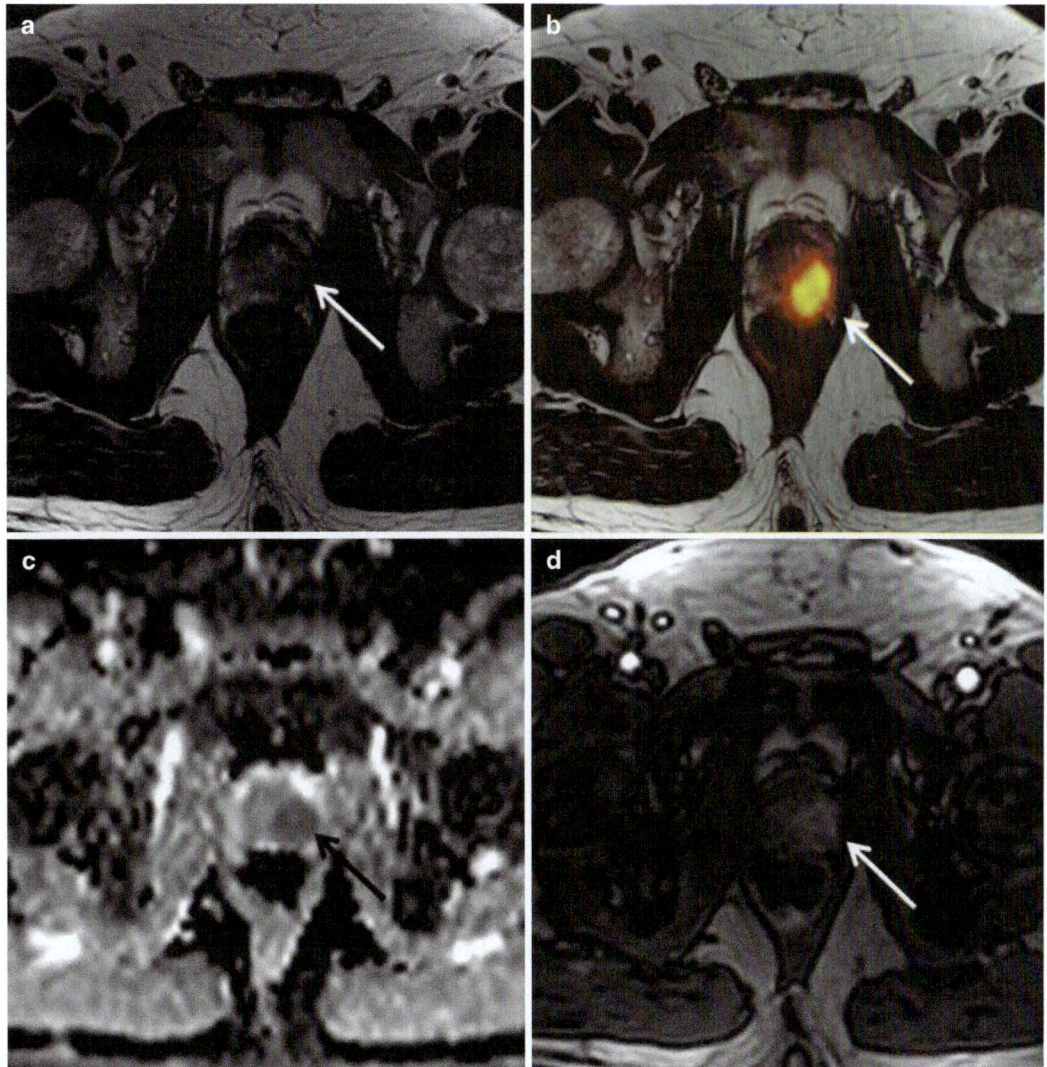

Fig. 4.1 ^{68}Ga PSMA-11 PET/MR images from a patient with biopsy-proven Gleason 4 + 4 prostate cancer at initial staging. The images demonstrate exemplarily the combination of multi-parametric MRI with PET. The prostate harbors a large hypo-intense lesion of the left peripheral and parts of the transitional zone (**a**) with increased ^{68}Ga PSMA-11 uptake (**b**), diffusion restriction, shown as a corresponding hypo-intensity in the ADC map (**c**), and pathological early enhancement in dynamic-contrast-enhanced imaging (**d**)

parametric MR examination combined with PET in a patient with a biopsy-proven prostate carcinoma.

4.5.2 Recurrent Prostate Cancer

Imaging of biochemical recurrence of prostate cancer is probably the most important field of PET imaging with choline derivatives or PSMA ligands. Especially precise imaging of the prostate bed after radical prostatectomy is challenging, as this anatomical region is complex due to scar tissue and postoperative changes as well as urine collection at the urethro-urethral anastomosis. As a result of this, both MR imaging and PET imaging are limited on their own, as scar

tissue might be misinterpreted as local recurrence in MRI, and a potential local recurrence might be overlooked in PET/CT due to limited soft tissue contrast. In this regard, integrated PET/MRI offers a solution, as unclear tracer accumulations in the prostate bed can be precisely assigned to anatomical structures and suspicious soft-tissue lesions. Moreover, the multiparametric approach including diffusion-weighted imaging and contrast-enhanced imaging allows for improved characterization of unclear PET positive lesions in the prostate bed (Lütje et al. 2017, Freitag et al. 2017). Figures 4.2 and 4.3 outline the additional value of mpMRI to PSMA-ligand PET and choline PET by using PET/MRI in patients with biochemical recurrent prostate cancer.

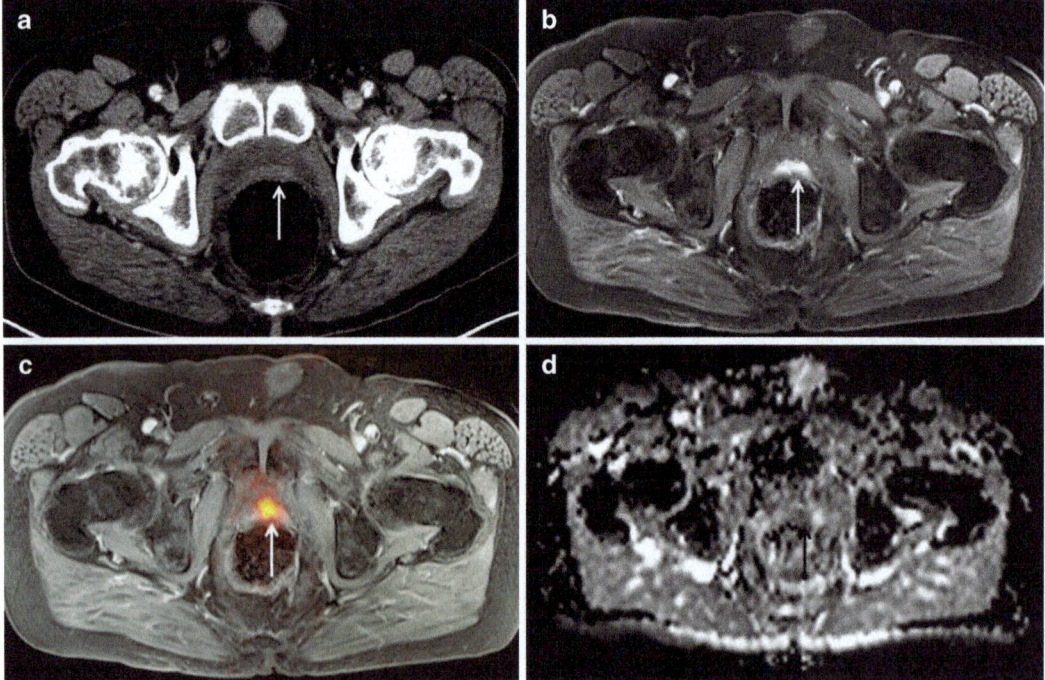

Fig. 4.2 Images from integrated ^{68}Ga PSMA-11 PET/MRI in a patient with biochemical recurrence after radical prostatectomy. PET/MRI identifies a soft-tissue lesion between the rectal and bladder wall diagnostic for local recurrence after radical prostatectomy (**b–d**). Due to the lack of soft-tissue contrast, it was regarded as part of the urinary bladder in PET/CT (**a**). Contrast-enhanced MRI demonstrates a clear soft-tissue mass (**b**) with[68]Ga PSMA-11 uptake (**c**) and a corresponding diffusion restriction (**d**)

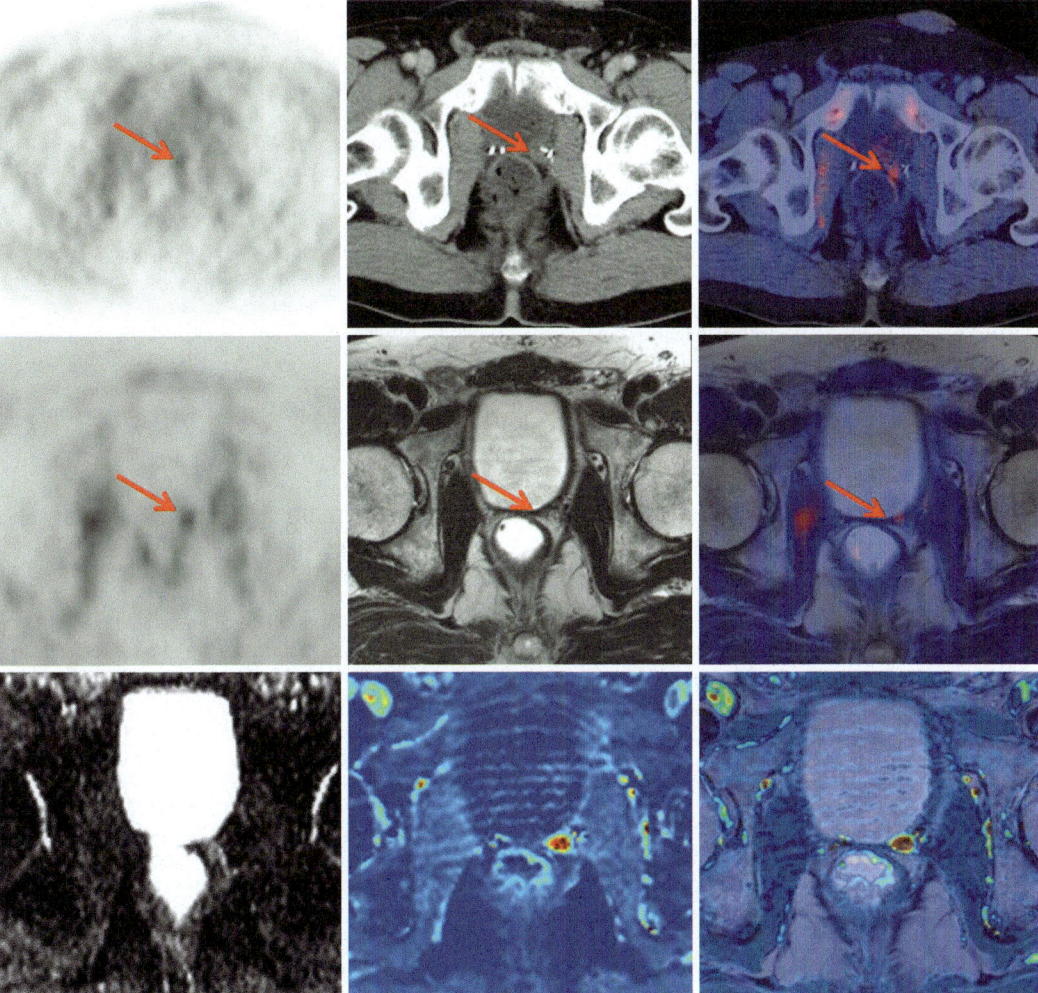

Fig. 4.3 ^{11}C-Choline PET/CT and PET/MR of a 79y/o patient with biochemical recurrence (PSA 1.7 ng/ml) after radical prostatectomy (*upper row*). PET/CT showed a faint choline uptake adjacent to the bladder on the left side which raised the suspicion for local recurrence but was judged as being unclear. PET/MR images demonstrated tracer uptake in a tiny tissue nodule (*middle row*). Additional information from the functional MR sequences showed a diffusion restriction in the ADC map (*left, lower row*). The iAUC60 derived from DCE (*middle, lower row*) and its fusion with T2w (*right, lower row*) demonstrated intense early contrast media influx. In conjunction with the choline uptake, the findings from functional MRI were highly indicative for a local recurrence

4.6 Outlook

Integrated PET/MRI in prostate cancer is a promising imaging modality for both primary and recurrent prostate cancer. For future key applications a clear benefit based on the combination of the molecular information from PET and excellent anatomical resolution as well as functional information from mpMRI is pertinent. Specific emerging applications include precise, imaging-based biopsy planning in primarily biopsy-negative patients with high suspicion for prostate cancer and detection of local recurrences in patients with biochemical recurrence after primary definitive treatment.

References

Afshar-Oromieh A, Babich JW, Kratochwil C, et al. The rise of PSMA ligands for diagnosis and therapy of prostate cancer. J Nucl Med. 2016;57(Suppl 3):79S–89S.

Afshar-Oromieh A, Haberkorn U, Schlemmer HP, et al. Comparison of PET/CT and PET/MRI hybrid systems using a ⁶⁸Ga-labelled PSMA ligand for the diagnosis of recurrent prostate cancer: initial experience. Eur J Nucl Med Mol Imaging. 2014;41:887–97.

Afshar-Oromieh A, Malcher A, Eder M, et al. PET imaging with a [⁶⁸Ga]gallium-labelled PSMA ligand for the diagnosis of prostate cancer: biodistribution in humans and first evaluation of tumour lesions. Eur J Nucl Med Mol Imaging. 2013;40:486–95.

Barentsz JO, Richenberg J, Clements R, et al. European Society of Urogenital Radiology: ESUR prostate MR guidelines 2012. Eur Radiol. 2012;22:746–57.

Brierley J, Gospodarowicz MK, Wittekind C. TNM classification of malignant tumors. 8th ed. Wiley-Blackwell; 2016.

Drzezga A, Souvatzoglou M, Eiber M, et al. First clinical experience with integrated whole-body PET/MR: comparison to PET/CT in patients with oncologic diagnoses. J Nucl Med. 2012;53:845–55.

Eiber M, Maurer T, Souvatzoglou M, et al. Evaluation of hybrid ⁶⁸Ga-PSMA ligand PET/CT in 248 patients with biochemical recurrence after radical prostatectomy. J Nucl Med. 2015;56:668–74.

Freitag MT, Radtke JP, Afshar-Oromieh A, et al. Local recurrence of prostate cancer after radical prostatectomy is at risk to be missed in ⁶⁸Ga-PSMA-11-PET of PET/CT and PET/MRI: comparison with mpMRI integrated in simultaneous PET/MRI. Eur J Nucl Med Mol Imaging. 2017;44:776–87.

Fütterer JJ, Engelbrecht MR, Jager GJ, et al. Prostate cancer localization with dynamic contrast-enhanced MR imaging and proton MR spectroscopic imaging. Radiology. 2006;241:449–58.

Giesel FL, Hadaschik B, Cardinale J, et al. F-18 labelled PSMA-1007: biodistribution, radiation dosimetry and histopathological validation of tumor lesions in prostate cancer patients. Eur J Nucl Med Mol Imaging. 2017;44:678–88.

Giovacchini G, Giovannini E, Leoncini R, Riondato M, Ciarmiello A. PET and PET/CT with radiolabeled choline in prostate cancer: a critical reappraisal of 20 years of clinical studies. Eur J Nucl Med Mol Imaging. 2017;44:1751–76.

Gleason DF. Classification of prostatic carcinomas. Cancer Chemother Rep. 1966;3:125–8.

Hamoen EH, de Rooij M, Witjes JA, Barentsz JO, Rovers MM. Use of the prostate imaging reporting and data system (PI-RADS) for prostate cancer detection with multiparametric magnetic resonance imaging: a diagnostic meta-analysis. Eur Urol. 2015;67:1112–21. Review

Hara T, Kosaka N, Kishi H. Development of (18) F-fluoroethylcholine for cancer imaging with PET: synthesis, biochemistry, and prostate cancer imaging. J Nucl Med. 2002;43:187–99.

Hara T, Kosaka N, Kishi H. PET imaging of prostate cancer using carbon-11-choline. J Nucl Med. 1998;39:990–5.

Hricak H, Williams RD, Spring DB, et al. Anatomy and pathology of the male pelvis by magnetic resonance imaging. AJR Am J Roentgenol. 1983;141:1101–10.

Lee MS, Cho JY, Kim SY, et al. Diagnostic value of integrated PET/MRI for detection and localization of prostate cancer: comparative study of multiparametric MRI and PET/CT. J Magn Reson Imaging. 2017;45:597–609.

Lütje S, Cohnen J, Gomez B, et al. Integrated ⁶⁸Ga-HBED-CC-PSMA-PET/MRI in patients with suspected recurrent prostate cancer. Nuklearmedizin. 2017;56:73–81.

Martinez-Möller A, Eiber M, Nekolla SG, et al. Workflow and scan protocol considerations for integrated wholebody PET/MRI in oncology. J Nucl Med. 2012;53:1415–26.

Morgan VA, Kyriazi S, Ashley SE, DeSouza NM. Evaluation of the potential of diffusion-weighted imaging in prostate cancer detection. Acta Radiol. 2007;48:695–703.

Partin AW, Yoo J, Carter HB, et al. The use of prostate specific antigen, clinical stage and Gleason score to predict pathological stage in men with localized prostate cancer. J Urol. 1993;150:110–4.

Pichler WHF, Kolb A, Judenhofer MS. Positron emission tomography/magnetic resonance imaging: the next generation of multimodality imaging? Semin Nucl Med. 2008;38:199–208.

Piert M, Montgomery J, Kunju LP, et al. ¹⁸F-Choline PET/MRI: the additional value of PET for MRI-guided transrectal prostate biopsies. J Nucl Med. 2016;57:1065–70.

Seith F, Gatidis S, Schmidt H, et al. Comparison of positron emission tomography quantification using magnetic resonance- and computed tomography-based attenuation correction in physiological tissues and lesions: a whole-body positron emission tomography/magnetic resonance study in 66 patients. Investig Radiol. 2016;51:66–71.

Souvatzoglou M, Eiber M, Takei T, et al. Comparison of integrated whole-body [11C] choline PET/MR with PET/CT in patients with prostate cancer. Eur J Nucl Med Mol Imaging. 2013;40:1486–99.

Sweat SD, Pacelli A, Murphy GP, Bostwick DG. Prostate-specific membrane antigen expression is greatest in prostate adenocarcinoma and lymph node metastases. Urology. 1998;52:637–40.

Torre LA, Bray F, Siegel RL, Ferlay J, Lortet-Tieulent J, Jemal A. Global cancer statistics, 2012. CA Cancer J Clin. 2015;65:87–108.

Weinreb JC, Barentsz JO, Choyke PL, et al. PI-RADS prostate imaging - reporting and data system: 2015, version 2. Eur Urol. 2016;69:16–40.

Wetter A, Lipponer C, Nensa F, et al. Evaluation of the PET component of simultaneous ^{18}F choline PET/MRI in prostate cancer: comparison with ^{18}F choline PET/CT. Eur J Nucl Med Mol Imaging. 2014;41:79–88.

Wetter A, Lipponer C, Nensa F, et al. Simultaneous ^{18}F choline positron emission tomography/magnetic resonance imaging of the prostate: initial results. Investig Radiol. 2013;48:256–62.

Female Pelvis

5

Johannes Grueneisen and Lale Umutlu

5.1 Introduction

Reliable and high quality diagnostics of gynecological cancers of the pelvis is of fundamental importance to determine disease extent which aids in the selection of the appropriate therapeutic strategy for each patient. Although clinical evaluation as well as surgical interventions still play an elementary part in the assessment of female pelvic malignancies, advanced imaging techniques have gained an increasing role for treatment planning and disease monitoring. Particularly magnetic resonance imaging (MRI) and positron emission tomography (PET) represent two important imaging techniques, which are frequently applied for primary tumor evaluation as well as the identification of potential tumor relapse. MRI has been shown useful for the assessment of malignant pathologies in the female pelvis, accompanied with the substantial advantage of the omission of ionizing radiation exposure (Beddy et al. 2012; Sala et al. 2013). Based on its high soft tissue contrast, MRI has been proven superior over other conventional imaging techniques for the determination of the local extent of primary tumors and for the differentiation between post therapeutic changes and tumor recurrences (Sala et al. 2013; Bipat et al. 2003, Weber et al. 1995).

Molecular imaging utilizing 18F-Fluorodeoxyglucose (18F-FDG) positron-emission-tomography (PET) provides an insight into tumor metabolism depending on the glycolytic activity of malignant cells (Hoh et al. 1993). As a part of hybrid imaging, 18F-FDG PET/CT has been proven highly accurate and superior to conventional imaging modalities for the detection of metastatic spread, due to the identification of hypermetabolic activity of malignant lesions (Choi et al. 2006, Selman et al. 2008; Antoch et al. 2003). Therefore, 18F-FDG PET/CT is frequently applied for staging a large number of different tumor entities, including gynecological cancers (Bollineni et al. 2016; Kitajima et al. 2008). After some major technical challenges were solved, integrated PET/MR scanners have been increasingly introduced into clinical use (Pichler et al. 2008). This new-generation hybrid imaging technology enables the simultaneous acquisition of PET- and MR-datasets, providing complementary metabolic, functional and morphologic information for image analysis (Cavaliere et al. 2017; Romeo et al. 2017; Lee et al. 2016). Hence, PET/MRI offers the diagnostic capability for an accurate and efficient tumor staging approach. The initial concerns about significantly extended examination times could be largely overcome due

J. Grueneisen (✉) • L. Umutlu
Department of Diagnostic and Interventional
Radiology and Neuroradiology, University Hospital
Essen, Essen, Germany
e-mail: Johannes.Grueneisen@uk-essen.de;
Lale.Umutlu@uk-essen.de

© Springer International Publishing AG 2018
L. Umutlu, K. Herrmann (eds.), *PET/MR Imaging: Current and Emerging Applications*,
https://doi.org/10.1007/978-3-319-69641-6_5

to a reasonable selection of suitable MR sequences as a part of whole-body staging protocols (Grueneisen et al. 2015). Nevertheless, the greatest benefit of integrated PET/MRI embodies the implementation of MRI into hybrid imaging itself, providing significant advantages over the CT-component in PET/CT. This fact raises the possibility for an expansion and change of the diagnostic spectrum. In addition to anatomical imaging, MRI enables the acquisition of certain functional and quantitative data facilitating a more comprehensive assessment of specific (soft-tissue) organs and pathologies. In combination with the metabolic information of 18F-FDG PET, quantitative multiparametric PET/MR imaging can be used for tissue characterization and response evaluation and may play a role in the management of targeted tumor therapies (Romeo et al. 2017; Lee et al. 2016).

5.2 PET/MR Imaging of the Female Pelvis

5.2.1 PET/MR Protocols

Optimal patient preparation as well as a precise selection of imaging parameters and protocols is mandatory to obtain high quality imaging results. For 18F-FDG PET data acquisition, patients should be instructed to fast for a period of at least 6 hours to ensure adequate blood glucose levels ($\leq$ 150 mg/dL) at the time of radiotracer injection, which is of particular importance to minimize competitive inhibition of 18F-FDG uptake. Therefore, baseline blood glucose levels should be checked prior to the administration of 18F-FDG and regular human insulin should be administered intraveniously if the levels are exceeded. 18F-FDG should be injected at least 60 min after insulin administration and endogenous glucose levels have to be checked again priorily. Then, a body-weight adapted dosage of 18F-FDG (4 MBq/kg body weight) can be applied intraveniously (Lartizien et al. 2002). However, new generation PET-detector systems containing lutetium oxyorthosilicate (LSO)-based avalanche photodiodes (APD), most frequently used in integrated PET/MRI scanners, have been shown

highly sensitive for PET-measurements (Delso et al. 2011). Accordingly, after attentive consideration of the correct duration for PET-data acquisition, reduced 18F-FDG doses of 2 MBq/kg bodyweight can be applied, while preserving adequate PET-image quality (Hartung-Knemeyer et al. 2013; Grueneisen et al. 2015). Simultaneous PET and MR imaging should be started approximately 1 hour thereafter. Within this uptake period, patients should experience thermal comfort as well as avoid increased physical activity. Furthermore, increased peristalsis of the small-but especially of the large-bowel is a well recognized potential cause for artifacts in abdominal MR imaging, potentially severely impeding image quality. Besides the previously mentioned fasting period, antiperistaltic agents (e.g. hyoscine butylbromide) can be applied in addition, to reduce bowel activity and limit the occurrence of motion artifacts (Johnson et al. 2007).

Whole-body PET/MRI scans for primary tumor evaluation as well as for restaging female pelvic malignancies are generally performed in supine position with arms placed next to the torso. Datasets are commonly obtained in 4-5 bed positions (usually from skull-base to mid-thigh), depending on the size of the patient. For whole-body MR data acquisition combined head and neck coils as well as phased-array radiofrequency body surface coils can be used, depending on the desired coverage.

As for the protocol set up, in terms of sequences and parameters, it is important to differentiate between tumor entities (e.g. cancer of the uterine cervix or endometrial cancer) as well as between (Beddy et al. 2012) primary local staging (pelvis only), (Sala et al. 2013) primary local and additional whole-body staging and (Bipat et al. 2003) whole-body restaging.

Primary staging of cancers of the female pelvis should comprise dedicated MR protocols for the female pelvis for accurate determination of the local extent of primary tumors in dependence of the imaged tumor entity (Table 5.1). In general, basic MR imaging protocols of the female pelvis include transversal T1-weighted images as well as high resolution T2-weighted images in transversal and sagittal planes. For optimal assessment of the different tumor entities protocol adaptations

Table 5.1 Parameters of the most commonly applied MR sequences for the assessment of the female pelvis

Parameters	Coronal T1w	Axial T1w	Sagittal T2w	Axial T2w/ Axial oblique T2w	Axial DWI	Sagittal T1w (fs)	Axial T2w (fs)
Sequence	Dixon-based VIBE	TSE	TSE	TSE	EPI	Dynamic VIBE[a]	TSE
Slice thickness (mm)	5	4	4	4	5	2.5	7
Echo time (ms)	1.23 (1st) and 2.46 (2nd)	12	101	114	82	1.69	97
Repetition time (ms)	3.6	495	4930	5820	9900	4.46	3120
Flip angle (°)	10	180	150	120	90	9	160
Field of view (mm)	500	400	300	400	420	300	380
Phase FoV (%)	65.6	75.0	78.1	75.0	75.0	68.8	75
Matrix size	192×79	512×230	512×240	512×192	160×90	512×240	512×202
b value (s/mm^2)	–	–	–	–	0, 500, 1000	–	–
Parallel imaging acceleration factor	n/a	2	2	2	2	2	2
Acquisition time (min:s)	0:13	3:53	4:08	2:33	2:48	0:26	1:16

Careful selection of suitable MR sequences is required for the assessment of each of the different pelvic cancer types

[a]For dynamic imaging three repetitive scans are acquired with a delay of 20, 60 and 90 s after the application of i.v. contrast agent

Abbreviations: VIBE volume interpolated breath-hold examination, *TSE* Turbo-spin echo; *DWI* Diffusion-weighted imaging, *EPI* Echo-planar imaging, *fs* Fat-saturated

are needed: Primary cancers of the uterine cervix should be examined with high-resolution T2-weighted sequences in axial oblique plane to identify potential tumor invasion in the parametria. For the evaluation of adnexal masses, contrast-enhanced T1w images as well as diffusion-weighted sequences are helpful for the identification of solid components of a suspect mass and the detection of peritoneal implants. In addition, fat-saturated T1-weighted sequences are useful for the differentiation between hemorrhage or fat-tissue. For the assessment of endometrial cancer, dynamic contrast-enhanced T1-weighted images in sagittal and transversal plane as well as diffusion-weighted sequences should be incorporated for improved determination of the depth of myometrial invasion and the occurrence of cervical tumor infiltration.

In addition to dedicated primary cancer staging of the female pelvis, integrated PET/MRI also facilitates the so-called "one-stop-shop imaging procedure", in terms of the combined assessment of local primary cancer imaging and whole-body imaging in one exam. First studies on this matter were published by Grueneisen et al, revealing the high diagnostic capability of integrated PET/MRI for local and whole-body staging in patients with cervical cancer (Grueneisen et al. 2015).

For restaging of patients with a suspected tumor relapse of a female pelvic malignancy, various studies could demonstrate a higher accuracy of hybrid imaging techniques for tumor detection than conventional imaging modalities (Kirchner et al. 2017; Kitajima et al. 2009). PET/CT provides a good diagnostic performance for whole-body restaging of gynecological cancers within a reasonable scan duration (Kirchner et al. 2017). In this context, the usage of extended study protocols in the majority of initial studies of integrated PET/MR imaging, comprising a substantial number of different MR-sequences, revealed a disadvantage of PET/MR imaging compared to PET/CT imaging. Causing potential patient discomfort accompanied by negative economic impact, the prolonged examination times applied in initial whole-body PET/MRI studies provoked the urge for optimization and implementation of well-adapted MRI protocols, dedicatedly established for certain tumor entities. Grueneisen et al. demonstrated the feasibility and clinical applicability of a "FAST"-PET/MR protocol for restaging female pelvic malignancies (Grueneisen et al. 2015). The reduction of the applied MR sequences to an inevitable minimum, encompassing non-enhanced T2w, post-contrast T1 sequences as well as diffusion-weighted imaging (Table 5.2), enabled a significant reduction in scan duration (from 44 min to 27.5 min), while providing an equivalent tumor detection rate compared to PET/CT. The identical study protocol has already been transferred for the assessment of other tumor types e.g. lymphomas (Grueneisen et al. 2016; Kirchner et al. 2017). Furthermore, the implementation of diffusion-weighted sequences as an additional functional parameter to exclusively morphologic MR imaging has been shown to facilitate a significant increase of sensitivity for identification of tumors and metastatic sites (Low et al. 2009; Gu et al. 2011; Michielsen et al. 2014). However, comparable to PET, diffusion-weighted imaging is commonly used as a searching-tool in MR staging protocols and the option of a quantification of resulting ADC values enables an improved differentiation between benign or malignant findings (Kovac et al. 2016; Lee et al. 2016; Liu et al. 2011). Accordingly, previous studies assessed the usefulness of DWI as a part of whole-body MR protocols for staging of cancer patients with integrated PET/MRI, yet, could not demonstrate a clear additional diagnostic benefit for tumor detection (Grueneisen et al. 2014, 2017; Buchbender et al. 2013). Hence, the omission DWI (from whole-body PET/MR protocols) enables a significant shortening of the examination time comparable to PET/CT acquisition times (18.5 ± 1 min. vs. 18.2 min), while preserving an equivalent diagnostic performance when compared to PET/CT (Kirchner et al. 2017; Grueneisen et al. 2017). The application of these fast or ultra-fast imaging protocols enables the utilization of PET/MR imaging as an efficient and high-quality staging tool for whole-body staging and/or whole-body restaging.

5.2.2 Cervical Cancer

Despite the successful introduction of preventive measures and reduced mortality rates in developed countries within the last decades, cervical carcinoma continues to be one of the leading causes of cancer-related death worldwide

Table 5.2 MR imaging parameters for whole-body PET/MR imaging based on the FAST-Protocol

Parameters	Coronal T1w	Axial T2w	Axial DWI	Axial T1w (fs) post-contrast
Sequence	Dixon-based VIBE	HASTE	EPI	VIBE
Slice thickness (mm)	5	5	5	3
Echo time (ms)	1.23 (1st) and 2.46 (2nd)	97	82	1.53
Repetition time (ms)	3.6	1500	9900	3.64
Flip angle (°)	10	160	90	9
Field of view (mm)	500	400	420	380
Phase FoV (%)	65.6	75.0	75.0	81.3
Matrix size	192×79	320×194	160×90	512×250
b value (s/mm^2)	–	–	0, 500, 1000	–
Parallel imaging acceleration factor	n/a	2	2	2
Acquisition time (min:s/bed position)	0:13	0:47	2:48	0:19

Abbreviations: *VIBE* Volume interpolated breath-hold examination, *HASTE* Half-Fourier acquisition single-shot turbo spin-echo, *DWI* Diffusion-weighted imaging, *EPI* Echo-planar imaging, *fs* fat-saturated

(Torre et al. 2015). For an efficient and appropriate patient management highly accurate assessment of primary cancers of the uterine cervix is mandatory. Initial diagnosis is usually made by histopathological sampling, delivering valuable information about tumor histology and tumor aggressiveness. But the choice of the initial therapeutic strategy highly depends on the local extent of the primary tumor as well as the occurrence of metastastic spread. Tumors confined to the uterine cervix are primarily treated by surgical resection, while patients with locally advanced tumor stages will undergo combined chemo-radiation therapy with a curative intent. Due to social epidemiological reasons, cervical cancers are usually clinically staged in accordance with the criteria as proposed by the International Federation of Gynecology and Obstetrics (FIGO) (Pecorelli et al. 2009). However, large discrepancies have been described between the results of primary clinical staging and operative evaluation, especially in the assessment of advanced tumor stages (Lagasse et al. 1980; Qin et al. 2009). Accordingly, the increasing role of advanced imaging techniques for primary tumor staging as well as the assessment of therapy response has been recognized within the last years. Based on its high soft tissue contrast, MRI is considered the most accurate imaging technique for the identification of tumor localization and tumor extent for tumors of the female pelvis (Sala et al. 2013; Bipat et al. 2003). Reported sensitivity, specificity and negative predictive value of MRI for the determination of parametrial tumor invasion vary between 75-100%, 96-99% and 94-100%, respectively (Mirpour et al. 2013; Sala et al. 2007; Zand et al. 2007). Therefore, MRI helps to triage patients towards surgery or radiochemotherapy and is now recommended for the assessment of primary cervical cancers and treatment planning in the revised FIGO staging system (Pecorelli et al. 2009).

Apart from assessment of the primary cancer, the identification of lymph node or distant metastases in cervical cancer patients is of particular importance and has high impact on the selection of a potentially multimodal therapeutic concept (Koh et al. 2013). The detection of pelvic lymph node metastases requires adjuvant radiation or radiochemotherapy, and potentially an extension of the radiation field, if metastatic paraaortic nodes can be verified (Koh et al. 2013). In addition, the presence of nodal metastases reflects one of the most important prognostic factors of cervical cancers regarding progression-free and overall survival (Delgado et al. 1990; Tinga et al. 1990; Stehman et al. 1991). Previous studies have demonstrated that survival rates significantly decrease from 85–91% to 50–55% in a patient cohort with early tumor stages (IB and IIA), if lymph node metastases are present (Piver and Chung 1975; Elliott et al. 1989). Currently, patients' nodal status is primarily assessed by pelvic and/or paraaortic lymphadenectomy. However, this invasive procedure may be associated with post-surgical complications.

Among the imaging techniques used for nodal staging, 18F-FDG PET and PET/CT have been shown to be more sensitive than CT and MRI for the identification of metastatic spread (Choi et al. 2010). In a review article, Grant et al. summarized the results of different meta-analyses and reported sensitivities and specificities of 75–84% and 95–98% for PET and PET/CT, 47–58% and 92% for CT as well as 54–56% and 91–96% for MRI, respectively (Grant et al. 2014). The majority of those studies comprised only limited patient cohorts and in addition, histopathological verification of the imaged nodes was not always present. However, a number of studies could demonstrate the effectiveness of the additional information provided by PET/CT, particularly in patients with locally advanced tumor stages, leading to substantial changes in treatment planning (Magne et al. 2008; Bjurberg and Brun 2013). This was mainly due to an improved assessment of extra-pelvic metastatic spread.

For some years now, integrated PET/MR scanners have been commercially available and the clinical applicability has been shown in numerous clinical trials (Nie et al. 2017; Nensa et al. 2014; Sotoudeh et al. 2016). These new imaging systems combine the diagnostic advantages of MRI, for highly efficient morphological and functional imaging, and the PET-component, delivering valuable metabolic information for tumor detection and characterization (Fig. 5.1). Kitajima and colleagues investigated the diagnostic potential of retrospectively fused

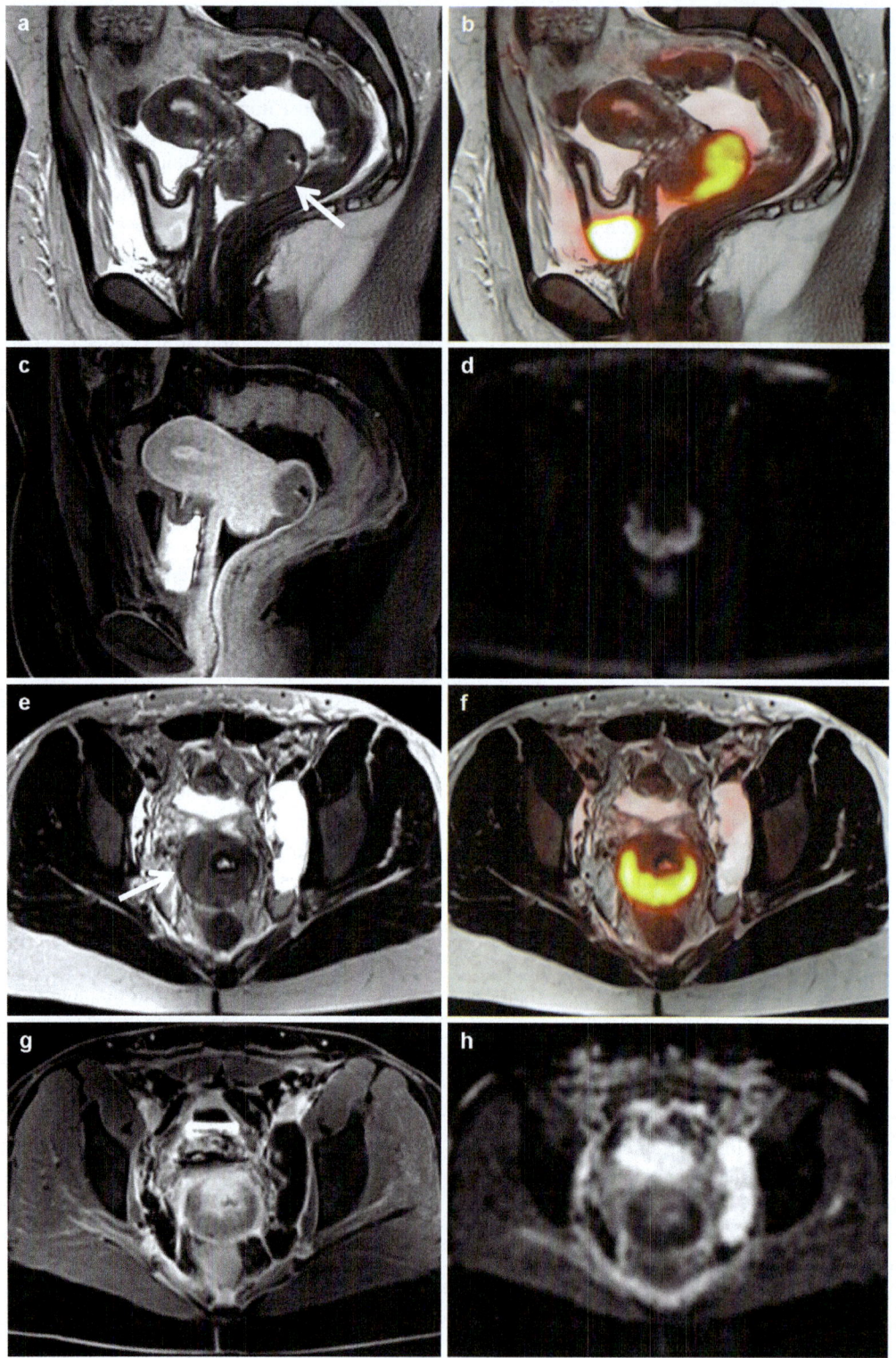

Fig. 5.1 Images of a 51 years-old patient with primary cervical cancer (Squamous cervical carcinoma). T2w TSE images (**a**, **e**) show an exophytic growing tumor of the uterine cervix (**a**, arrow), which does not invades the parametria (**e**, arrow). Fused 18F-FDG PET/MR images (**b**, **f**) reveal a pathologically increased glucose metabolism of the tumor manifestation, which nicely correlates with parts of the tumor displaying a wash-out phenomenon (**c**, **g**; T1w VIBE post-contrast) as well as restricted diffusivity on diffusion-weighted images (**d**, DWI: **b** -1000; **h**, ADC-map).

18F-FDG PET- and MR-data for the evaluation of locoregional tumor extent as well as nodal staging in cervical cancer patients (Kitajima et al. 2014). They could show a significantly higher accuracy of fused PET/MRI and contrast-enhanced MRI for the determination of the T-stage in comparison to PET/CT (83.3% vs. 53.3%). For the identification of nodal positive patients PET/MRI and PET/CT revealed a higher sensitivity and accuracy than MRI alone (92.3, 88.2 and 90.0% vs. 69.2, 100 and 86.7%). These findings go in line with the results from a study by Queiroz and colleagues, investigating the diagnostic ability for tumor staging of cervical cancer with a sequential trimodality PET/CT-MR system (Queiroz et al. 2015). The authors reported a higher accuracy of PET/MRI for the delineation of pelvic tumor extent when compared to PET/CT, whereas both imaging techniques performed equivalently well for the detection of metastatic spread. In a recently published preliminary study comprising 27 patients, Grueneisen et al. assessed the diagnostic utility of integrated PET/MRI for primary whole-body staging of cervical cancers (Grueneisen et al. 2015). Besides a good performance for the identification of the local tumor extent, PET/MRI revealed high sensitivity, specificity and accuracy rates (91, 94 and 93%) for the detection of lymph node metastases. In addition, the authors could show significant correlations between PET- and MR-derived functional parameters (SUVs and ADC values) and the differentiation grade of primary cervical carcinomas. Numerous studies have demonstrated the predictive value of the quantification of metabolic activity and tissue cellularity of cervical cancers, revealing significant correlations with treatment response as well as patient survival (Nakamura et al. 2012; Kidd et al. 2010; Kuang et al. 2013; Park et al. 2014). Nakamura et al. could predict a shorter overall and disease-free survival in patients with cervical cancer, exhibiting a higher SUVmax in combination with lower ADCmin values (Nakamura et al. 2012). Two further studies found significant inverse correlations between SUV and ADC values of primary cancers of the uterine cervix (Grueneisen et al. 2014; Brandmaier et al. 2015). Accordingly, apart from the interpretation of tumor morphology, inte-grated PET/MRI bears the potential of quantitative multiparametric data analysis in a single examination approach. Hence, the simultaneous generation of a large number of morphologic, metabolic and functional imaging features may contribute to a more comprehensive non-invasive evaluation and characterization of tumor biology. Moreover, quantitative analysis of certain functional parameters can be utilized for therapy response assessment based on changes during primary systemic therapy (Romeo et al. 2017; Deuschl et al. 2017; Kelly-Morland et al. 2017).

The extraction and collection of numerous quantitative imaging features, potentially reflecting the underlying pathophysiology, has been introduced as Radiomics (Lambin et al. 2012; Gillies et al. 2016) (Fig. 5.2). Regarding the increasing role of personalized and precision medicine, a multitude of data can be obtained from medical imaging, providing complementary information to other sources (e.g. epidemiology, histopathology). The integration of these data may help for improvements in clinical decision support due to increased precision in diagnosis and more reliable assessment of prognosis. Based on its widespread availability and frequent use in the field of cancer management, the information from CT images are most widely used for radiomics analyses so far, providing anatomical and structural tumor information (Coroller et al. 2015; van Timmeren et al. 2017; Huynh et al. 2016). Some studies could already demonstrate that CT-based radiomic features can function as predictors for early tumor recurrences of hepatocellular carcinoma and capture information which can be applied as prognostic biomarkers for the occurrence of distant metastases and overall survival of lung cancer patients (Coroller et al. 2015; Zhou et al. 2017; Aerts et al. 2014). In this context, PET/MR enables an extension of the diagnostic spectrum, providing additional functional data, reflecting physiological and pathophysiological processes such as perfusion (DCE-MRI), cellularity (DWI) and metabolic activity (18F-FDG PET) of healthy tissues and neoplasms (Yin et al. 2017). Accordingly, joint texture-based multivariable models derived from simultaneously and pretherapeutical obtained 18F-FDG PET and MRI data may enhance the understanding of

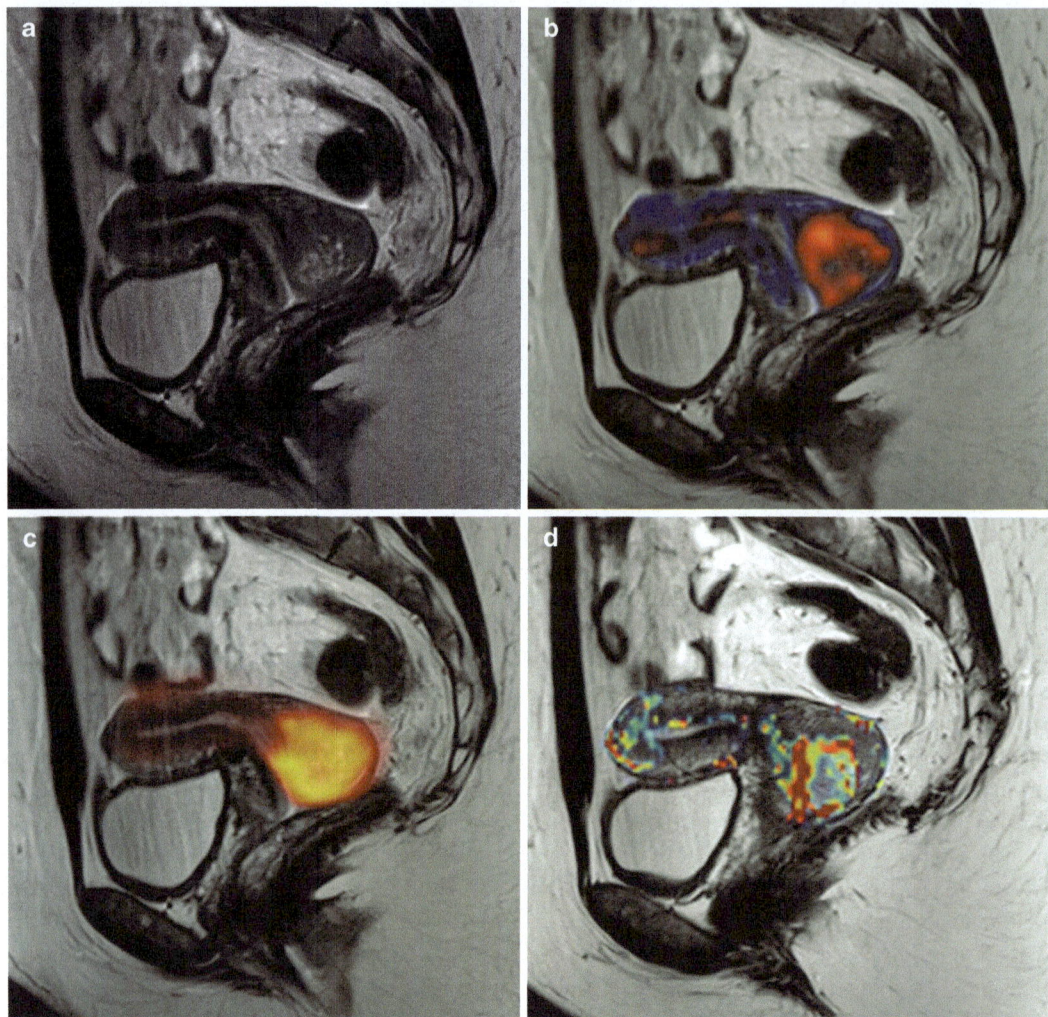

Fig. 5.2 35 years-old patient with tumor manifestation at the posterior lip of the uterine cervix on T2w MR images (**a**, T2w TSE). In addition to morphological tumor evaluation, integrated PET/MRI enables simultaneous acquisi-tion of different quantitative parameters: (**b**) T2w TSE fused with ADC-values, (**c**) T2w TSE fused with PET-data and (**d**) T2w TSE fused with perfusion parameters (k^{trans})

tumor biology and enable the selection of more personalized and optimized treatment strategies for cervial cancers patients. Moreover, these data may deliver valuable additional information, which may assist to predict prognosis and potentially help to improve patient survival.

Approximately one third of cervical cancer patients suffer from tumor relapse with a majority of the cases occurring within the first two years after initial treatment (Friedlander et al. 2002; Bellone et al. 2007). In most cases tumor recurrences are confined to the female pelvis or manifest as lymph node metastases. However, due to the

more frequent application of successful pelvic radiation or radiochemotherapy especially in advanced tumor stages, reducing locoregional tumor recurrence, the number of distant metastases has relatively increased (Fulcher et al. 1999; Kavanagh et al. 1997). Currently, CT or MRI are considered the standard imaging procedures for the evaluation of a potential tumor relapse. While CT is widely established for whole-body staging strategies, MRI is frequently used for the assessment of potential local tumor relapse within the female pelvis. But numerous studies already demonstrated the superiority of hybrid imaging, in terms of

PET/CT, over conventional cross-sectional imaging modalities, providing more accurate primary and restaging of several different tumor types (Antoch et al. 2003, 2003; Kitajima et al. 2009; Bar-Shalom et al. 2003). One of the major challenges of "pure" morphological assessment lies in the differentiation between post-therapeutic changes or local tumor recurrences (Vesselle and Miraldi 1998). Therefore, 18F FDG-PET provides valuable additional metabolic information, which facilitates improved detection of tumor relapse and the distinction to scar tissue.

Kitajima and colleagues investigated the staging performance of 18F-FDG PET/CT in comparison to 18F-FDG PET alone and contrast-enhanced CT alone in a study comprising 90 patients with a suspected tumor recurrence of cervical or endometrial cancer (Kitajima et al. 2009). The authors found a significantly higher accuracy of PET/CT for the detection of recurrent cancers, leading to changes in subsequent treatment recommendations in 42% of the patients. Furthermore, Grueneisen and colleagues demonstrated the diagnostic advantage of combined 18F-FDG PET/MRI over MRI alone, enabling a higher detection rate as well as higher confidence for the identification of recurrences of cervical and ovarian cancer (Grueneisen et al. 2014). A number of studies have investigated and compared the staging performance of integrated PET/MRI and PET/CT for the depiction of tumor recurrences of female pelvic malignancies. Apart from an overall equivalent diagnostic ability for tumor detection, only minor differences have been described, regarding the delineation of suspect lesions in dependence of their localization (Grueneisen et al. 2015). Previous studies reported a higher detection rate of pulmonary lesions with PET/CT in comparison to PET/MRI (Fig. 5.3), particularly for lesions smaller than 10 mm (Sawicki et al. 2016a, b). On the other hand, PET/MRI has been shown to offer a higher accuracy for the identification and characterization of liver metastases and better detectability of

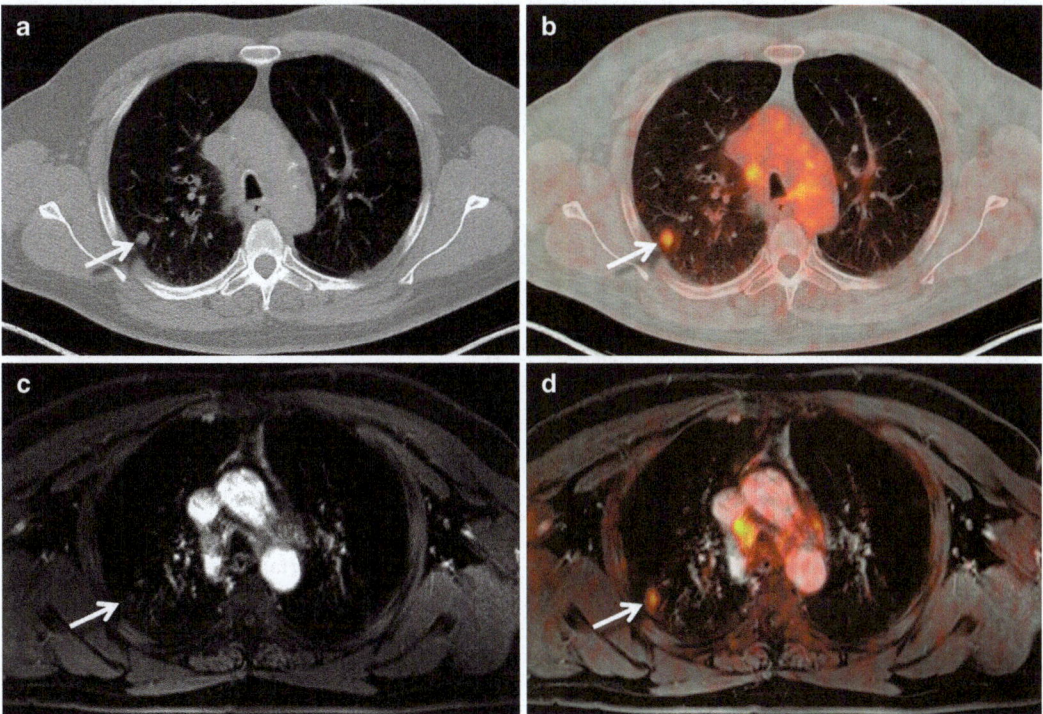

Fig. 5.3 Images of a 47 years-old patient with a subpleural metastasis in the right lung (arrows), clearly detectable on CT images (**a**), which shows a pathologically increased glucose metabolism in PET/CT (**b**). The identical lesion is barely visible on contrast-enhanced MR-images (**c**, T1w VIBE) and the diagnosis of a pulmonary metastasis has been made in PET/MRI (**d**), due to the additional information provided by 18F-FDG PET

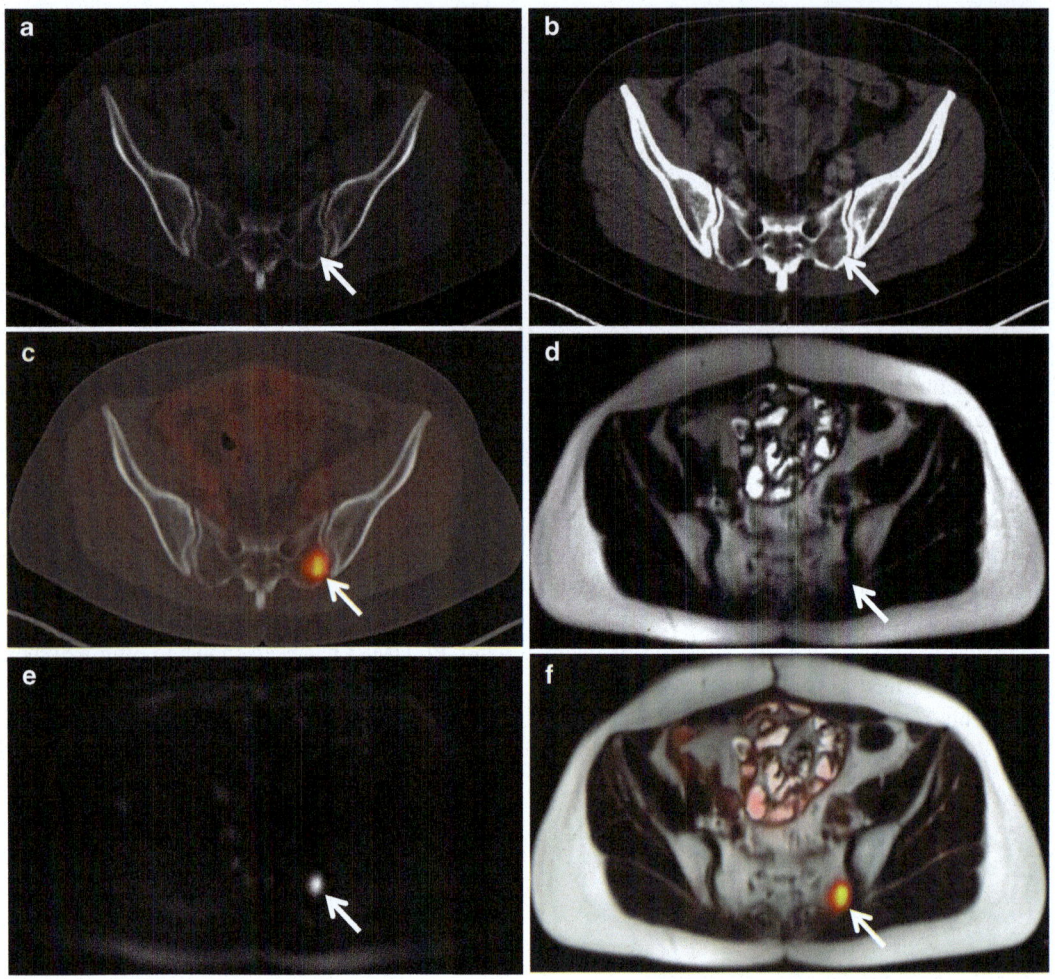

Fig. 5.4 Images of a 43 years-old patient with a 18F-FDG PET-positive sacral metastasis of cervical cancer (arrows). The tumor manifestation cannot be clearly identified on CT images (**a**, **b**) but reveals a pathologic glucose metabolism after image fusion in PET/CT (**c**). Corresponding MR-images, acquired with one hour delay, show a T2-hypointense sacral lesion (**d**, T2w HASTE) with restricted diffusivity on diffusion-weighted images (**e**, DWI: b-1000), highly suspicious for malignancy. Finally, the diagnosis of a bone metastasis could be made with a higher confidence after image fusion in PET/MRI (**f**)

bone metastases when compared to PET/CT (Fig. 5.4) (Beiderwellen et al. 2013, 2014, 2015; Eiber et al. 2014). Moreover, based on its high soft-tissue contrast, the MR-component as part of a hybrid imaging technique, might be beneficial for a more accurate delineation of local tumor recurrences as well as for the determination of tumor extent within the female pelvis.

Another advantage of integrated PET/MR imaging lies in the opportunity of a significant reduction of potentially harmful ionizing radiation exposure when compared to PET/CT (Schafer et al. 2014). Reported radiation dose savings of PET/MRI amount to 73–77% in comparison to a full-dose PET/CT scan and even of 29% when applied as an alternative to low-dose PET/CT imaging (Grueneisen et al. 2016). This is of particular importance considering the application of repetitive follow-up examinations in cancer patients and a young peak age of cervical cancer patients. Regarding a markedly reduced radiation exposure, PET/MR epitomizes a valuable alternative staging tool for cervical cancer patients within a reasonable scan duration as demonstrated in recent publications by Grueneisen and Kirchner et al. (2015; 2017).

5.2.3 Ovarian Cancer

Ovarian cancers are one of the most common neoplasms of the female pelvis and a leading cause of cancer-related deaths in western countries (Siegel et al. 2014). Despite radical/extensive surgical treatments as well as improvements in therapeutic strategies, patients' prognosis remains poor when compared to other gynecological malignancies, as the diagnosis of ovarian cancer is frequently made at advanced tumor stages due to the asymptomatic nature of early disease.

In cases of a suspected manifestation of ovarian cancer, clinical evaluation and the determination of tumor markers (e.g. cancer antigen (CA)-125) are initially applied (Forstner et al. 2010). In addition, ultrasound examinations are performed for the identification and characterization of ovarian masses. For primary tumor staging CT is most frequently used for the assessment of local tumor spread and the detection of metastatic disease, which aids in the selection of a surgical or a systemic treatment approach. As demonstrated for most tumors of the female pelvis, previous studies have shown that MR imaging enables a more reliable differentiation between benign and malignant ovary lesions than CT as well as a more accurate determination of the extent of primary tumors (Hricak et al. 2000; Forstner et al. 1995; Kinkel et al. 2005).

In case of advanced tumor stages, thus, tumor spread beyond the female pelvis, the prognosis of ovarian cancer patients is highly dependent on an optimal cytoreduction during primary surgery. Older studies found a comparable predictability to achieve maximal tumor debulking based on the information derived from CT or MRI (Forstner et al. 1995; Qayyum et al. 2005). Due to technical innovations and the introduction of diffusion-weighted imaging techniques, the diagnostic accuracy of MRI for tumor detection has significantly improved over the past few years (Low et al. 2009; Fujii et al. 2008). Michielsen and colleagues reported a higher accuracy of whole-body MRI including diffusion-weighted sequences than CT for the detection of peritoneal carcinomatosis (91% vs. 75%), retroperitoneal lymph node metastases (87% vs. 71%) as well as for the definition of the correct tumor stage (94% vs. 56%)

(Michielsen et al. 2014). Furthermore, the potential role of PET/CT for staging ovarian cancer has been assessed in several studies and promising results have been demonstrated, especially for the identification of metastatic spread (Kitajima et al. 2008; Murakami et al. 2006; Mangili et al. 2007). A meta-analysis investigated the diagnostic value of 18F-FDG PET imaging for the identification of lymph node metastases in ovarian cancer patients (Yuan et al. 2012). The authors reported a higher sensitivity and specificity of PET or PET/CT (73.2% and 96.7%) when compared to CT (42.6% and 95%) and MRI (54.7% and 88.3%) (Yuan et al. 2012). Schmidt et al. compared 18F-FDG PET/CT and MRI for detection of peritoneal carcinomatosis in patients with ovarian cancer and found a higher sensitivity of MRI (98% vs. 95%) and higher specificity of PET/CT (96% vs. 84%) (Schmidt et al. 2015). Fiaschetti and colleagues assessed the potential of retrospectively fused PET and MRI datasets for the characterization of suspicious ovarian lesions (Fiaschetti et al. 2011). In their study PET/MRI revealed a higher sensitivity, specificity and negative predictive value (94%, 100%, 83%) than PET/CT (74%, 80% and 44%) and MRI alone (84%, 60%, 50%) for the identification of ovarian tumor manifestations (Fiaschetti et al. 2011). In a previously mentioned study, Queiroz et al. directly compared PET/CT and PET/MRI for staging female pelvic malignancies, comprising 12/26 (46%) patients with ovarian cancer (Queiroz et al. 2015). While both modalities showed equivalent results for the identification of abdominal and regional lymph node metastases, PET/MRI enabled better determination of the local tumor extent in 5 out of the 12 cases. These findings illustrate the diagnostic potential by combining the complementary information of PET and MRI for more accurate primary evaluation of ovarian cancers. Accordingly, integrated PET/MRI may help to triage the patient towards the most appropriate treatment strategy (e.g. primary surgery vs. neoadjuvant chemotherapy) as well as to predict the option of an optimal cytoreductive surgical intervention.

Approximately, two thirds of ovarian cancer patients develop tumor relapse. In general, patient follow-up comprises clinical examination, transvaginal ultrasound as well as determination of tumor marker levels. However, for therapy planning and the selection of patients who will benefit from a surgical treatment approach, reliable information about the extent and distribution of tumor manifestations are required. In case of a suspected tumor recurrence, the use of CT and MRI is widely established (Forstner et al. 2010). For PET and PET/CT higher sensitivities for the detection of recurrent ovarian cancer have been shown (Kitajima et al. 2008; Gu et al. 2009). Hence in case of suspicion of tumor relapse, these modalities should be applied even in case of negative or inconclusive findings in conventional cross-sectional imaging. In a meta-analysis by Gu et al., the authors reported a pooled sensitivity, specificity and AUC of 91%, 88% and 0.96 for PET/CT, 75%, 78% and 0.80 for MRI, 79%, 84% and 0.88 for CT as well as 69%, 93% and 0.92 for CA-125 for the identification of recurrent disease (Gu et al. 2009). Menzel et al. could demonstrate a high accuracy of PET for tumor detection, especially in high-risk patients which showed elevated CA-125 levels (Menzel et al. 2004). Furthermore, Murakami et al. found a sensitivity of 97.8% for the detection of recurrent ovarian cancer by combining the information of PET data and CA-125 (Murakami et al. 2006).

In a mixed population of 34 women with a suspected recurrence of a female pelvic malignancy, Grueneisen and colleagues assessed and compared the performance of whole-body MRI and PET/MRI for restaging female pelvic malignancies (Grueneisen et al. 2014). PET/MRI enabled correct identification of 25/25 (100%) patients with cancer recurrence, while MRI alone detected 23/25 (92%) patients correctly. In addition, PET/MRI provided a higher detection rate of malignant lesions, when compared to MRI alone (98.9% vs. 88.8%). A number of studies have compared the diagnostic value of PET/MRI and PET/CT for whole-body restaging of female pelvic cancers (Grueneisen et al. 2015; Kirchner et al. 2017; Beiderwellen et al. 2015). In general, the authors found comparable to equivalent detection rates of tumor recurrence on a per-patient- and per-lesion basis, while minor differences were shown between the two imaging modalities for lesion detection in dependence of their localization. Beiderwellen

et al. reported a higher diagnostic confidence for the determination of local tumor recurrences and lymph node metastases using PET/MRI (Beiderwellen et al. 2015). These early study results of integrated PET/MR imaging indicate the high diagnostic potential of this emerging hybrid imaging technique to facilitate improved detection and delineation of ovarian cancer recurrences and provide useful information for the definition of resectable/unresectable disease extent (Figure 5.5).

5.2.4 Endometrial Cancer

Endometrial cancer is the most frequently diagnosed gynecological malignancy in developed countries (Torre et al. 2015). Typical clinical symptoms such as abnormal or postmenopausal bleeding usually occur at an early stage of the disease, which results in good survival rates, when appropriate diagnostic and therapeutic measures are initiated. In symptomatic patients, clinical examination and transvaginal ultrasound are applied for primary tumor evaluation. Since endometrcial cancers are surgically staged, further preoperative imaging is not generally recommended. Important prognostic determinants are the local tumor extent, the occurrence of lymph node and distant metastases as well as the histologic subtype (Beddy et al. 2012). Based on its high soft-tissue contrast, the utilization of dynamiccontrast-enhancedimaginganddiffusion-weighted sequences, MRI is considered highly accurate for the determination of local tumor extent within the female pelvis (Beddy et al. 2012; Sala et al. 2007). MRI has been shown superior to CT or ultrasound for the assessment of the depth of myometrial tumor invasion, representing one of the most important prognostic factors (Sala et al. 2007; Kinkel et al. 1999; Kim et al. 1995). Previous studies could demonstrate that the presence of lymph node metastases increased from 3% in cases with superficial myometrial tumor infiltration to 46%, when tumor invasion extended > 50% of myometrial depth (Larson et al. 1996; Berman et al. 1980). Reported sensitivities and specificities of MRI for the determination of the depth of myometrial tumor

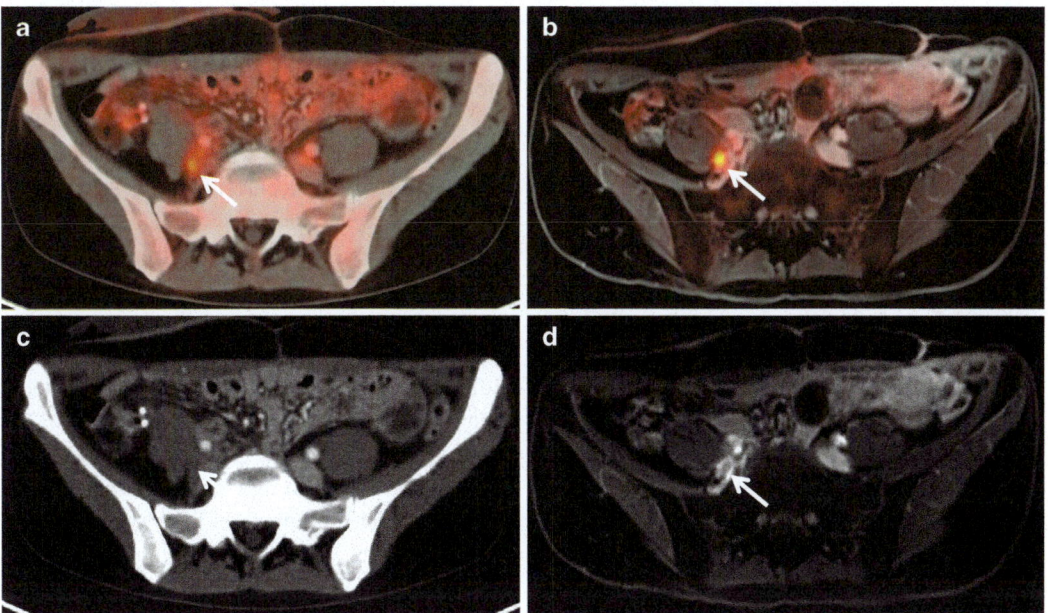

Fig. 5.5 Images of a 25 years-old patient with a tumor recurrence of ovarian cancer adjacent to the right psoas muscle (arrows), which shows a focally increased tracer uptake in PET/CT and PET/MRI (**a**, **b**). When compared to the CT-component (**c**), MRI (**d**) enables better detection and delineation of the tumor manifestation, based on a higher soft-tissue contrast

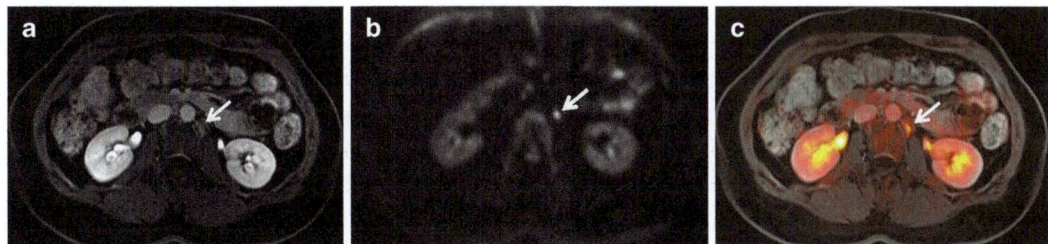

Fig. 5.6 Images of a morphologically inconspicuous paraaortic lymph node (**a**, T1w VIBE), displaying slighty increased signal intensity in diffusion-weighted images (**b**, DWI: b-1000). The diagnosis of a lymph node metastasis has been made due to the identification of a pathologically increased glucose metabolism after image fusion in PET/MRI (**c**)

invasion vary between 70–95% and 80–95%, respectively (Sala et al. 2013). Moreover, MRI offers an excellent accuracy for the identification of cervical involvement, which requires modifications in surgical treatment, in terms of more extensive tumor resection (Sala et al. 2013; Murakami et al. 1995; Freeman et al. 2012). Furthermore, increasing evidence has underlined the added value of presurgical treatment planning via MRI, yielding valuable information in case of high grade tumors and advance tumor stage at the time of diagnosis (Kinkel et al. 2009; Querleu et al. 2011).

The presence of pelvic and/or paraaortic lymph node metastases in endometrial cancer has impact on surgical treatment and adjuvant therapeutic strategies and designates the patient to a stage IIIC or higher (Freeman et al. 2012; Creutzberg et al. 2000; Kim et al. 2016). Morphological criteria, as most commonly applied in conventional cross-sectional imaging modalities, have not been proven sufficient for the correct identification of lymph node involvement (Fig. 5.6) (Rockall et al. 2007; Park et al. 2008). Rockall and colleagues reported a sensitivity and specificity of 44% and 98%, respectively, for the identification of lymph node metastases using MRI (Rockall et al. 2007). In another study comprising 287 patients, Kim and colleagues investigated the staging performance of MRI and PET/CT in the detection of nodal positive patients (Kim et al. 2016). The authors found a significantly higher sensitivity, specificity, PPV, NPV and accuracy of PET/CT (70.0, 95.4, 74.4, 94.3 and 91.3%) in comparison to MRI (34.0, 95.0, 58.6, 87.2 and 84.3%). In addition, PET/CT showed a high sensitivity, specificity and NPV (92.9, 98.9 and 99.6%) for the detection of distant metastases (Kim et al. 2016). Furthermore, Kitajima and colleagues analyzed the diagnostic value of a retrospective fusion of pelvic MR- and 18F-FDG PET-datasets for locoregional tumor staging of primary endometrial carcinoma in comparison to MR alone and PET/CT (Kitajima et al. 2013). Fused PET/MRI was most effective for the determination of the local tumor extent and pelvic lymph node staging. An initial study on a trimodality PET/CT-MR system reported similar results, yet, comprising a mixed study population with only four patients diagnosed with endometrial cancer (Queiroz et al. 2015). Based on these initial results on hybrid imaging in endometrial cancer, integrated PET/MRI bears the potential to provide valuable information for initial treatment planning and the definition of a multimodal therapeutic concept, particularly in high risk patients and or advanced tumor stages, thus, being inherently associated to an increased risk of metastatic spread.

Approximately, 15% of primarily treated endometrial cancer patients develop recurrent disease (Creutzberg et al. 2000; Todo et al. 2010). Almost 90% of tumor recurrences occur within 3 years after initial treatment and the most common sites are lymph nodes or the vaginal vault (Sohaib et al. 2007). If tumor manifestations are still confined to the female pelvis, they are preferentially treated with surgical resection or pelvic radiation. However, if distant metastases are present, the therapeutic options are limited. CT, MRI and PET/CT are frequently applied imaging modalities for the assessment of a suspected tumor relapse. MRI is considered helpful for the evaluation of surgical resectability of local recurrences within the female pelvis. Furthermore, CT is widely established for a whole-body restaging approach to detect recurrent pelvic and distant disease. However, previous studies have found a significantly higher sensitivity of PET/CT than CT for the identification of disease recurrences, which had a substantial effect on further treatment planning (Kitajima et al. 2009; Belhocine et al. 2002). A systematic review article reported a pooled sensitivity and specificity of 95.8% and 92.5% of 18F-FDG PET/CT for the depiction and localization of recurrences in post-therapeutical follow-up of endometrial cancer patients (Kadkhodayan et al. 2013). A few initial studies compared the diagnostic capability of integrated PET/MRI and PET/CT for restaging female pelvic malignances and found comparable results for tumor detection comparable to other tumors of the female pelvis (Grueneisen et al. 2015; Kirchner et al. 2017; Beiderwellen et al. 2015). Accordingly, PET/MRI bears the potential for highly accurate evaluation of endometrial cancer patients with a suspected tumor recurrence and may provide useful information, especially for further treatment planning of intrapelvic tumor manifestations.

Conclusion

Cancers of the female pelvis represent one of the most appreciative application fields of integrated PET/MR imaging, as the inherently high soft-tissue contrast of MRI, as well as the combined analysis of morphologic, functional and metabolic data bear the potential for improved detection of potential primary, metastatic or recurrent cancerous lesions in a "one-stop-shop-imaging" setting. Emerging applications of radiomics analyses are awaited to leverage hybrid imaging to improved understanding of tumor biology and contingently result in ameliorated targeted/personalized treatment.

References

Aerts HJ, Velazquez ER, Leijenaar RT, Parmar C, Grossmann P, Carvalho S, et al. Decoding tumour phenotype by noninvasive imaging using a quantitative radiomics approach. Nat Commun. 2014;5:4006.

Antoch G, Stattaus J, Nemat AT, Marnitz S, Beyer T, Kuehl H, et al. Non-small cell lung cancer: dual-modality PET/CT in preoperative staging. Radiology. 2003;229(2):526–33.

Antoch G, Vogt FM, Freudenberg LS, Nazaradeh F, Goehde SC, Barkhausen J, et al. Whole-body dual-modality PET/CT and whole-body MRI for tumor staging in oncology. JAMA. 2003;290(24): 3199–206.

Bar-Shalom R, Yefremov N, Guralnik L, Gaitini D, Frenkel A, Kuten A, et al. Clinical performance of PET/CT in evaluation of cancer: additional value for diagnostic imaging and patient management. J Nucl Med. 2003;44(8):1200–9.

Beddy P, O'Neill AC, Yamamoto AK, Addley HC, Reinhold C, Sala E. FIGO staging system for endometrial cancer: added benefits of MR imaging. Radiographics. 2012;32(1):241–54.

Beiderwellen K, Geraldo L, Ruhlmann V, Heusch P, Gomez B, Nensa F, et al. Accuracy of [18F]FDG PET/MRI for the detection of liver metastases. PLoS One. 2015;10(9):e0137285.

Beiderwellen K, Gomez B, Buchbender C, Hartung V, Poeppel TD, Nensa F, et al. Depiction and characterization of liver lesions in whole body [(1)(8)F]-FDG PET/MRI. Eur J Radiol. 2013;82(11):e669–75.

Beiderwellen K, Grueneisen J, Ruhlmann V, Buderath P, Aktas B, Heusch P, et al. [(18)F]FDG PET/MRI vs. PET/CT for whole-body staging in patients with recurrent malignancies of the female pelvis: initial results. Eur J Nucl Med Mol Imaging. 2015;42(1):56–65.

Beiderwellen K, Huebner M, Heusch P, Grueneisen J, Ruhlmann V, Nensa F, et al. Whole-body [(1)(8)F] FDG PET/MRI vs. PET/CT in the assessment of bone lesions in oncological patients: initial results. Eur Radiol. 2014;24(8):2023–30.

Belhocine T, De Barsy C, Hustinx R, Willems-Foidart J. Usefulness of (18)F-FDG PET in the post-therapy surveillance of endometrial carcinoma. Eur J Nucl Med Mol Imaging. 2002;29(9):1132–9.

Bellone S, Pecorelli S, Cannon MJ, Santin AD. Advances in dendritic-cell-based therapeutic vaccines for cervical cancer. Expert Rev Anticancer Ther. 2007;7(10):1473–86.

Berman ML, Ballon SC, Lagasse LD, Watring WG. Prognosis and treatment of endometrial cancer. Am J Obstet Gynecol. 1980;136(5):679–88.

Bipat S, Glas AS, van der Velden J, Zwinderman AH, Bossuyt PM, Stoker J. Computed tomography and magnetic resonance imaging in staging of uterine cervical carcinoma: a systematic review. Gynecol Oncol. 2003;91(1):59–66.

Bjurberg M, Brun E. Clinical impact of 2-deoxy-2-[18F]fluoro-D-glucose (FDG)-positron emission tomography (PET) on treatment choice in recurrent cancer of the cervix uteri. Int J Gynecol Cancer. 2013;23(9):1642–6.

Bollineni VR, Ytre-Hauge S, Bollineni-Balabay O, Salvesen HB, Haldorsen IS. High diagnostic value of 18F-FDG PET/CT in endometrial cancer: systematic review and meta-analysis of the literature. J Nucl Med. 2016;57(6):879–85.

Brandmaier P, Purz S, Bremicker K, Hockel M, Barthel H, Kluge R, et al. Simultaneous [18F]FDG-PET/MRI: correlation of Apparent Diffusion Coefficient (ADC) and Standardized Uptake Value (SUV) in primary and recurrent cervical cancer. PLoS One. 2015;10(11):e0141684.

Buchbender C, Hartung-Knemeyer V, Beiderwellen K, Heusch P, Kuhl H, Lauenstein TC, et al. Diffusion-weighted imaging as part of hybrid PET/MRI protocols for whole-body cancer staging: does it benefit lesion detection? Eur J Radiol. 2013;82(5):877–82.

Cavaliere C, Romeo V, Aiello M, Mesolella M, Iorio B, Barbuto L, et al. Multiparametric evaluation by simultaneous PET-MRI examination in patients with histologically proven laryngeal cancer. Eur J Radiol. 2017;88:47–55.

Choi HJ, Ju W, Myung SK, Kim Y. Diagnostic performance of computer tomography, magnetic resonance imaging, and positron emission tomography or positron emission tomography/computer tomography for detection of metastatic lymph nodes in patients with cervical cancer: meta-analysis. Cancer Sci. 2010;101(6):1471–9.

Choi HJ, Roh JW, Seo SS, Lee S, Kim JY, Kim SK, et al. Comparison of the accuracy of magnetic resonance imaging and positron emission tomography/computed tomography in the presurgical detection of lymph node metastases in patients with uterine cervical carcinoma: a prospective study. Cancer. 2006;106(4): 914–22.

Coroller TP, Grossmann P, Hou Y, Rios Velazquez E, Leijenaar RT, Hermann G, et al. CT-based radiomic signature predicts distant metastasis in lung adenocarcinoma. Radiother Oncol. 2015;114(3):345–50.

Creutzberg CL, van Putten WL, Koper PC, Lybeert ML, Jobsen JJ, Warlam-Rodenhuis CC, et al. Surgery and postoperative radiotherapy versus surgery alone for patients with stage-1 endometrial carcinoma: multicentre randomised trial. PORTEC Study Group Post Operative Radiation Therapy in Endometrial Carcinoma. Lancet. 2000;355(9213):1404–11.

Delgado G, Bundy B, Zaino R, Sevin BU, Creasman WT, Major F. Prospective surgical-pathological study of disease-free interval in patients with stage IB squamous cell carcinoma of the cervix: a Gynecologic Oncology Group study. Gynecol Oncol. 1990;38(3):352–7.

Delso G, Furst S, Jakoby B, Ladebeck R, Ganter C, Nekolla SG, et al. Performance measurements of the

Siemens mMR integrated whole-body PET/MR scanner. J Nucl Med. 2011;52(12):1914–22.

Deuschl C, Moenninghoff C, Goericke S, Kirchner J, Koppen S, Binse I, et al. Response assessment of bevacizumab therapy in GBM with integrated 11C-MET-PET/MRI: a feasibility study. Eur J Nucl Med Mol Imaging. 2017;

Eiber M, Takei T, Souvatzoglou M, Mayerhoefer ME, Furst S, Gaertner FC, et al. Performance of whole-body integrated 18F-FDG PET/MR in comparison to PET/CT for evaluation of malignant bone lesions. J Nucl Med. 2014;55(2):191–7.

Fuller AF, Jr., Elliott N, Kosloff C, Hoskins WJ, Lewis JL, Jr. Determinants of increased risk for recurrence in patients undergoing radical hysterectomy for stage IB and IIA carcinoma of the cervix. Gynecol Oncol 1989;33(1):34-39.

Erfanian Y, Grueneisen J, Kirchner J, Wetter A, Podleska LE, Bauer S, et al. Integrated 18F-FDG PET/MRI compared to MRI alone for identification of local recurrences of soft tissue sarcomas: a comparison trial. Eur J Nucl Med Mol Imaging. 2017;

Fiaschetti V, Calabria F, Crusco S, Meschini A, Nucera F, Schillaci O, et al. MR-PET fusion imaging in evaluating adnexal lesions: a preliminary study. Radiol Med. 2011;116(8):1288–302.

Forstner R, Hricak H, Occhipinti KA, Powell CB, Frankel SD, Stern JL. Ovarian cancer: staging with CT and MR imaging. Radiology. 1995;197(3):619–26.

Forstner R, Sala E, Kinkel K, Spencer JA. European Society of Urogenital R. ESUR guidelines: ovarian cancer staging and follow-up. Eur Radiol. 2010;20(12):2773–80.

Freeman SJ, Aly AM, Kataoka MY, Addley HC, Reinhold C, Sala E. The revised FIGO staging system for uterine malignancies: implications for MR imaging. Radiographics. 2012;32(6):1805–27.

Friedlander M, Grogan M, Force USPST. Guidelines for the treatment of recurrent and metastatic cervical cancer. Oncologist. 2002;7(4):342–7.

Fujii S, Matsusue E, Kanasaki Y, Kanamori Y, Nakanishi J, Sugihara S, et al. Detection of peritoneal dissemination in gynecological malignancy: evaluation by diffusion-weighted MR imaging. Eur Radiol. 2008;18(1):18–23.

Fulcher AS, O'Sullivan SG, Segreti EM, Kavanagh BD. Recurrent cervical carcinoma: typical and atypical manifestations. Radiographics. 1999;19. Spec No:S103-16; quiz S264-5

Gillies RJ, Kinahan PE, Hricak H. Radiomics: images are more than pictures, they are data. Radiology. 2016;278(2):563–77.

Grant P, Sakellis C, Jacene HA. Gynecologic oncologic imaging with PET/CT. Semin Nucl Med. 2014;44(6):461–78.

Grueneisen J, Beiderwellen K, Heusch P, Buderath P, Aktas B, Gratz M, et al. Correlation of standardized uptake value and apparent diffusion coefficient in integrated whole-body PET/MRI of primary and recurrent cervical cancer. PLoS One. 2014;9(5):e96751.

Grueneisen J, Beiderwellen K, Heusch P, Gratz M, Schulze-Hagen A, Heubner M, et al. Simultaneous positron emission tomography/magnetic resonance imaging for whole-body staging in patients with recurrent gynecological malignancies of the pelvis: a comparison to whole-body magnetic resonance imaging alone. Investig Radiol. 2014;49(12):808–15.

Grueneisen J, Sawicki LM, Schaarschmidt BM, Suntharalingam S, von der Ropp S, Wetter A, et al. Evaluation of a fast protocol for staging lymphoma patients with integrated PET/MRI. PLoS One. 2016;11(6):e0157880.

Grueneisen J, Sawicki LM, Wetter A, Kirchner J, Kinner S, Aktas B, et al. Evaluation of PET and MR datasets in integrated 18F-FDG PET/MRI: a comparison of different MR sequences for whole-body restaging of breast cancer patients. Eur J Radiol. 2017;89: 14–9.

Grueneisen J, Schaarschmidt BM, Beiderwellen K, Schulze-Hagen A, Heubner M, Kinner S, et al. Diagnostic value of diffusion-weighted imaging in simultaneous 18F-FDG PET/MR imaging for whole-body staging of women with pelvic malignancies. J Nucl Med. 2014;55(12):1930–5.

Grueneisen J, Schaarschmidt BM, Heubner M, Aktas B, Kinner S, Forsting M, et al. Integrated PET/MRI for whole-body staging of patients with primary cervical cancer: preliminary results. Eur J Nucl Med Mol Imaging. 2015;42(12):1814–24.

Grueneisen J, Schaarschmidt BM, Heubner M, Suntharalingam S, Milk I, Kinner S, et al. Implementation of FAST-PET/MRI for whole-body staging of female patients with recurrent pelvic malignancies: a comparison to PET/CT. Eur J Radiol. 2015;84(11): 2097–102.

Gu J, Chan T, Zhang J, Leung AY, Kwong YL, Khong PL. Whole-body diffusion-weighted imaging: the added value to whole-body MRI at initial diagnosis of lymphoma. AJR Am J Roentgenol. 2011;197(3):W384–91.

Gu P, Pan LL, Wu SQ, Sun L, Huang G. CA 125, PET alone, PET-CT, CT and MRI in diagnosing recurrent ovarian carcinoma: a systematic review and meta-analysis. Eur J Radiol. 2009;71(1):164–74.

Hartung-Knemeyer V, Beiderwellen KJ, Buchbender C, Kuehl H, Lauenstein TC, Bockisch A, et al. Optimizing positron emission tomography image acquisition protocols in integrated positron emission tomography/magnetic resonance imaging. Investig Radiol. 2013;48(5):290–4.

Hoh CK, Hawkins RA, Glaspy JA, Dahlbom M, Tse NY, Hoffman EJ, et al. Cancer detection with whole-body PET using 2-[18F]fluoro-2-deoxy-D-glucose. J Comput Assist Tomogr. 1993;17(4):582–9.

Hricak H, Chen M, Coakley FV, Kinkel K, KK Y, Sica G, et al. Complex adnexal masses: detection and characterization with MR imaging – multivariate analysis. Radiology. 2000;214(1):39–46.

Huynh E, Coroller TP, Narayan V, Agrawal V, Hou Y, Romano J, et al. CT-based radiomic analysis of stereotactic body radiation therapy patients with lung cancer. Radiother Oncol. 2016;120(2):258–66.

Johnson W, Taylor MB, Carrington BM, Bonington SC, Swindell R. The value of hyoscine butylbromide in pelvic MRI. Clin Radiol. 2007;62(11):1087–93.

Kadkhodayan S, Shahriari S, Treglia G, Yousefi Z, Sadeghi R. Accuracy of 18-F-FDG PET imaging in the follow up of endometrial cancer patients: systematic review and meta-analysis of the literature. Gynecol Oncol. 2013;128(2):397–404.

Kavanagh BD, Gieschen HL, Schmidt-Ullrich RK, Arthur D, Zwicker R, Kaufman N, et al. A pilot study of concomitant boost accelerated superfractionated radiotherapy for stage III cancer of the uterine cervix. Int J Radiat Oncol Biol Phys. 1997;38(3):561–8.

Kelly-Morland C, Rudman S, Nathan P, Mallett S, Montana G, Cook G, et al. Evaluation of treatment response and resistance in metastatic renal cell cancer (mRCC) using integrated 18F-Fluorodeoxyglucose (18F-FDG) positron emission tomography/magnetic resonance imaging (PET/MRI); The REMAP study. BMC Cancer. 2017;17(1):392.

Kidd EA, Siegel BA, Dehdashti F, Grigsby PW. Pelvic lymph node F-18 fluorodeoxyglucose uptake as a prognostic biomarker in newly diagnosed patients with locally advanced cervical cancer. Cancer. 2010;116(6):1469–75.

Kim HJ, Cho A, Yun M, Kim YT, Kang WJ. Comparison of FDG PET/CT and MRI in lymph node staging of endometrial cancer. Ann Nucl Med. 2016;30(2):104–13.

Kim SH, Kim HD, Song YS, Kang SB, Lee HP. Detection of deep myometrial invasion in endometrial carcinoma: comparison of transvaginal ultrasound, CT, and MRI. J Comput Assist Tomogr. 1995;19(5):766–72.

Kinkel K, Forstner R, Danza FM, Oleaga L, Cunha TM, Bergman A, et al. Staging of endometrial cancer with MRI: guidelines of the European Society of Urogenital Imaging. Eur Radiol. 2009;19(7):1565–74.

Kinkel K, Kaji Y, KK Y, Segal MR, Lu Y, Powell CB, et al. Radiologic staging in patients with endometrial cancer: a meta-analysis. Radiology. 1999;212(3):711–8.

Kinkel K, Lu Y, Mehdizade A, Pelte MF, Hricak H. Indeterminate ovarian mass at US: incremental value of second imaging test for characterization – meta-analysis and Bayesian analysis. Radiology. 2005;236(1):85–94.

Kirchner J, Deuschl C, Schweiger B, Herrmann K, Forsting M, Buchbender C, et al. Imaging children suffering from lymphoma: an evaluation of different 18F-FDG PET/MRI protocols compared to whole-body DW-MRI. Eur J Nucl Med Mol Imaging. 2017;

Kirchner J, Sawicki LM, Suntharalingam S, Grueneisen J, Ruhlmann V, Aktas B, et al. Whole-body staging of female patients with recurrent pelvic malignancies: Ultra-fast 18F-FDG PET/MRI compared to 18F-FDG PET/CT and CT. PLoS One. 2017;12(2):e0172553.

Kitajima K, Murakami K, Yamasaki E, Domeki Y, Kaji Y, Fukasawa I, et al. Performance of integrated FDG-PET/contrast-enhanced CT in the diagnosis of recurrent ovarian cancer: comparison with integrated FDG-PET/non-contrast-enhanced CT and enhanced CT. Eur J Nucl Med Mol Imaging. 2008;35(8):1439–48.

Kitajima K, Murakami K, Yamasaki E, Domeki Y, Kaji Y, Morita S, et al. Performance of integrated FDG-PET/contrast-enhanced CT in the diagnosis of recurrent uterine cancer: comparison with PET and enhanced CT. Eur J Nucl Med Mol Imaging. 2009;36(3): 362–72.

Kitajima K, Murakami K, Yamasaki E, Kaji Y, Fukasawa I, Inaba N, et al. Diagnostic accuracy of integrated FDG-PET/contrast-enhanced CT in staging ovarian cancer: comparison with enhanced CT. Eur J Nucl Med Mol Imaging. 2008;35(10):1912–20.

Kitajima K, Suenaga Y, Ueno Y, Kanda T, Maeda T, Makihara N, et al. Value of fusion of PET and MRI in the detection of intra-pelvic recurrence of gynecological tumor: comparison with 18F-FDG contrast-enhanced PET/CT and pelvic MRI. Ann Nucl Med. 2014;28(1):25–32.

Kitajima K, Suenaga Y, Ueno Y, Kanda T, Maeda T, Takahashi S, et al. Value of fusion of PET and MRI for staging of endometrial cancer: comparison with (1)(8)F-FDG contrast-enhanced PET/CT and dynamic contrast-enhanced pelvic MRI. Eur J Radiol. 2013;82(10):1672–6.

Koh WJ, Greer BE, Abu-Rustum NR, Apte SM, Campos SM, Chan J, et al. Cervical cancer. J Natl Compr Cancer Netw. 2013;11(3):320–43.

Kovac JD, Terzic M, Mirkovic M, Banko B, Dikic-Rom A, Maksimovic R. Endometrioid adenocarcinoma of the ovary: MRI findings with emphasis on diffusion-weighted imaging for the differentiation of ovarian tumors. Acta Radiol. 2016;57(6):758–66.

Kuang F, Ren J, Zhong Q, Liyuan F, Huan Y, Chen Z. The value of apparent diffusion coefficient in the assessment of cervical cancer. Eur Radiol. 2013;23(4):1050–8.

Lagasse LD, Creasman WT, Shingleton HM, Ford JH, Blessing JA. Results and complications of operative staging in cervical cancer: experience of the Gynecologic Oncology Group. Gynecol Oncol. 1980;9(1):90–8.

Lambin P, Rios-Velazquez E, Leijenaar R, Carvalho S, van Stiphout RG, Granton P, et al. Radiomics: extracting more information from medical images using advanced feature analysis. Eur J Cancer. 2012;48(4):441–6.

Larson DM, Connor GP, Broste SK, Krawisz BR, Johnson KK. Prognostic significance of gross myometrial invasion with endometrial cancer. Obstet Gynecol. 1996;88(3):394–8.

Lartizien C, Comtat C, Kinahan PE, Ferreira N, Bendriem B, Trebossen R. Optimization of injected dose based on noise equivalent count rates for 2- and 3-dimensional whole-body PET. J Nucl Med. 2002;43(9):1268–78.

Lee DH, Kim SH, Im SA, DY O, Kim TY, Han JK. Multiparametric fully-integrated 18-FDG PET/MRI of advanced gastric cancer for prediction of chemotherapy response: a preliminary study. Eur Radiol. 2016;26(8):2771–8.

Lee SY, Jee WH, Jung JY, Park MY, Kim SK, Jung CK, et al. Differentiation of malignant from benign soft tissue tumours: use of additive qualitative and quantitative diffusion-weighted MR imaging to standard MR imaging at 3.0 T. Eur Radiol. 2016;26(3):743–54.

Liu Y, Liu H, Bai X, Ye Z, Sun H, Bai R, et al. Differentiation of metastatic from non-metastatic lymph nodes in patients with uterine cervical cancer using diffusion-weighted imaging. Gynecol Oncol. 2011;122(1):19–24.

Low RN, Sebrechts CP, Barone RM, Muller W. Diffusion-weighted MRI of peritoneal tumors: comparison with conventional MRI and surgical and histopathologic findings – a feasibility study. AJR Am J Roentgenol. 2009;193(2):461–70.

Magne N, Chargari C, Vicenzi L, Gillion N, Messai T, Magne J, et al. New trends in the evaluation and treatment of cervix cancer: the role of FDG-PET. Cancer Treat Rev. 2008;34(8):671–81.

Mangili G, Picchio M, Sironi S, Vigano R, Rabaiotti E, Bornaghi D, et al. Integrated PET/CT as a first-line re-staging modality in patients with suspected recurrence of ovarian cancer. Eur J Nucl Med Mol Imaging. 2007;34(5):658–66.

Menzel C, Dobert N, Hamscho N, Zaplatnikov K, Vasvatekis S, Matic V, et al. The influence of CA 125 and CEA levels on the results of (18)F-deoxyglucose positron emission tomography in suspected recurrence of epithelial ovarian cancer. Strahlenther Onkol. 2004;180(8):497–501.

Michielsen K, Vergote I, Op de Beeck K, Amant F, Leunen K, Moerman P, et al. Whole-body MRI with diffusion-weighted sequence for staging of patients with suspected ovarian cancer: a clinical feasibility study in comparison to CT and FDG-PET/CT. Eur Radiol. 2014;24(4):889–901.

Mirpour S, Mhlanga JC, Logeswaran P, Russo G, Mercier G, Subramaniam RM. The role of PET/CT in the management of cervical cancer. AJR Am J Roentgenol. 2013;201(2):W192–205.

Murakami M, Miyamoto T, Iida T, Tsukada H, Watanabe M, Shida M, et al. Whole-body positron emission tomography and tumor marker CA125 for detection of recurrence in epithelial ovarian cancer. Int J Gynecol Cancer. 2006;16(Suppl 1):99–107.

Murakami T, Kurachi H, Nakamura H, Tsuda K, Miyake A, Tomoda K, et al. Cervical invasion of endometrial carcinoma – evaluation by parasagittal MR imaging. Acta Radiol. 1995;36(3):248–53.

Nakamura K, Joja I, Kodama J, Hongo A, Hiramatsu Y. Measurement of SUVmax plus ADCmin of the primary tumour is a predictor of prognosis in patients with cervical cancer. Eur J Nucl Med Mol Imaging. 2012;39(2):283–90.

Nensa F, Beiderwellen K, Heusch P, Wetter A. Clinical applications of PET/MRI: current status and future perspectives. Diagn Interv Radiol. 2014;20(5):438–47.

Nie J, Zhang J, Gao J, Guo L, Zhou H, Hu Y, et al. Diagnostic role of 18F-FDG PET/MRI in patients with gynecological malignancies of the pelvis: a systematic review and meta-analysis. PLoS One. 2017;12(5):e0175401.

Park JJ, Kim CK, Park SY, Simonetti AW, Kim E, Park BK, et al. Assessment of early response to concurrent chemoradiotherapy in cervical cancer: value of diffusion-weighted and dynamic contrast-enhanced MR imaging. Magn Reson Imaging. 2014;32(8):993–1000.

Park JY, Kim EN, Kim DY, Suh DS, Kim JH, Kim YM, et al. Comparison of the validity of magnetic resonance imaging and positron emission tomography/computed tomography in the preoperative evaluation of patients with uterine corpus cancer. Gynecol Oncol. 2008;108(3):486–92.

Pecorelli S, Zigliani L, Odicino F. Revised FIGO staging for carcinoma of the cervix. Int J Gynaecol Obstet. 2009;105(2):107–8.

Pichler BJ, Wehrl HF, Kolb A, Judenhofer MS. Positron emission tomography/magnetic resonance imaging: the next generation of multimodality imaging? Semin Nucl Med. 2008;38(3):199–208.

Piver MS, Chung WS. Prognostic significance of cervical lesion size and pelvic node metastases in cervical carcinoma. Obstet Gynecol. 1975;46(5):507–10.

Qayyum A, Coakley FV, Westphalen AC, Hricak H, Okuno WT, Powell B. Role of CT and MR imaging in predicting optimal cytoreduction of newly diagnosed primary epithelial ovarian cancer. Gynecol Oncol. 2005;96(2):301–6.

Qin Y, Peng Z, Lou J, Liu H, Deng F, Zheng Y. Discrepancies between clinical staging and pathological findings of operable cervical carcinoma with stage IB-IIB: a retrospective analysis of 818 patients. Aust N Z J Obstet Gynaecol. 2009;49(5):542–4.

Queiroz MA, Kubik-Huch RA, Hauser N, Freiwald-Chilla B, von Schulthess G, Froehlich JM, et al. PET/MRI and PET/CT in advanced gynaecological tumours: initial experience and comparison. Eur Radiol. 2015;25(8):2222–30.

Querleu D, Planchamp F, Narducci F, Morice P, Joly F, Genestie C, et al. Clinical practice guidelines for the management of patients with endometrial cancer in France. Recommendations of the Institut National du Cancer and the Societe Francaise d'Oncologie Gynecologique. Int J Gynecol Cancer. 2011;21(5):945–50.

Rockall AG, Meroni R, Sohaib SA, Reynolds K, Alexander-Sefre F, Shepherd JH, et al. Evaluation of endometrial carcinoma on magnetic resonance imaging. Int J Gynecol Cancer. 2007;17(1):188–96.

Romeo V, D'Aiuto M, Frasci G, Imbriaco M, Nicolai E. Simultaneous PET/MRI assessment of response to cytotoxic and hormone neo-adjuvant chemotherapy in breast cancer: a preliminary report. Med Oncol. 2017;34(2):18.

Sala E, Rockall AG, Freeman SJ, Mitchell DG, Reinhold C. The added role of MR imaging in treatment stratification of patients with gynecologic malignancies:

what the radiologist needs to know. Radiology. 2013;266(3):717–40.

Sala E, Wakely S, Senior E, Lomas D. MRI of malignant neoplasms of the uterine corpus and cervix. AJR Am J Roentgenol. 2007;188(6):1577–87.

Sawicki LM, Grueneisen J, Buchbender C, Schaarschmidt BM, Gomez B, Ruhlmann V, et al. Evaluation of the outcome of lung nodules missed on 18F-FDG PET/MRI compared with 18F-FDG PET/CT in patients with known malignancies. J Nucl Med. 2016a;57(1):15–20.

Sawicki LM, Grueneisen J, Buchbender C, Schaarschmidt BM, Gomez B, Ruhlmann V, et al. Comparative performance of 18F-FDG PET/MRI and 18F-FDG PET/CT regarding detection and characterization of pulmonary lesions in 121 oncologic patients. J Nucl Med. 2016b;

Schafer JF, Gatidis S, Schmidt H, Guckel B, Bezrukov I, Pfannenberg CA, et al. Simultaneous whole-body PET/MR imaging in comparison to PET/CT in pediatric oncology: initial results. Radiology. 2014;273(1):220–31.

Schmidt S, Meuli RA, Achtari C, Prior JO. Peritoneal carcinomatosis in primary ovarian cancer staging: comparison between MDCT, MRI, and 18F-FDG PET/CT. Clin Nucl Med. 2015;40(5):371–7.

Selman TJ, Mann C, Zamora J, Appleyard TL, Khan K. Diagnostic accuracy of tests for lymph node status in primary cervical cancer: a systematic review and meta-analysis. CMAJ. 2008;178(7):855–62.

Siegel R, Ma J, Zou Z, Jemal A. Cancer statistics, 2014. CA Cancer J Clin. 2014;64(1):9–29.

Sohaib SA, Houghton SL, Meroni R, Rockall AG, Blake P, Reznek RH. Recurrent endometrial cancer: patterns of recurrent disease and assessment of prognosis. Clin Radiol. 2007;62(1):28–34. discussion 5-6

Sotoudeh H, Sharma A, Fowler KJ, McConathy J, Dehdashti F. Clinical application of PET/MRI in oncology. J Magn Reson Imaging. 2016;44(2):265–76.

Stehman FB, Bundy BN, DiSaia PJ, Keys HM, Larson JE, Fowler WC. Carcinoma of the cervix treated with radiation therapy. I. A multi-variate analysis of prognostic variables in the Gynecologic Oncology Group. Cancer. 1991;67(11):2776–85.

Tinga DJ, Timmer PR, Bouma J, Aalders JG. Prognostic significance of single versus multiple lymph node metastases in cervical carcinoma stage IB. Gynecol Oncol. 1990;39(2):175–80.

Todo Y, Kato H, Kaneuchi M, Watari H, Takeda M, Sakuragi N. Survival effect of para-aortic lymphadenectomy in endometrial cancer (SEPAL study): a retrospective cohort analysis. Lancet. 2010;375(9721):1165–72.

Torre LA, Bray F, Siegel RL, Ferlay J, Lortet-Tieulent J, Jemal A. Global cancer statistics, 2012. CA Cancer J Clin. 2015;65(2):87–108.

van Timmeren JE, Leijenaar RTH, van Elmpt W, Reymen B, Oberije C, Monshouwer R, et al. Survival prediction of non-small cell lung cancer patients using radiomics analyses of cone-beam CT images. Radiother Oncol. 2017;

Vesselle HJ, Miraldi FD. FDG PET of the retroperitoneum: normal anatomy, variants, pathologic conditions, and strategies to avoid diagnostic pitfalls. Radiographics. 1998;18(4):805–23. discussion 23-4

Weber TM, Sostman HD, Spritzer CE, Ballard RL, Meyer GA, Clark-Pearson DL, et al. Cervical carcinoma: determination of recurrent tumor extent versus radiation changes with MR imaging. Radiology. 1995;194(1):135–9.

Yin Q, Hung SC, Wang L, Lin W, Fielding JR, Rathmell WK, et al. Associations between tumor vascularity, vascular endothelial growth factor expression and PET/MRI radiomic signatures in primary clear-cell-renal-cell-carcinoma: proof-of-concept study. Sci Rep. 2017;7:43356.

Yuan Y, ZX G, Tao XF, Liu SY. Computer tomography, magnetic resonance imaging, and positron emission tomography or positron emission tomography/computer tomography for detection of metastatic lymph nodes in patients with ovarian cancer: a meta-analysis. Eur J Radiol. 2012;81(5):1002–6.

Zand KR, Reinhold C, Abe H, Maheshwari S, Mohamed A, Upegui D. Magnetic resonance imaging of the cervix. Cancer Imaging. 2007;7:69–76.

Zhou Y, He L, Huang Y, Chen S, Wu P, Ye W, et al. CT-based radiomics signature: a potential biomarker for preoperative prediction of early recurrence in hepatocellular carcinoma. Abdom Radiol. 2017;42(6):1695–704.

PET/MRI and Molecular Imaging in Breast Cancer

Amy Melsaether, Roy Raad, Thomas Helbich, Linda Moy, and Katja Pinker

6.1 PET/MRI of the Breast

MRI is an indispensable tool in breast imaging with multiple established indications (Sardanelli et al. 2010, 2017; D'Orsi et al. 2013). Dynamic contrast-enhanced MRI (DCE-MRI) is the back-bone of any standard MRI breast protocol and the most sensitive method for breast cancer detection with sensitivities ranging up to 98–100%, but variable specificities ranging from 47–97% (Sardanelli et al. 2010; D'Orsi et al. 2013; Pinker et al. 2009;

Pinker-Domenig et al. 2012; Morris 2007; Morrow et al. 2011; Mann et al. 2015). The effectiveness of DCE-MRI relies on its ability not only to provide high-resolution morphological information about a given tumor but also functional information about tumor neo-angiogenesis as a cancer specific hallmark. In their multi-step development, cancers acquire several other hallmark capabilities such as proliferative signaling, evading growth suppressors, resisting cell death, enabling replicative immortality and activating invasion and metastasis (Hanahan and Weinberg 2000; 2011). To over-come the limitations of DCE regarding its specificity, multiple other functional MRI parameters such as diffusion-weighted imaging (DWI), proton magnetic spectroscopic imaging (^{1}H-MRSI), phosphorus MRSI, sodium imaging or chemical change saturation transfer imaging (CEST) have been developed and investigated to interrogate more cancer hallmarks in breast imaging, revealing encouraging results (Dorrius et al. 2014; Baltzer et al. 2012; Schmitt et al. 2011; Zaric et al. 2016; Bogner et al. 2009, 2012; Gruber et al. 2011, 2016; Pinker et al. 2012). Despite challenges unique to the individual MRI parameters, some of these parameters, e.g. DWI or ^{1}H-MRSI have been successfully translated from experimental to clinical breast imaging. Their combined application with DCE-MRI is defined as multiparametric MRI (mpMRI) of the breast and data indicate that mpMRI of the breast improves diagnostic accuracy in breast cancer, obviates unneces-

A. Melsaether, M.D. (✉) • R. Raad, M.D.
L. Moy, M.D.
Department of Radiology, NYU Center for Advanced Imaging and Innovation, NYU School of Medicine, New York, NY, USA
e-mail: amy.melsaether@nyumc.org; roy.raad@nyumc.org; linda.moy@nyumc.org

T. Helbich, M.D.
Division of Molecular and Gender Imaging, Department of Biomedical Imaging and Image-guided Therapy, Medical University of Vienna, Vienna, Austria
e-mail: thomas.helbich@meduniwien.ac.at

K. Pinker, M.D., Ph.D., E.B.B.I.
Division of Molecular and Gender Imaging, Department of Biomedical Imaging and Image-guided Therapy, Medical University of Vienna, Vienna, Austria

Department of Radiology, Memorial Sloan Kettering Cancer Center, New York, NY, USA
e-mail: pinkerdk@mskcc.org; katja.pinker-domenig@meduniwien.ac.at

© Springer International Publishing AG 2018
L. Umutlu, K. Herrmann (eds.), *PET/MR Imaging: Current and Emerging Applications*, https://doi.org/10.1007/978-3-319-69641-6_6

sary breast biopsies, and enables an improved assessment and prediction of response to neoadjuvant therapy (Rahbar et al. 2011; Minarikova et al. 2017; Pinker et al. 2013, 2014a, b, 2016; Spick et al. 2014; Rahbar and Partridge 2016; Schmitz et al. 2015; Baltzer et al. 2016; Ei Khouli et al. 2010; Yabuuchi et al. 2008, 2010).

PET is a well-established diagnostic nuclear medicine imaging method that enables the assessment of physiological processes using different radiotracers. However, PET alone provides limited anatomical information and has a low spatial resolution, which results in difficulties in lesion localization and the assessment of potential tumor infiltration into adjacent organs. Therefore, PET is commonly performed in conjunction with other imaging modalities such computed tomography (CT). The most commonly used radiotracer in oncology is [^{18}F]Fluorodeoxyglucose ([^{18}F]FDG). [^{18}F]FDG PET allows the interrogation of another cancer hallmark- reprogramming of energy metabolism- by the assessment of tissue glycolysis, which is typically increased in cancer. In breast imaging [^{18}F]FDG PET/CT has emerged as a valuable tool and is indicated in the local, regional, and axillary staging of locally advanced metastatic or recurrent breast cancer and in the response evaluation of locally advanced and metastatic breast cancer to treatment (Koolen et al. 2012; Moy et al. 2007a; Yutani et al. 1999; Avril and Adler 2007). However, [^{18}F]FDG PET/CT is limited in the detection of small lesions and low grade cancers with sensitivities ranging from 80–87% and specificities ranging from 73–100%, which is inferior to MRI. It is therefore currently not recommended as the method of choice for local staging of known or suspected primary breast malignancies when MRI is available (Samson et al. 2002; Fletcher et al. 2008).

In efforts to combine the advantages of MRI and PET, the concept of PET/MRI has been explored. Several clinical studies evaluated the potential of fused [^{18}F]FDG PET and DCE-MRI for breast cancer diagnosis (Moy et al. 2007a, b, Moy et al. 2010; Garcia-Velloso et al. 2017; Domingues et al. 2009). Moy et al. compared prone [^{18}F]FDG PET and fused [^{18}F]FDG PET/MRI. The authors demonstrated that prone [^{18}F]

FDG PET scans were suitable for fusion with DCE-MRI of the breast and increased the confidence of the readers in lesion assessment (Koolen et al. 2012; Yutani et al. 1999; Moy et al. 2007b; Bitencourt et al. 2014a). Domingues et al. investigated fused PET/MRI using [^{18}F]FDG and DCE-MRI and concluded that [^{18}F]FDG PET/MRI provides accurate morphological and functional data for an improved diagnostic accuracy in breast cancer (Domingues et al. 2009). Bitencourt et al. extended the protocol to include DWI for the assessment of breast tumors and reported that mpPET/MRI using three parameters showed good diagnostic accuracy for breast cancer diagnosis (Bitencourt et al. 2014b). To fully exploit the potential of mpPET/MRI, Pinker et al. used a protocol including multiple functional MRI parameters, i.e. DCE-MRI, DWI, ^{1}H-MRSI, and [^{18}F]FDG for the assessment of breast tumors (Pinker et al. 2014b). Mp [^{18}F]FDG PET/MRI provided an improved differentiation of benign and malignant breast tumors when several MRI and PET parameters were combined without missing any cancers (Figs. 6.1 and 6.2). In addition, the authors concluded that [^{18}F]FDG PET/MRI may lead to an up to 50% reduction of unnecessary breast biopsies.

Most recently integrated PET/MRI systems have been developed and introduced into clinical routine. These PET/MRI scanners allow the simultaneous assessment of the multiple hallmark processes in cancer development and progression at multiple levels and therefore can provide a plethora of morphologic, functional, metabolic, and molecular information on breast tumors. To date hybrid PET/MRI data in breast imaging is still scarce. However, initial results for different indications are promising and encourage further research.

6.1.1 Differentiation of Benign and Malignant Breast Tumors

In an initial study Pace et al. compared whole-body [^{18}F]FDG PET/MRI to [^{18}F]FDG PET/CT of the breast and demonstrated that integrated whole-body PET/MRI is feasible in a clinical setting

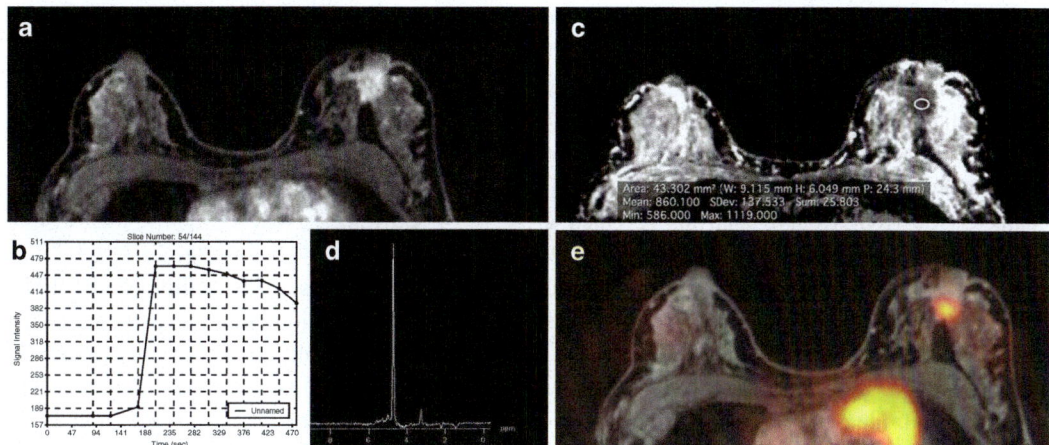

Fig. 6.1 Invasive ductal carcinoma grade 3 (IDC) in the left breast in a 55-year-old woman. The irregular shaped and spiculated mass lesion demonstrates (**a**) initial strong enhancement heterogenous enhancement followed by a wash-out (**b**). DWI shows a restricted diffusivity with low apparent diffusion coefficient (ADC) values (0.86×10^{-3} mm^2/s) (**c**). On proton magnetic resonance spectroscopic imaging, there was a choline peak at 3.2 ppm (dashed arrow) (**d**). The lesion is highly [^{18}F]FDG-avid with an SUVmax of 5.35 further hinting at malignancy (**e**). Multiparametric PET/MRI accurately classified the lesion as BI-RADS 5 (highly suggestive of malignancy)

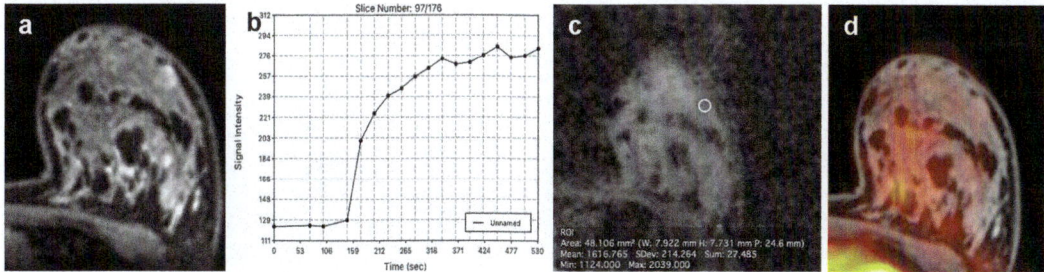

Fig. 6.2 Fibroadenoma in a 39-year-old woman, laterally in the left breast. The slightly irregularly shaped and marginated mass (**a**) demonstrated a heterogeneous medium/persistent contrast enhancement (**b**) and was classified as BI-RADS 4 in DCE-MRI. On diffusion-weighted imaging (DWI), the ADC values (1.616×10^{-3} mm^2/s) (**f**) were well above the threshold for malignancy (**c**) and the lesion is not ^{18}[F]FDG avid (**d**) thus allowing an accurate classification as a benign finding (BI-RADS 3- probably benign) with mp [^{18}F]FDG PET/MRI

with high quality and in a short examination time (Pace et al. 2014). Botsikas investigated sequential [^{18}F]FDG PET/MRI for the detection and primary staging of breast cancer (Botsikas et al. 2016). In a sequential PET/ MRI system, the MRI and the PET are located in the same room at a certain distance and share a common rotating table. The patient is first scanned on one device (MRI), after which the table rotates and the patient is scanned on the second device (PET). This approach also allows PET/MRI the acquisition of automatically co-registered sequentially acquired PET and MR images. In this study the authors reported areas under the curve (AUC) for breast cancer detection of 0.9558, 0.8347 and 0.8855 with MRI, qualitative and quantitative [^{18}F]FDG PET/MRI, respectively ($p = 0.066$). The specificity for MRI and [^{18}F]FDG PET/MRI for primary cancers was 67 and 100% ($p = 0.03$) and for lymph nodes 98% and 100% ($p = 0.25$). The authors conclude that in breast cancer patients, MRI alone has the highest diagnostic accuracy for primary tumors, yet for the assessment of nodal metastases both MRI and [^{18}F]FDG PET/MRI are highly specific.

Jena et al. focused on the reliability of pharmacokinetic DCE-MRI parameters (Ktrans, Kep, ve) derived as part of a routine high resolution breast MRI protocol when using a simultaneous [^{18}F]FDG PET/MRI system for the differentiation of benign and malignant lesions. The results suggest that a reliable measurement of pharmacokinetic parameters with reduced acquisition time is feasible. In this study receiver operating characteristic (ROC) curve analysis revealed a cut off value for Ktrans, Kep, ve as 0.50, 2.59, 0.15 respectively, which reliably distinguished benign and malignant breast lesions. There was an overall diagnostic accuracy of 94.50%, 79.82% and 87.16% for Ktrans, Kep, ve respectively. The introduction of native T1 normalization with an externally placed phantom enabled a

higher accuracy than without native T1 normalization (93.50% vs. 94.50%) with an increase in specificity of 87% vs. 84% (Jena et al. 2017).

6.1.2 Primary Staging of Breast Cancer

Tanjea et al. assessed the utility of [^{18}F]FDG PET/MRI in the initial staging of breast carcinoma (Taneja et al. 2014). In this study 36 patients with breast cancer underwent dedicated breast primary and nodal as well as whole body staging (Fig. 6.3). The study showed a sensitivity

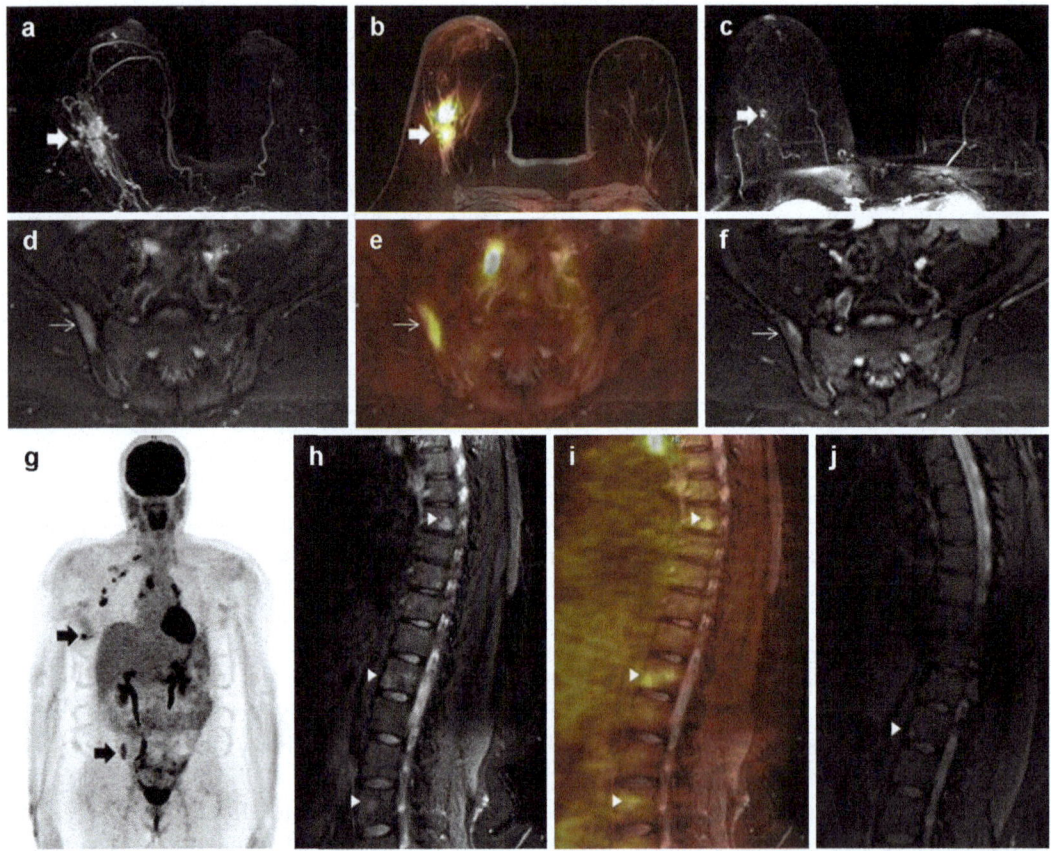

Fig. 6.3 Invasive ductal cancer in the right breast (thick arrows). 1 min subtraction MIP image (**a**) [^{18}F]FDG PET/MRI fused axial (**b**) show a metabolically active mass with satellite lesions. STIR axial (**d**) and [^{18}F]FDG PET/MRI fused axial (**e**) showing [^{18}F]FDG avid marrow lesion in the right iliac bone (thin arrows in (**d**) and (**e**)). [^{18}F]FDG PET/MRI MIP image (**g**) shows multiple focal hypermetabolic areas (thick arrows). STIR sagittal (**h**) and [^{18}F]FDG PET/MRI fused sagittal (**i**) show multiple mildly [^{18}F]FDG avid marrow lesions in vertebrae (arrow heads). 1 min subtraction MIP image (**c**) STIR axial (**f**) and STIR sagittal (**j**) show marked regression of primary breast as well as osseous lesions after chemotherapy. *Reprinted with permission from:* Taneja S, Jena A, Goel R, Sarin R, Kaul S. Simultaneous whole-body ^{18}F-FDG PET-MRI in primary staging of breast cancer: a pilot study. Eur J Radiol. 2014;83(12):2231–9

of 60% and 93.3% for PET and MRI. In the detection of axillary lymph nodes metastases there was a specificity of 91% for both and a false-negative rate of 6.7% on MRI and 40% on [^{18}F]FDG PET. [^{18}F]FDG PET/MRI increased diagnostic confidence for nodal involvement. Distant metastases were found in 22% of patients at the time of diagnosis. Overall [^{18}F]FDG PET/MRI led to a change in management in 12 (33.3%) patients. The authors conclude that in this pilot study simultaneous [^{18}F]FDG PET/MRI has been useful in whole-body initial staging of breast cancer patients. Eun-Jung Kong et al. investigated the application of combined whole-body and dedicated [^{18}F]FDG PET/MRI of the breast in 42 breast cancer patients (Kong et al. 2014). They authors conclude that such a "one-stop-shopping" examination is feasible and facilitates the benefits of combining high-resolution local breast and whole-body staging with metabolic images. They found that [^{18}F]FDG breast PET/MRI utilizing a dedicated coil is still necessary to enable an accurate diagnosis and staging of invasive carcinomas that are less than 1 cm in size.

6.1.3   Assessment of Tumor Aggressiveness

Margolis et al. investigated the feasibility of dedicated [^{18}F]FDG PET/MRI of the breast to assess the synergy of MR pharmacokinetic and [^{18}F] FDG uptake data to determine tumor aggressiveness in terms of metastatic burden and Ki67 status (Fig. 6.4) (Margolis et al. 2016). In this study patients with systemic metastases showed significantly lower kep values compared to patients with local disease (0.45 vs. 0.99 min^{-1}, $p = 0.011$). Metastatic burden was positively correlated with Ktrans and standardized uptake values (SUV), and negatively with kep. Ki67 positive tumors showed a significantly greater Ktrans compared to Ki67 negative tumors (0.29 vs. 0.45 min^{-1}, $p = 0.03$). These preliminary data suggest that MRI pharmacokinetic and [^{18}F]FDG PET parameters may aid in the assessment of tumor aggressiveness and metastatic potential.

6.1.4   Therapy Monitoring

In a case-report study of four patients with locally advanced breast cancer, Romeo et al. evaluated the response to neoadjuvant cytotoxic and endocrine therapy with mp [^{18}F]FDG PET/MRI using DCE-MRI with pharmacokinetic modelling, DWI and maximum standard up-take values (SUVmax) (Romeo et al. 2017) (Fig. 6.5). Therapy monitoring in both types of neoadjuvant treatment with mp [^{18}F]FDG PET/MRI was successfully performed and the authors conclude another potential application for [^{18}F]FDG PET/MRI in breast cancer care might be the concurrent evaluation of breast tumor extension, nodal involvement, for the detection of distant metastasis, and for treatment monitoring.

6.1.5   Breast Cancer Recurrence

Grueneisen et al. investigated whole-body mp [^{18}F]FDG PET/MRI for the detection of local, regional and distant recurrences of breast cancer (Grueneisen et al. 2017). mpPET/MRI readings showed a significantly higher accuracy and higher confidence levels for the detection of recurrent breast cancer lesions when compared to MRI alone ($p < 0.05$). Although for the detection of local recurrences dedicated mpMRI of the breast is most likely sufficient, combined whole body and dedicated [^{18}F]FDG PET/MRI of the breast has an inherent benefit of simultaneous accurate regional and distant staging.

6.1.6   Future Developments and Potential Applications: Specific Radiotracers

PET/MRI of the breast is currently mainly performed using the radiotracer [^{18}F]FDG. [^{18}F]FDG is a very sensitive, yet not very specific radiotracer and there is a significant overlap in the uptake behavior of benign and malignant lesions. To overcome these limitations, more specific radiotracers to target hallmark processes involved in cancer development and progression are continuously being

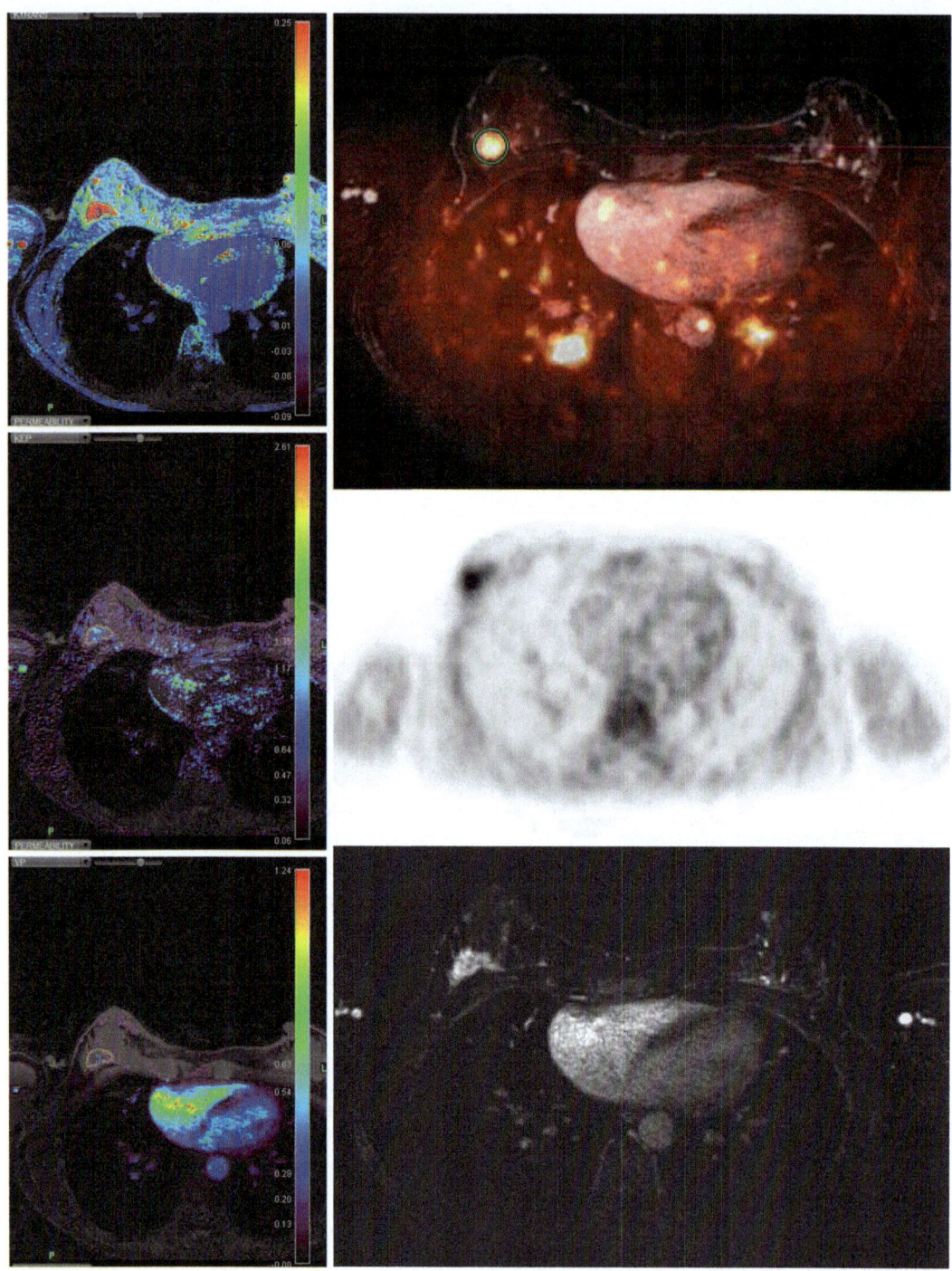

Fig. 6.4 39 year old female with ER, PR, and HER2 positive right breast cancer. Left top to bottom: MR PET Fusion, PET, and MR axial radial VIBE images. Right top to bottom: Ktrans, KEP, and VP color maps. Regions of interest have been drawn over the enhancing area of the tumor as depicted by the radial VIBE sequence *Reprinted with permission from*: Margolis NE, Moy L, Sigmund EE et al. Assessment of aggressiveness of breast cancer using simultaneous 18F-FDG-PET and DCE-MRI: preliminary observation. Clin Nucl Med. 2016;41(8):e355–61

developed such as ^{18}F-fluorodeoxythymidine ([^{18}F] FLT) and ^{18}F-deoxyfluoroarabinofuranosylthymine ([^{18}F]FMAU) for DNA synthesis and cell proliferation; [^{18}F-fluoromisonidazole ([^{18}F]FMISO) for the assessment of tumor hypoxia, or ^{18}F-fluoroestradiol ([^{18}F]FES) or ^{18}F-fluorodihydrotestosterone ([^{18}F] FDHT) for the assessment of receptor status and are also being investigated for breast imaging:

Although these specific radiotracers currently play a greater role in whole body staging and ther-

apy monitoring of advanced breast cancer, their application has also been investigated for primary breast lesions. A promising application seems to be the assessment of tumor hypoxia as one of the most pervasive tumor microenvironmental factors and a feature of most solid tumors (Grueneisen et al. 2017). Conclusive research has shown that tumor hypoxia is one of the key factors in inducing the development of cell clones with an aggressive and treatment-resistant phenotype that leads

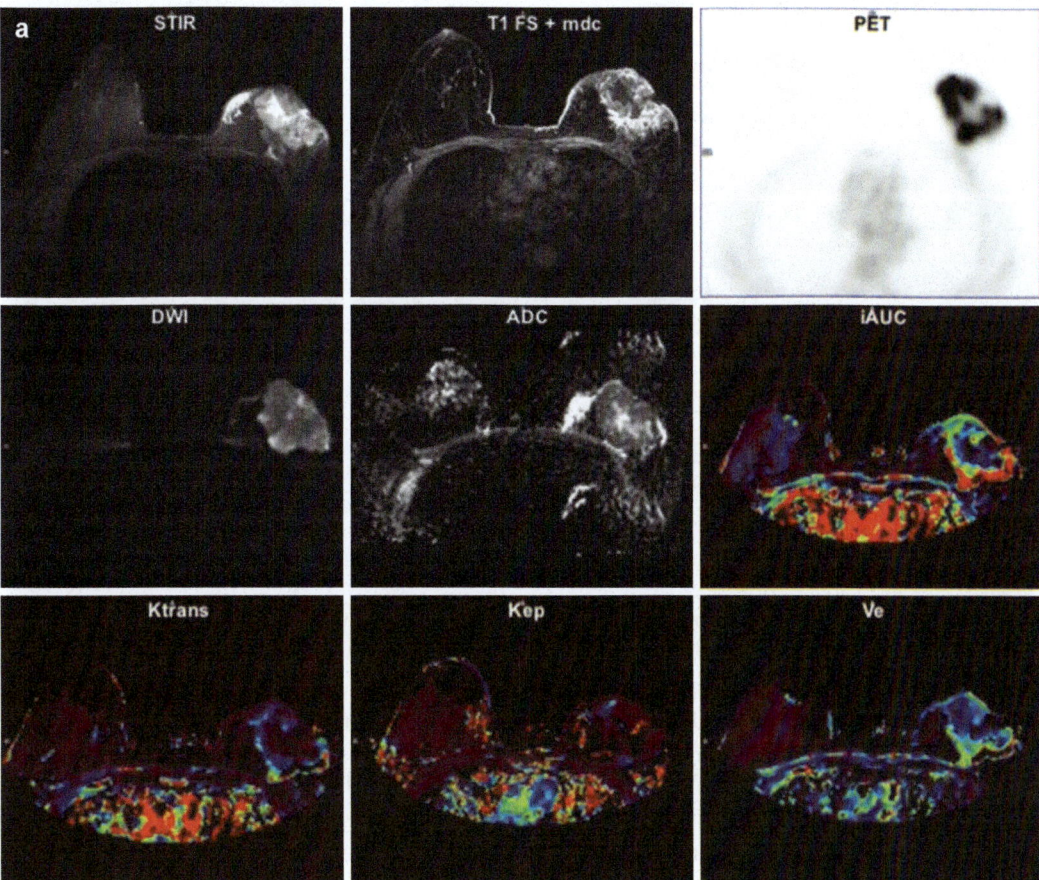

Fig. 6.5 (**a**) Invasive ductal/lobular cancer in a 54-year old female. Multiparametric evaluation of morphological (STIR and DCE), metabolic (PET) and functional (DWI, ADC, iAUC, Ktrans, kep, Ve) parameters before cytotoxic chemotherapy. A large tumoral mass with significant post-contrast enhancement, increased of [^{18}F]FDG uptake, restricted diffusivity and increased perfusion is appreciated. (**b**) Multiparametric evaluation of morphological (STIR and DCE), metabolic (PET) and functional (DWI, ADC, iAUC, Ktrans, kep, Ve) parameters after the second cycle of cytotoxic chemotherapy. A significant reduction of tumor volume, [^{18}F]FDG, perfusion and an increased diffusivity are now detected compared to the pre-treatment evaluation. *Reprinted with permission from:* Romeo V, D'Aiuto M, Frasci G, Imbriaco M, Nicolai E. Simultaneous PET/MRI assessment of response to cytotoxic and hormone neo-adjuvant chemotherapy in breast cancer: a preliminary report. Med Oncol. 2017;34(2):18

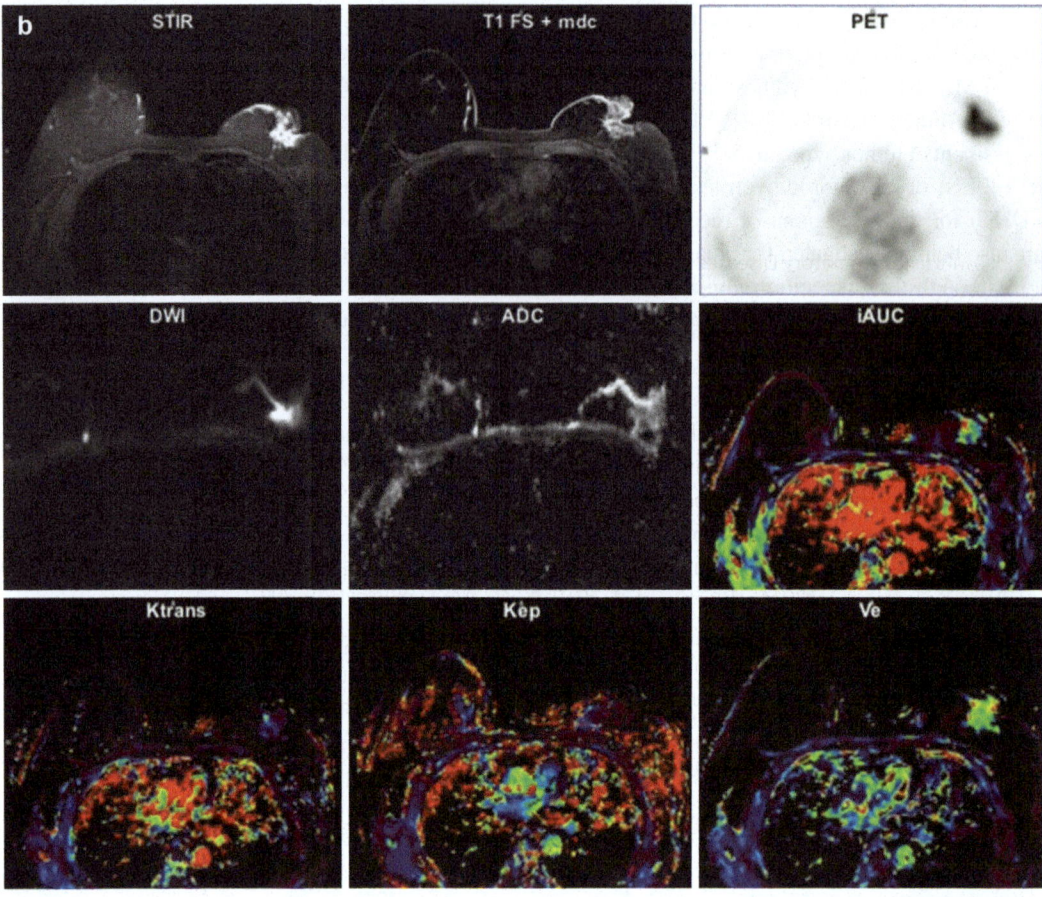

Fig. 6.5 (continued)

to rapid progression and a poor prognosis (Ruan et al. 2009; Vaupel 2008; Hockel et al. 1996a, b; Hockel and Vaupel 2001a, b; Okunieff et al. 2003; Tatum et al. 2006; Vaupel et al. 2002). The radiotracer [18F]FMISO has a high affinity to hypoxic cells with active nitroreductase enzymes and accumulates in activated tumor cells, but not necrotic cells. Cheng et al. investigated whether [18F]FMISO PET/CT can predict primary resistance to endocrine therapy in estrogen-receptor-positive breast cancer, and found a significantly positive correlation between baseline [18F]FMISO uptake and clinical outcomes after ≥3 months of primary endocrine therapy with letrozole. These preliminary results indicate that [18F]FMISO PET/CT may be an effective method for early monitoring of response to neo-endocrine therapy (Cheng et al. 2013). In a recent feasibility study,

Pinker et al. investigated fused mp PET/MRI of breast tumors with DCE-MRI, DWI, [18F]FDG, and [18F]FMISO in eight patients (Fig. 6.6). MRI and PET parameters were correlated with pathological features, grading, proliferation-rate (ki67), immuno-histochemistry, and the clinical endpoints: metastasis and death (Pinker et al. 2015). There were several moderate-to-excellent correlations between quantitative imaging markers, grading, receptor status, and proliferation rate. DCE-MRI, [18F]FDG-, and [18F]FMISO-avidity strongly correlated with the presence of metastases [$r = 0.75$ ($p < 0.01$), 0.63 ($p = 0.212$), and 0.58 ($p = 0.093$)], and patients' death [$r = 0.60$ ($p = 0.09$), 0.62 ($p = 0.08$), 0.56 ($p = 0.11$)]. These initial data suggest that mp[18F]FDG /[18F]FMISO PET/MRI might be able to provide quantitative prognostic information in breast cancer patients.

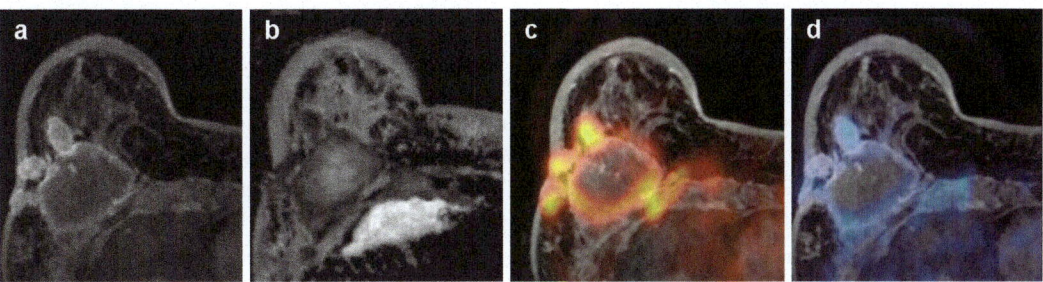

Fig. 6.6 Invasive ductal carcinoma triple-negative grade 3 (IDC) with ki-67 90% in the right breast in a 70-year-old woman. The irregular shaped and marginated mass lesion demonstrates (**a**) a strong enhancement rim with central necrosis and several satellite nodules in the immediate vicinity. DWI shows a restricted diffusivity with low apparent diffusion coefficient (ADC) values (0.665×10^{-3} mm²/s) (**b**). The enhancing part of the lesion and especially the satellites are highly [^{18}F]FDG-avid indicating increased tissue glycolysis (**c**) and ^{18}[F]MISO-avid indicating tumor hypoxia as a prognostic bad indicator (**d**)

In summary, mpPET/MRI of the breast with different functional MRI parameters visualizes and quantifies processes of cancer development and progression at multiple levels, and provides specific information about the hallmarks of cancer. Initial results indicate that mp[^{18}F]FDG-, PET/MRI of the breast can improve diagnostic accuracy in breast cancer and obviate unnecessary breast biopsies. It can be expected that in the future the role of PET/MRI will further increase through application of specific radiotracers and that it might play a major role as part of precision medicine in breast cancer.

6.2 Molecular Breast Imaging Tools BSGI and PEM

Two molecular breast imaging tools—breast-specific gamma imaging (BSGI)/molecular breast imaging (MBI) and positron emission mammography (PEM) have been introduced recently. Both exams use dedicated breast-specific gamma technology to detect increased blood flow to cancerous cells in the breasts. While BSGI/MBI is based on the assessment of Tc-99 m sestamibi uptake, PEM uses F18-fluorodeoxyglucose (FDG). The benefit of both exams is that they have a higher spatial resolution than PET/CT and may detect small breast tumors that are below the resolution of conventional PET equipment. A drawback is that these imaging studies do not evaluate anatomy. Hence, they differ from conventional breast imaging studies such as mammography, ultrasound and MRI, where the anatomy is clearly depicted. Another limitation is that both tests only facilitate local staging of the breast and axilla and do not enable assessment of distant metastases.

One of the commercially available BSGI systems, the Dilon 6800 system (Dilon Technologies, Newport News, Va), uses a single 15 × 20-cm detector plate composed of an array of 3 × 3-mm sodium iodide crystals. Similar to mammography, the breast is compressed between the detector plate and a compression paddle. The images obtained are in projections similar to conventional mammographic views. PEM uses a pair of dedicated gamma radiation detectors placed above and below the breast and mild breast compression to detect coincident gamma rays after administration of 18F-FDG.

Small single center studies have compared BSGI to mammography in asymptomatic high risk women with dense breasts in the screening setting. They found that BSGI detects mammographically occult breast cancers and is unaffected by dense breast tissue, a major drawback of conventional mammography (Brem et al. 2002, 2005, 2008; Rechtman et al. 2014). Rhodes et al. demonstrated that BSGI had a breast cancer detection rate three times that of mammography (9.6 per 1000 vs. 3.2 per 1000) when a dose of 740 MBq (20 mCi) of 99mTc-sestamibi was injected (Rhodes et al. 2011). However, there are concerns about the radiation risk from BSGI as a screening tool (Hendrick and Tredennick 2016). In 2015, Rhodes published a follow up study where a lower dose of 300 MBq (8 mCi) was used. The results revealed a higher cancer detection rate of BSGI (10.7 per 1000) compared to mammography alone (3.2 per 1000) despite using a lower dose (Rhodes et al. 2015). The cancer detection rate for mammography combined with BSGI was 12.0 per 1000 (Rhodes et al. 2015). Additional studies are necessary to determine if the reduced-dose BSGI may be an appropriate supplemental breast cancer screening tool in women with dense breasts given the radiation risk (Hendrick and Tredennick 2016). Comparable to BSGI systems, PEM is also commercially available. However, the clinical utility of PEM has yet to be demonstrated, restricting its successful establishment into clinical imaging.

6.3   Whole Body PET/MRI in Breast Cancer

PET/MRI is particularly exciting in the context of whole body imaging for breast cancer patients, facilitating a single, thorough exam with high sensitivity in typical sites of metastasis. At present, there is no uniform recommendation for body imaging in newly diagnosed breast cancer patients. If performed, body imaging is non-standardized and may consist of a PET/CT or of a mix of radionuclide bone scan, chest radiograph, abdominal and pelvic CT, and brain MRI, depending on a patient's symptoms. Notably, in patients with breast cancers 2 cm or greater, whole body imaging has been shown to detect clinically occult distant metastases in approximately 6–10% of patients (Bernsdorf et al. 2012; Groheux et al. 2008) and clinically occult non-axillary nodal metastases in up to 22% of patients (Taneja et al. 2014; Groheux et al. 2008). Detection of early, still isolated organ metastases, especially in the brain and liver, is important because local treatment of early metastatic disease has been shown to improve local control and thereby, quality and length of life (Selzner et al. 2000; Mack et al. 2004; Patchell et al. 1990; De Ieso et al. 2015).

Shortcomings that hinder broader implementation of whole body imaging at the time of diagnosis likely include a lack of uniform recommendations and, in case of PET/CT, a relatively high radiation dose of up to approximately 32 mSv. The Lifetime Attributable Risk (LAR) of radiation induced breast cancer due to a single 18FDG-PET/CT has been estimated at up to 0.25%, or 2.5/1000 patients in 30–60 year old women (Huang et al. 2009; Brix et al. 2005). Moreover, PET scans can show high physiologic uptake of FDG in the brain and liver that may obscure underlying lesions (Moon et al. 1998; Gallowitsch et al. 2003).

PET/MRI is a whole body examination that requires significantly less radiation PET/CT (Melsaether et al. 2016) and provides high sensitivity in lymph nodes, bone, liver, and brain via its novel ability to acquire MR data concurrently with metabolic PET data. Early studies specifically in breast cancer patients typically compare PET/MRI with PET/CT and are encouraging, suggesting that replacing CT with MRI does provide some gains in the search for metastatic disease. In general, small studies consistently show that PET/MR detects the same or a few more systemic metastases than PET/CT or PET alone (Pace et al. 2014; Taneja et al. 2014). In assessing bone metastases, Catalano et al. (2015), showed that PET/MRI found not only more osseous metastases, but also more osseous metastases in more patients as compared with PET/CT. One concern is that PET/MRI may miss lung metastases. Raad et al. demonstrated that while PET/MRI did miss small lung nodules in oncologic patients, 97% of the missed nodules were stable at follow-up, suggesting that the missed nodules may be clinically unimportant (Raad et al. 2016). Melsaether et al. found that PET/MRI detected liver, lymph node, bone, and brain metastases not seen on PET/CT. While some of these differences in detection were significant at the lesion level, none reached significance at the patient level, likely because larger patient cohorts would be needed (Melsaether et al. 2016). Finally, Grueneisen et al. looked at PET/MR another way and, rather than comparing PET/MR to PET/CT, showed that adding PET to whole body MR increases sensitivity and overall accuracy in breast cancer patients (Grueneisen et al. 2017). In that same vein, Heusner et al. demonstrated that adding PET to DWI greatly improves the specificity of DWI in whole body imaging (Heusner et al. 2010).

One of the strengths of PET/MRI is that it is highly customizable. The acquired MR sequences can be varied and adapted accordingly to the request of each of the 6–7 bed positions involving the thighs to the vertex that comprise a PET/MR examination. For example, one could run a T2 weighted post-contrast fluid attenuated inversion recovery (FLAIR) sequence during the brain station to look for leptomeningeal disease and diffusion weighted imaging (DWI) during the liver station in the interest of characterizing liver lesions. Research as to which sequences are the most useful overall and at each station is ongoing. Grueneisen et al. found similar sensitivities for PET combined with MR half-fourier acquisition single-shot turbo spin-echo (HASTE) and DWI, PET combined with MR HASTE and T1-post contrast imaging, and PET combined with MR HASTE, DWI, and T1-post contrast imaging (Grueneisen et al. 2017). They noted that reader confidence was significantly higher when a T1-post contrast sequence was included, as would be expected because of the superior anatomic imaging this sequence provides. Melsaether et al. looked at individual organ systems and found that the post-contrast T1-weighted sequence detected more breast, lung, pleural, and brain metastases (Figs. 6.7 and 6.8) than DWI

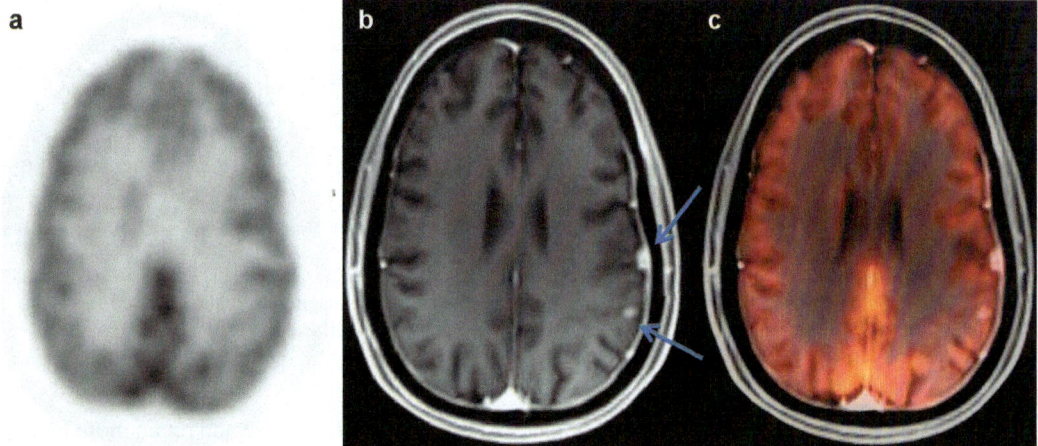

Fig. 6.7 37 year-old female with right breast cancer. An axial PET image (**a**) shows no evidence of metastases while T1 post-contrast (**b**) and fusion (**c**) images demonstrate two adjacent enhancing lesions in the left parietal lobe (arrows), consistent with leptomeningeal metastases

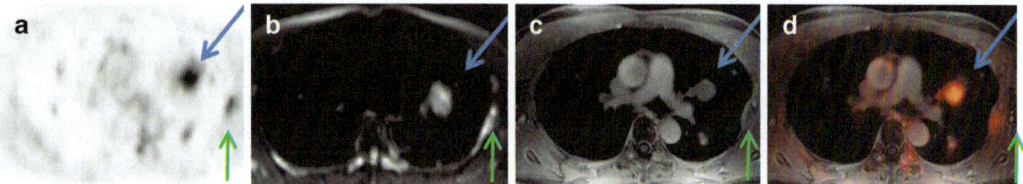

Fig. 6.8 48 year-old female with history of metastatic breast cancer. Axial PET (**a**) , DWI (**b**), T1 post-contrast (**c**), and fusion (**d**) images demonstrate a hypermetabolic 2.5-cm enhancing nodule in the left upper lobe (blue arrow) with restricted diffusion (ADC map not shown), consistent with a lung metastasis. Note the presence of additional lung metastases are best seen on the T1-post-contrast image (**c**), while a hypermetabolic osseous metastasis in a left rib (green arrow), is most conspicuous on the DWI image (**b**)

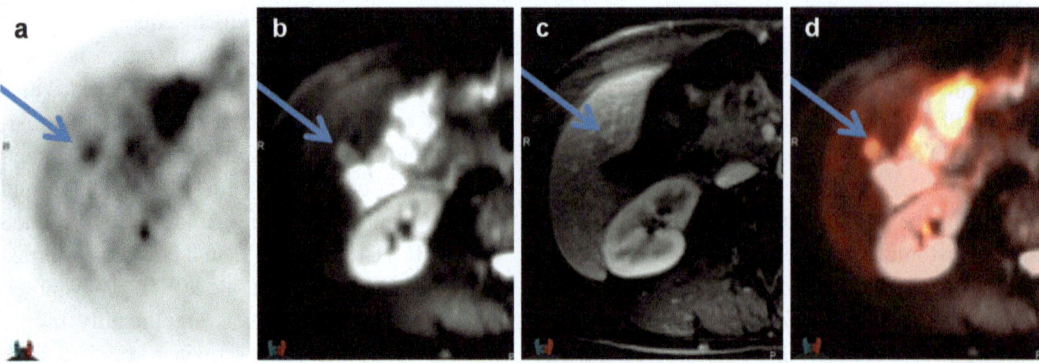

Fig. 6.9 48 year-old female with history of metastatic breast cancer. Axial PET (**a**) and DWI (**b**) images demonstrate a hypermetabolic lesion (**a**) with restricted diffusion (**b**) (ADC map not pictured) in hepatic segment VI (arrow), consistent with a liver metastasis. The lesion is barely visualized on the T1 post-contrast image (**c**), but can be seen on fused images due to increased FDG uptake (**d**)

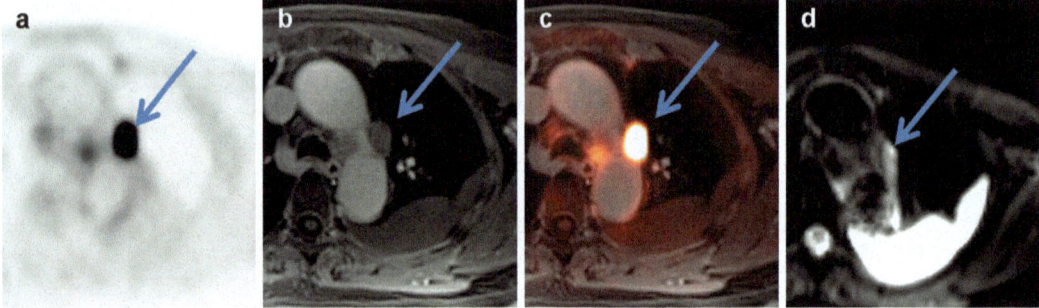

Fig. 6.10 76 year-old female with history of metastatic breast cancer. Axial PET (**a**) , DWI (**b**), Tq post-contrast (**c**) , and fusion (**d**) images demonstrate a hypermetabolic lymph node metastasis in the AP window of the mediastinum (arrow), which is more conspicuous on DWI than on post-contrast T1 imaging. Note the presence of a layering small left pleural effusion

while DWI detected more liver, bone, and nodal lesions than post-contrast T1-weighted imaging (Melsaether et al. 2016) (Figs. 6.9 and 6.10). While the capacity to customize individual stations within a PET/MR examination has not yet been fully explored in the literature, we look forward to what might be on the horizon. Ongoing work will hopefully be able to cut exam time and to improve diagnostic accuracy by finding the most efficient sequences for each station.

In addition to customizing MR sequences, radiotracers beyond ^{18}F-FDG can be administered, either alone or together with ^{18}F-FDG. In breast cancer, ^{18}F-FDG is effective at demonstrating both primary lesions and metastases in any organ because breast cancer cells are typically more metabolically active than surrounding tissue, and, as such, take up and retain more labeled glucose, allowing for lesion detection (Lim et al. 2007). There is some debate as to whether the bone specific radiotracer ^{18}F sodium fluoride (Na-F) outperforms ^{18}F-FDG for detecting osseous metastases, the most common metastases in breast cancer patients. While ^{18}F-NaF imaging finds more osseous lesions, (Piccardo et al. 2015), it is questionable whether lesions seen by ^{18}F-NaF but not by ^{18}F-FDG provide an accurate picture of the disease burden. Specifically, Piccardo et al. (2015) found that no patients with lesions on ^{18}F-NaF, but not ^{18}F-FDG, progressed during their study period and that ^{18}F-FDG parameters, but not ^{18}F-NaF parameters were associated with overall survival. These findings may reflect that ^{18}F-FDG more closely tracks biologically active breast cancer than does ^{18}F-NaF, whose uptake is tied to osseous blood flow and bony remodeling (Czernin et al. 2010) rather than directly to breast cancer cells.

The next step for functional PET imaging may be to accurately image the characteristics of breast cancer metastases. Primary breast cancers are not uniform throughout. They are heterogeneous, dynamic, and characterized by genomic instability (Marino et al. 2013). In the same way, metastases differ from their index lesion, from one another, and even from themselves over time, especially in response to treatments. Imaging with radio-ligands targeted to molecules that influence therapy would provide a way to non-invasively assess appropriateness of certain therapeutic agents and to reassess when treatment response appears to stall.

Breast cancer biopsy and surgical specimens are commonly assessed histologically for estrogen and progesterone receptors and for human epidermal growth factor receptor 2 (HER2) because these receptors determine whether certain treatments can be effective. Tracers targeting steroid receptors are under development and include the estrogen analog 16a-[18]F-17B-estradiol (Katzenellenbogen 1995), as well as fluorine labeled progesterone receptor ligands (Gemignani et al. 2013). Zirconium labeled human epidermal growth factor receptor 2 (HER2) receptor tracers including 89Zr-trastuzumab have also been developed (Dijkers et al. 2010; Ulaner et al. 2016). Recently, Ulaner et al. showed that 89Zr-trastuzumab PET can detect HER2 positive metastases in patients with HER2 negative primary breast cancers (Ulaner et al. 2016). This study underlines how functional imaging of metastases, which typically are not biopsied, can provide additional information and potentiate personalized treatment options. Further studies may be able to establish standardized SUV levels that correlate to histologic levels of receptor expression and therapeutic efficacy. Future PET/MRI directions may ultimately include radiolabeled therapies coupled with dynamic PET imaging, which could enable the physician to see in real time whether therapeutic drugs are delivered to and retained within their targets.

References

Avril N, Adler LP. F-18 fluorodeoxyglucose-positron emission tomography imaging for primary breast cancer and loco-regional staging. Radiol Clin N Am. 2007;45(4):645–57. vi

Baltzer PA, Dietzel M, Kaiser WA. MR-spectroscopy at 1.5 tesla and 3 tesla. Useful? A systematic review and meta-analysis. Eur J Radiol. 2012;81(Suppl 1):S6–9.

Baltzer A, Dietzel M, Kaiser CG, Baltzer PA. Combined reading of contrast enhanced and diffusion weighted magnetic resonance imaging by using a simple sum score. Eur Radiol. 2016;26(3):884–91.

Bernsdorf M, Berthelsen AK, Wielenga VT, et al. Preoperative PET/CT in early-stage breast cancer. Ann Oncol. 2012;23(9):2277–82.

Bitencourt AG, Lima EN, Chojniak R, et al. Can 18F-FDG PET improve the evaluation of suspicious breast lesions on MRI? Eur J Radiol. 2014a;83(8):1381–6.

Bitencourt AG, Lima EN, Chojniak R, et al. Multiparametric evaluation of breast lesions using PET-MRI: initial results and future perspectives. Medicine (Baltimore). 2014b;93(22):e115.

Bogner W, Gruber S, Pinker K, et al. Diffusion-weighted MR for differentiation of breast lesions at 3.0 T: how does selection of diffusion protocols affect diagnosis? Radiology. 2009;253(2):341–51.

Bogner W, Pinker-Domenig K, Bickel H, et al. Readout-segmented echo-planar imaging improves the diagnostic performance of diffusion-weighted MR breast examinations at 3.0 T. Radiology. 2012;263(1):64–76.

Botsikas D, Kalovidouri A, Becker M, et al. Clinical utility of 18F-FDG-PET/MR for preoperative breast cancer staging. Eur Radiol. 2016;26(7):2297–307.

Brem RF, Schoonjans JM, Kieper DA, Majewski S, Goodman S, Civelek C. High-resolution scintimammography: a pilot study. J Nucl Med. 2002;43(7):909–15.

Brem RF, Rapelyea JA, Zisman G, et al. Occult breast cancer: scintimammography with high-resolution breast-specific gamma camera in women at high risk for breast cancer. Radiology. 2005;237(1):274–80.

Brem RF, Floerke AC, Rapelyea JA, Teal C, Kelly T, Mathur V. Breast-specific gamma imaging as an adjunct imaging modality for the diagnosis of breast cancer. Radiology. 2008;247(3):651–7.

Brix G, Lechel U, Glatting G, et al. Radiation exposure of patients undergoing whole-body dual-modality 18F-FDG PET/CT examinations. J Nucl Med. 2005;46(4):608–13.

Catalano OA, Nicolai E, Rosen BR, et al. Comparison of CE-FDG-PET/CT with CE-FDG-PET/MR in the evaluation of osseous metastases in breast cancer patients. Br J Cancer. 2015;112:1452–60.

Cheng J, Lei L, Xu J, et al. 18F-fluoromisonidazole PET/CT: a potential tool for predicting primary endocrine therapy resistance in breast cancer. J Nucl Med. 2013;54(3):333–40.

Czernin J, Satyamurthy N, Schiepers C. Molecular mechanisms of bone 18F-NaF deposition. J Nucl Med. 2010;51:1826–9.

D'Orsi CJ, Sickles EA, Mendelson EB, et al. ACR BI-RADS® Atlas, Breast Imaging Reporting and Data System. 5th ed. Reston, VA: American College of Radiology; 2013.

De Ieso PB, Schick U, Rosenfelder N, Mohammed K, Ross GM. Breast cancer brain metastases: a 12 year review of treatment outcomes. Breast. 2015;24(4):426–33.

Dijkers EC, Oude Munnink TH, Kosterink JG, et al. Biodistribution of 89Zr-trastuzumab and PET imaging of HER2-positive lesions in patients with metastatic breast cancer. Clin Pharmacol Ther. 2010;87:586–92.

Domingues RC, Carneiro MP, Lopes FC, da Fonseca LM, Gasparetto EL. Whole-body MRI and FDG PET fused images for evaluation of patients with cancer. AJR Am J Roentgenol. 2009;192(4):1012–20.

Dorrius MD, Dijkstra H, Oudkerk M, Sijens PE. Effect of b value and pre-admission of contrast on diagnostic accuracy of 1.5-T breast DWI: a systematic review and meta-analysis. Eur Radiol. 2014;24(11):2835–47.

Ei Khouli RH, Jacobs MA, Mezban SD, et al. Diffusion-weighted imaging improves the diagnostic accuracy of conventional 3.0-T breast MR imaging. Radiology. 2010;256(1):64–73.

Fletcher JW, Djulbegovic B, Soares HP, et al. Recommendations on the use of 18F-FDG PET in oncology. J Nucl Med. 2008;49(3):480–508.

Gallowitsch HJ, Kresnik E, Gasser J, et al. F-18 fluorodeoxyglucose positron-emission tomography in the diagnosis of tumor recurrence and metastases in the follow-up of patients with breast carcinoma: a comparison to conventional imaging. Investig Radiol. 2003;38(5):250–6.

Garcia-Velloso MJ, Ribelles MJ, Rodriguez M, et al. MRI fused with prone FDG PET/CT improves the primary tumour staging of patients with breast cancer. Eur Radiol. 2017;27(8):3190–8.

Gemignani ML, Patil S, Seshan VE, et al. Feasibility and predictability of perioperative PET and estrogen receptor ligand in patients with invasive breast cancer. J Nucl Med. 2013;54:1697–702.

Groheux D, Moretti JL, Baillet G, et al. Effect of (18)F-FDG PET/CT imaging in patients with clinical Stage II and III breast cancer. Int J Radiat Oncol Biol Phys. 2008;71(3):695–704.

Gruber S, Debski BK, Pinker K, et al. Three-dimensional proton MR spectroscopic imaging at 3 T for the differentiation of benign and malignant breast lesions. Radiology. 2011;261(3):752–61.

Gruber S, Minarikova L, Pinker K, et al. Diffusion-weighted imaging of breast tumours at 3 Tesla and 7 Tesla: a comparison. Eur Radiol. 2016;26(5):1466–73.

Grueneisen J, Sawicki LM, Wetter A, et al. Evaluation of PET and MR datasets in integrated 18F-FDG PET/MRI: a comparison of different MR sequences for whole-body restaging of breast cancer patients. Eur J Radiol. 2017;89:14–9.

Hanahan D, Weinberg RA. The hallmarks of cancer. Cell. 2000;100(1):57–70.

Hanahan D, Weinberg RA. Hallmarks of cancer: the next generation. Cell. 2011;144(5):646–74.

Hendrick RE, Tredennick T. Benefit to Radiation risk of breast-specific gamma imaging compared with mammography in screening asymptomatic women with dense breasts. Radiology. 2016;281(2):583–8.

Heusner TA, Kuemmel S, Koeninger A, et al. Diagnostic value of diffusion-weighted magnetic resonance imaging (DWI) compared to FDG PET/CT for whole-body breast cancer staging. Eur J Nucl Med Mol Imaging. 2010;37:1077–86.

Hockel M, Vaupel P. Biological consequences of tumor hypoxia. Semin Oncol. 2001a;28(2 Suppl 8):36–41.

Hockel M, Vaupel P. Tumor hypoxia: definitions and current clinical, biologic, and molecular aspects. J Natl Cancer Inst. 2001b;93(4):266–76.

Hockel M, Schlenger K, Aral B, Mitze M, Schaffer U, Vaupel P. Association between tumor hypoxia and malignant progression in advanced cancer of the uterine cervix. Cancer Res. 1996a;56(19):4509–15.

Hockel M, Schlenger K, Mitze M, Schaffer U, Vaupel P. Hypoxia and radiation response in human tumors. Semin Radiat Oncol. 1996b;6(1):3–9.

Huang B, Law MW, Khong PL. Whole-body PET/CT scanning: estimation of radiation dose and cancer risk. Radiology. 2009;251(1):166–74.

Jena A, Taneja S, Singh A, Negi P, Mehta SB, Sarin R. Role of pharmacokinetic parameters derived with high temporal resolution DCE MRI using simultaneous PET/MRI system in breast cancer: a feasibility study. Eur J Radiol. 2017;86:261–6.

Katzenellenbogen JA. Designing steroid receptor-based radiotracers to image breast and prostate tumors. J Nucl Med. 1995;36:8S–13S.

Kong EJ, Chun KA, Bom HS, Lee J, Lee SJ, Cho IH. Initial experience of integrated PET/MR mammography in patients with invasive ductal carcinoma. Hell J Nucl Med. 2014;17(3):171–6.

Koolen BB, Vogel WV, Vrancken Peeters MJ, Loo CE, Rutgers EJ, Valdes Olmos RA. Molecular imaging in breast cancer: from whole-body PET/CT to dedicated breast PET. J Oncol. 2012;2012:438647.

Lim HS, Yoon W, Chung TW, Kim JK, Park JG, Kang HK, Bom HS, Yoon JH. FDG PET/CT for the detection and evaluation of breast diseases: usefulness and limitations. Radiographics. 2007;27(Suppl 1):S197–213.

Mack MG, Straub R, Eichler K, Söllner O, Lehnert T, Vogl TJ. Breast cancer metastases in liver: laser-induced interstitial thermotherapy—local tumor control rate and survival data. Radiology. 2004;233(2):400–9.

Mann RM, Balleyguier C, Baltzer PA, et al. Breast MRI: EUSOBI recommendations for women's information. Eur Radiol. 2015;25(12):3669–78.

Margolis NE, Moy L, Sigmund EE, et al. Assessment of aggressiveness of breast cancer using simultaneous 18F-FDG-PET and DCE-MRI: preliminary observation. Clin Nucl Med. 2016;41(8):e355–61.

Marino N, Woditschka S, Reed LT, Nakayama J, Mayer M, Wetzel M, Steeg PS. Breast cancer metastasis issues for the personalization of its prevention and treatment. Am J Pathol. 2013;183(4):1084–95.

Melsaether AN, Raad RA, Pujara AC, et al. Comparison of whole-body (18)F FDG PET/MR imaging and whole-body (18)F FDG PET/CT in terms of lesion detection and radiation dose in patients with breast cancer. Radiology. 2016;281(1):193–202.

Minarikova L, Bogner W, Pinker K, et al. Investigating the prediction value of multiparametric magnetic resonance imaging at 3 T in response to neoadjuvant chemotherapy in breast cancer. Eur Radiol. 2017;27(5):1901–11.

Moon DH, Maddahi J, Silverman DH, et al. Accuracy of whole-body fluorine-18-FDG PET for the detection of recurrent or metastatic breast carcinoma. J Nucl Med. 1998;39(3):431–5.

Morris EA. Diagnostic breast MR imaging: current status and future directions. Radiol Clin N Am. 2007;45(5):863–80. vii

Morrow M, Waters J, Morris E. MRI for breast cancer screening, diagnosis, and treatment. Lancet. 2011;378(9805):1804–11.

Moy L, Noz ME, Maguire GQ, et al. Prone mammoPET acquisition improves the ability to fuse MRI and PET breast scans. Clin Nucl Med. 2007a;32(3):194–8.

Moy L, Ponzo F, Noz ME, et al. Improving specificity of breast MRI using prone PET and fused MRI and PET 3D volume datasets. J Nucl Med. 2007b;48(4):528–37.

Moy L, Noz ME, Maguire GQ, et al. Role of fusion of prone FDG-PET and magnetic resonance imaging of the breasts in the evaluation of breast cancer. Breast J. 2010;16(4):369–76.

Okunieff P, Ding I, Vaupel P, Hockel M. Evidence for and against hypoxia as the primary cause of tumor aggressiveness. Adv Exp Med Biol. 2003;510:69–75.

Pace L, Nicolai E, Luongo A, et al. Comparison of whole-body PET/CT and PET/MRI in breast cancer patients: lesion detection and quantitation of 18F-deoxyglucose uptake in lesions and in normal organ tissues. Eur J Radiol. 2014;83(2):289–96.

Patchell RA, Tibbs PA, Walsh JW, et al. A randomized trial of surgery in the treatment of single metastases to the brain. N Engl J Med. 1990;322(8):494–500.

Piccardo A, Puntoni M, Morbelli S, et al. 18F-FDG PET/CT is a prognostic biomarker in patients affected by bone metastases from breast cancer in comparison with 18F-NaF PET/CT. Nuklearmedizin. 2015;54:163–72.

Pinker K, Grabner G, Bogner W, et al. A combined high temporal and high spatial resolution 3 Tesla MR imaging protocol for the assessment of breast lesions: initial results. Investig Radiol. 2009;44(9):553–8.

Pinker K, Stadlbauer A, Bogner W, Gruber S, Helbich TH. Molecular imaging of cancer: MR spectroscopy and beyond. Eur J Radiol. 2012;81(3):566–77.

Pinker K, Bickel H, Helbich T, et al. Combined contrast enhanced magnetic resonance and diffusion weighted imaging reading adapted to the "Breast Imaging Reporting and Data System" for multiparametric 3 T imaging of breast lesions. Eur Radiol. 2013;23(7):1791–802.

Pinker K, Bogner W, Baltzer P, et al. Improved diagnostic accuracy with multiparametric magnetic resonance imaging of the breast using dynamic contrast-enhanced magnetic resonance imaging, diffusion-weighted imaging, and 3-dimensional proton magnetic resonance spectroscopic imaging. Investig Radiol. 2014a;49(6):421–30.

Pinker K, Bogner W, Baltzer P, et al. Improved differentiation of benign and malignant breast tumors with multiparametric 18fluorodeoxyglucose positron emission tomography magnetic resonance imaging: a feasibility study. Clin Cancer Res. 2014b;20(13):3540–9.

Pinker K, Baltzer P, Andrzejewski P, et al. eds. Dual Tracer PET/MRI of Breast Tumors: Insights Into Tumor Biology. In: Archives of The World Molecular Imaging Conference. Honolulu, HI. World Molecular Imaging Society; 2015.

Pinker K, Helbich TH, Morris EA. The potential of multiparametric MRI of the breast. Br J Radiol. 2016:20160715.

Pinker-Domenig K, Bogner W, Gruber S, et al. High resolution MRI of the breast at 3 T: which BI-RADS(R) descriptors are most strongly associated with the diagnosis of breast cancer? Eur Radiol. 2012;22(2):322–30.

Raad RA, Friedman KP, Heacock L, Ponzo F, Melsaether A, Chandarana H. Outcome of small lung nodules missed on hybrid PET/MRI in patients with primary malignancy. J Magn Reson Imaging. 2016;43(2):504–11.

Rahbar H, Partridge SC. Multiparametric MR imaging of breast cancer. Magn Reson Imaging Clin N Am. 2016;24(1):223–38.

Rahbar H, Partridge SC, Eby PR, et al. Characterization of ductal carcinoma in situ on diffusion weighted breast MRI. Eur Radiol. 2011;21(9):2011–9.

Rechtman LR, Lenihan MJ, Lieberman JH, et al. Breast-specific gamma imaging for the detection of breast cancer in dense versus nondense breasts. AJR Am J Roentgenol. 2014;202(2):293–8.

Rhodes DJ, Hruska CB, Phillips SW, Whaley DH, O'Connor MK. Dedicated dual-head gamma imaging for breast cancer screening in women with mammographically dense breasts. Radiology. 2011;258(1):106–18.

Rhodes DJ, Hruska CB, Conners AL, et al. Journal club: molecular breast imaging at reduced radiation dose for supplemental screening in mammographically dense breasts. AJR Am J Roentgenol. 2015;204(2):241–51.

Romeo V, D'Aiuto M, Frasci G, Imbriaco M, Nicolai E, Simultaneous PET. MRI assessment of response to cytotoxic and hormone neo-adjuvant chemotherapy in breast cancer: a preliminary report. Med Oncol. 2017;34(2):18.

Ruan K, Song G, Ouyang G. Role of hypoxia in the hallmarks of human cancer. J Cell Biochem. 2009;107(6):1053–62.

Samson DJ, Flamm CR, Pisano ED, Aronson N. Should FDG PET be used to decide whether a patient with an abnormal mammogram or breast finding at physical examination should undergo biopsy? Acad Radiol. 2002;9(7):773–83.

Sardanelli F, Boetes C, Borisch B, et al. Magnetic resonance imaging of the breast: recommendations from the EUSOMA working group. Eur J Cancer. 2010;46(8):1296–316.

Sardanelli F, Aase HS, Alvarez M, et al. Position paper on screening for breast cancer by the European Society of Breast Imaging (EUSOBI) and 30 national breast radiology bodies from Austria, Belgium, Bosnia and Herzegovina, Bulgaria, Croatia, Czech Republic, Denmark, Estonia, Finland, France, Germany, Greece, Hungary, Iceland, Ireland, Italy, Israel, Lithuania, Moldova, The Netherlands, Norway, Poland, Portugal, Romania, Serbia, Slovakia, Spain, Sweden, Switzerland and Turkey. Eur Radiol. 2017;27(7):2737–43.

Schmitt B, Zamecnik P, Zaiss M, et al. A new contrast in MR mammography by means of chemical exchange saturation transfer (CEST) imaging at 3 Tesla: preliminary results. Rofo. 2011;183(11):1030–6.

Schmitz AM, Veldhuis WB, Menke-Pluijmers MB, et al. Multiparametric MRI with dynamic contrast enhancement, diffusion-weighted imaging, and 31-phosphorus spectroscopy at 7 T for characterization of breast cancer. Investig Radiol. 2015;50(11):766–71.

Selzner M, Morse MA, Vredenburgh JJ, Meyers WC, Clavien PA. Liver metastases from breast cancer: long-term survival after curative resection. Surgery. 2000;127(4):383–9.

Spick C, Pinker-Domenig K, Rudas M, Helbich TH, Baltzer PA. MRI-only lesions: application of diffusion-weighted imaging obviates unnecessary MR-guided breast biopsies. Eur Radiol. 2014;24(6):1204–10.

Taneja S, Jena A, Goel R, Sarin R, Kaul S. Simultaneous whole-body (1)(8)F-FDG PET-MRI in primary staging of breast cancer: a pilot study. Eur J Radiol. 2014;83(12):2231–9.

Tatum JL, Kelloff GJ, Gillies RJ, et al. Hypoxia: importance in tumor biology, noninvasive measurement by imaging, and value of its measurement in the management of cancer therapy. Int J Radiat Biol. 2006;82(10):699–757.

Ulaner GA, Hyman DM, Ross DS, et al. Detection of HER2-positive metastases in patients with HER2-negative primary breast cancer using [89]Zr-trastuzumab PET/CT. J Nucl Med. 2016;57(10):1523–8.

Vaupel P. Hypoxia and aggressive tumor phenotype: implications for therapy and prognosis. Oncologist. 2008;13(Suppl 3):21–6.

Vaupel P, Briest S, Hockel M. Hypoxia in breast cancer: pathogenesis, characterization and biological/therapeutic implications. Wien Med Wochenschr. 2002;152(13–14):334–42.

Yabuuchi H, Matsuo Y, Okafuji T, et al. Enhanced mass on contrast-enhanced breast MR imaging: Lesion characterization using combination of dynamic contrast-enhanced and diffusion-weighted MR images. J Magn Reson Imaging. 2008;28(5):1157–65.

Yabuuchi H, Matsuo Y, Kamitani T, et al. Non-mass-like enhancement on contrast-enhanced breast MR imaging: lesion characterization using combination of dynamic contrast-enhanced and diffusion-weighted MR images. Eur J Radiol. 2010;75(1):e126–32.

Yutani K, Tatsumi M, Uehara T, Nishimura T. Effect of patients' being prone during FDG PET for the diagnosis of breast cancer. AJR Am J Roentgenol. 1999;173(5):1337–9.

Zaric O, Pinker K, Zbyn S, et al. Quantitative sodium MR imaging at 7 T: initial results and comparison with diffusion-weighted imaging in patients with breast tumors. Radiology. 2016;280(1):39–48.

Neurodegeneration Imaging

7

Henryk Barthel and Osama Sabri

7.1 Introduction

Progressive and chronic loss of neural tissue in different brain systems is the core feature of neurodegenerative diseases. This group of diseases comprises dementia disorders, Parkinsonian syndromes (PS), Huntington's disease, amyotrophic lateral sclerosis (ALS), and prion diseases. Although these diseases are all accompanied by neuronal cell loss, they are characterised and distinguished by specific pathogens, neurotransmitter deficiencies, genetic background and different clinical phenotypes.

In current clinical praxis, neurodegenerative diseases are often primarily diagnosed at the symptomatic stage by using clinical criteria. This is, in some cases, accompanied by biomarkers as obtained by brain imaging, cerebrospinal fluid analysis and other techniques. In suspected neurodegenerative disease, magnetic resonance imaging (MRI) represents the standard imaging tool for morphologic assessment. MRI is primarily utilized in this context to exclude other causes for the symptoms observed, like vascular disease, brain tumours, traumatic or inflammatory changes. In addition, atrophy patterns may supplement the clinical diagnosis of certain neurodegenerative diseases. PET imaging increasingly supports respective diagnostic workups. PET can with high sensitivity visualize and quantify the imaging targets on a molecular level. As such, PET promises a more sensitive and/or earlier diagnosis particularly in neurodegenerative disorders.

Until recently, the sequentially acquired PET and MRI data were often analysed side-by-side or *post hoc*-coregistered for multimodal brain image data analysis. As an alternative, hybrid PET/MRI has been investigated in neurodegenerative diseases for the past 5 years: The published literature covers PET/MRI studies in dementia disorders, PS, and ALS. In this chapter, the current state of knowledge and future perspectives for the use of PET/MRI in neurodegenerative disorders will be discussed.

7.2 General Considerations

In general, all PET/MR imaging protocols to investigate patients with suspected neurodegenerative disorders are designed to fully combine state-of-the-art MR protocols with sophisticated PET procedures. One example of a state-of-the-art PET/MRI protocol for hybrid amyloid imaging is demonstrated in Fig. 7.1 which shows the standard hybrid amyloid PET/MRI protocol as it is employed by our group in patients with cognitive decline to support/exclude the suspicion

H. Barthel (✉) • O. Sabri
Department of Nuclear Medicine,
University Hospital of Leipzig, Leipzig, Germany
e-mail: henryk.barthel@medizin.uni-leipzig.de

© Springer International Publishing AG 2018
L. Umutlu, K. Herrmann (eds.), *PET/MR Imaging: Current and Emerging Applications*,
https://doi.org/10.1007/978-3-319-69641-6_7

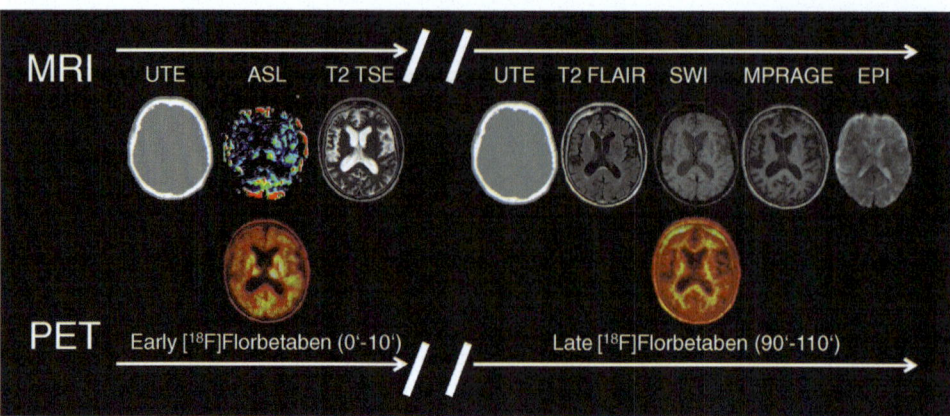

Fig. 7.1 Standard amyloid PET/MRI protocol as employed at the Department of Nuclear Medicine, Leipzig University (Leipzig, Germany) in suitable subjects with cognitive decline to support/exclude the suspicion of underlying Alzheimer's disease. The early after tracer administration PET data are used as neurodegeneration biomarker (Tiepolt et al. 2016)

of underlying Alzheimer's disease. For this purpose, [18F]Florbetaben is used as PET tracer (Barthel et al. 2011; Sabri et al. 2015). Here, the standard amyloid load PET imaging time-window of 90–110 min post tracer injection is accompanied by an early (0–10 min p.i.) PET data acquisition time-window. This double-imaging protocol is performed as early data acquisition has been shown to provide additional neurodegeneration biomarker readouts (in addition to the amyloid pathology biomarker information) (Tiepolt et al. 2016). Simultaneously to both PET imaging time-windows, the following standard neurodegeneration diagnosis MR sequences are acquired: T2 TSE, T2 FLAIR, SWI, T1 MPRAGE. This is accompanied by UTE for attenuation correction of the PET data, arterial spin labelling (ASL) for blood flow information for research purposes, and EPI for scientific resting-state fMRI. The entire protocol is completed within 10 + 20 min total acquisition time (Fig. 7.1).

One major methodological point of discussion associated with the PET/MRI technology relates to the fact that the first-generation algorithm to correct the PET data for attenuation effects, namely the Dixon approach, does not consider the relevantly attenuating bone. Thus, with regard to brain PET/MRI, a number of alternative approaches have been developed and tested over the last years. A recent multicentre study of more than 300 brain PET/MRI scans compared the quantification accuracy of eleven different attenuation correction approaches, taking the CT-based approach as standard of truth. In this study, the UTE which is the current vendor-provided approach yielded a quantitation error of −5%, while at least six either segmentation-based or template/atlas-based approaches provided error-less results (Fig. 7.2) (Ladefoged et al. 2017). As a consequence, it can be concluded that this methodological question is technically solved for PET/MR imaging of the brain.

The scientific community is rigerously searching for potential improvements of the diagnostic quality of hybrid PET/MRI as compared to sequentially acquired PET and MRI data. This is by taking advantage of the simultaneous data acquisition in perfect spatial fit, and with high sensitivity/spatial resolution (for the PET component often higher than that of state-of-the art stand-alone PET or PET/CT). For imaging of the brain, particularly in neurodegenerative disease, it is believed that there is potential for improved data and diagnostic quality on both sides of this bimodality technology (Fig. 7.3). Examples in this regard concerning PET advancement relate to (1) improved anatomical localisationof PET signals, also to small structures, (2) the possibility of online motion correction of the PET data (Chun et al. 2012),

Fig. 7.2 Deviation of brain PET signal from the gold standard by using eleven different attenuation correction approaches as obtained in a multi-centre study. Figure taken from (Ladefoged et al. 2017) with permission from Elsevier

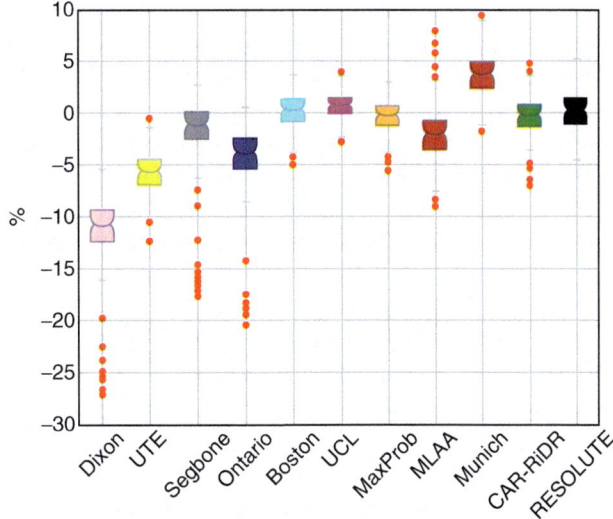

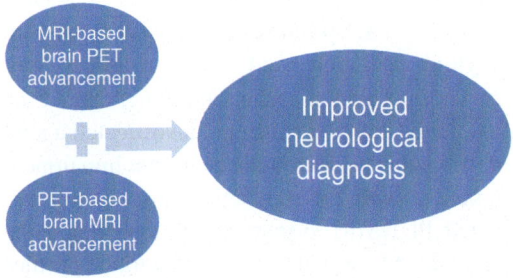

Fig. 7.3 Incremental value of hybrid PET/MRI for improved brain imaging diagnosis

(3) improved partial volume effect correction of the PET data which are most often compromised in neurodegenerative disorders by atrophy, (4) improved PET tracer uptake quantification (Jochimsen et al. 2015), and (5) the possibility to derive a non-invasive arterial input function (Jochimsen et al. 2016). Examples concerning both PET and MRI advancement refer to the fact that it is now possible to cross-evaluate novel imaging approaches in situations in which the complementing imaging modality is able to deliver the gold standard readout at the same time, under identical pathophysiological conditions. This aspect particularly concerns novel brain perfusion sequences, like ASL MRI against $[^{15}O]H_2O$ PET (Werner et al. 2016a), the imaging of amyloid-associated iron by QSM MRI against amyloid PET (Acosta-Cabronero

et al. 2013), or the testing of novel myelin-binding PET tracers for white matter imaging against DTI MRI (Matías-Guiu et al. 2016).

7.3   PET/MRI in Dementia Disorders

Amongst all brain diseases the use and utilization of imaging biomarkers is most advanced in dementia disorders, particularly in Alzheimer's disease (AD). Specific categories of amyloid pathology biomarkers (amyloid PET) and neuronal injury biomarkers (structural MRI showing hippocampal atrophy, $[^{18}F]$FDG PET, in the future potentially tau PET) have been defined for AD in the past few years (McKhann et al. 2011).

Multimodal image analysis based on sequentially acquired and separately or via *post hoc* coregistration analysed PET and MRI data has been demonstrated to have a great potential to supplement clinical testing in early and differential diagnosis of dementia disorders (Teipel et al. 2015). The positive state of use of imaging biomarkers in dementia disorders has channelled the focus of scientific and clinical studies on integrated PET/MRI on the assessment of neurodegenerative diseases: From 2012 onwards, nine respective publications comprising more than 300 subjects have been published, with most of these studies employing [^{18}F]FDG PET in combination with structural/functional MRI.

In initial feasibility studies of PET/MRI in dementia patients it was demonstrated that the quality of both, PET and the MRI data, obtained from this hybrid technology in a simultaneous fashion is as high as that from respective stand-alone systems (Jena et al. 2014; Schwenzer et al. 2012). Subsequently, the impact of the first-generation attenuation correction techniques provided by the vendors in the initial years after the merge of the PET/MRI technology on the clinical diagnosis in dementia disorders was investigated. A number of studies on [^{18}F]FDG and amyloid PET imaging in dementia patients showed that, despite certain quantification errors depending on the particular algorithms used, clinical diagnosis is not relevantly affected in most applications (Hitz et al. 2014; Su et al. 2016; Werner et al. 2016b).

With regard to [^{18}F]FDG PET/MRI in dementia disorders, recent data point to a potential gain in pathophysiology clarification and even differential diagnosis accuracy by the combined evaluation of metabolism, atrophy, and functional connectivity. Moodley et al. investigated 24 patients with AD dementia or frontotemporal dementia by means of [^{18}F]FDG PET/MRI and compared regional glucose consumption with atrophy as determined by T1-weighted MR imaging. They found that hypometabolism and atrophy patterns may differ in certain dementia forms

(Moodley et al. 2015). As a further advancement, Tahmasian et al. implemented resting-state fMRI into the diagnostic workup. By investigating 61 subjects with mild cognitive impairment or AD dementia and comparing them with 26 healthy control subjects, it was reported that hippocampal metabolism is negatively correlated with functional hippocampus-precuneus connectivity in AD dementia (Tahmasian et al. 2015). Extending these studies, the same group recently published their results, obtained in 40 AD dementia/frontotemporal lobar degeneration patients, demonstrating that this triple read-out approach (metabolism, atrophy, functional connectivity) may have the potential to improve differential dementia diagnosis (Tahmasian et al. 2016).

The use of amyloid PET tracers represents another promising option in dementia PET/MRI, as this approach promises the acquisition of both amyloid pathology and neuronal injury biomarker information at the same time. One of the first publications on this topic investigated a total of 100 subjects with mild cognitive impairment or patients with different dementias with an integrated PET/MRI system and demonstrated the potential to provide dual biomarker profiles (Fig. 7.4) known from sequential imaging studies. Of similar importance, patient/caregiver as well as referring doctor surveys showed that this was accomplished with increased comfort to the parties interviewed (Schütz et al. 2016).

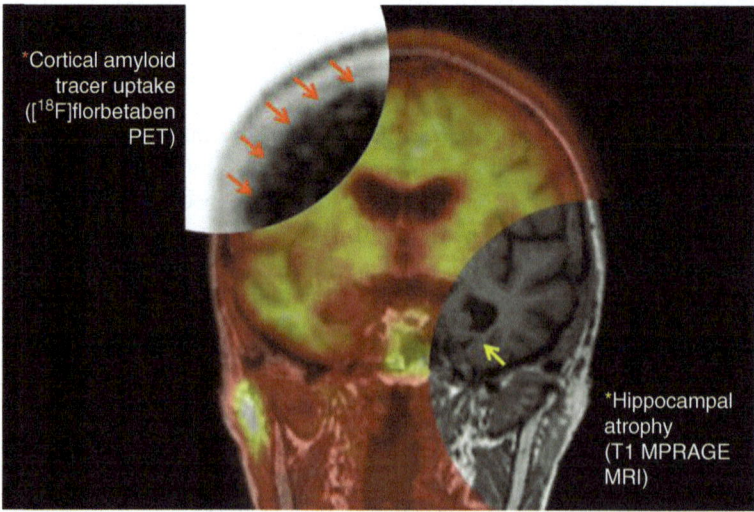

Fig. 7.4 One-stop shop dual (amyloid pathology and neuronal injury) biomarker delivery in Alzheimer's disease by hybrid PET/MRI

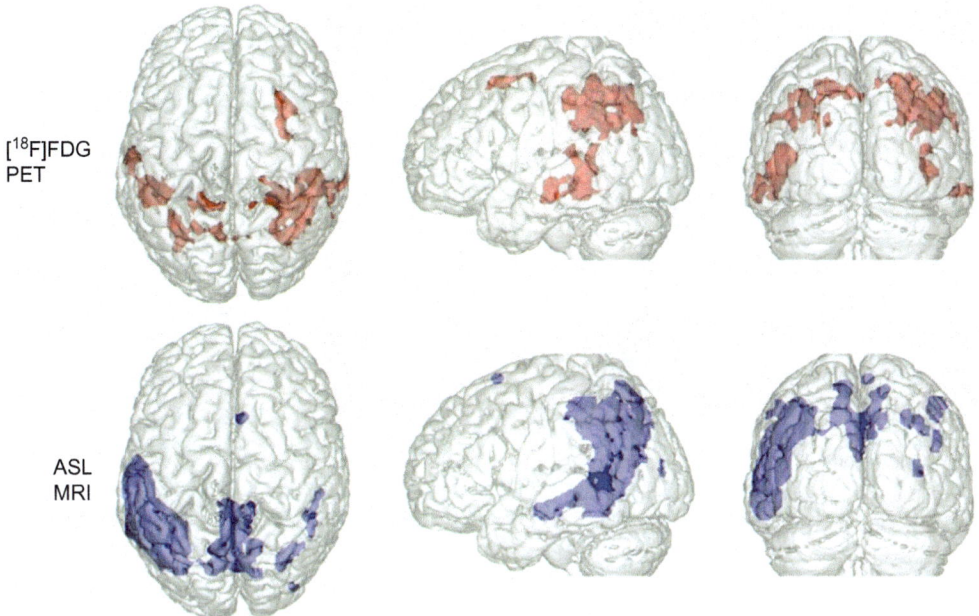

Fig. 7.5 Arterial spin labelling (ASL) MRI as a potential substitute for [^{18}F]FDG PET in dementia imaging. Voxelwise group comparisons between patients with AD dementia and non-AD dementias for both imaging modalities as acquired simultaneously by PET/MRI

Our group currently also investigates the potential of parallel arterial spin labelling (ASL) MRI in the context of dementia PET/MRI. ASL is a contrast media-free MRI method to obtain brain perfusion images, which—as neurodegeneration leads to more or less concordant perfusion and metabolism defects—might provide an [^{18}F]FDG-like neuronal injury AD biomarker information. We have investigated this feature by performing simultaneous [^{18}F]FDG PET/ASL MR imaging in dementia patients. Figure 7.5 shows voxelwise group comparisons between patients with AD dementia and non-AD dementias for both imaging modalities. It was found that the typical bilateral temporoparietal AD pattern known for [^{18}F]FDG PET can be reproduced to a large extent by ASL MRI (Fig. 7.5).

7.4 PET/MRI in Parkinsonian Syndromes

In Parkinson (PS) patients, the concept of supporting clinical diagnosis by imaging biomarkers is not yet as advanced as in dementia disorder. MRI is the first-line imaging tool, and is mainly used to exclude other pathologies as well as to reveal potential different atrophy patterns in different atypical PSs (Tolosa et al. 2006). PET imaging, based on the utilization of dopamine precursor [^{18}F]FDOPA or dopamine transporter ligands like [^{18}F]FP-CIT, represents another imaging option in the primary diagnosis of PSs. Furthermore, the glucose metabolism marker [^{18}F]FDG is utilized for differential PET diagnosis of PSs (Tolosa et al. 2006). For multimodal analyses, the data of both modalities have been mainly *post hoc* coregistered so far.

To date six PET/MRI studies have been published in patients with suspected PS: Like in dementia disorders, it was shown by Schwenzer et al. in nine patients with PS for [^{18}F]FDG and standard neurodegeneration MR sequences that the data are obtainable in full diagnostic quality via the simultaneous acquisition technology (Schwenzer et al. 2012). Furthermore, again comparable to dementia disorders, studies utilizing the suboptimal first-generation attenuation

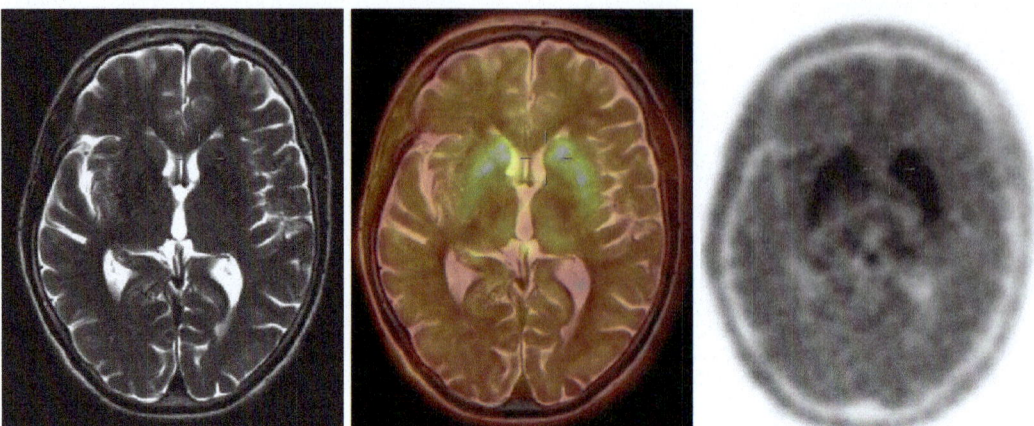

Fig. 7.6 [^{18}F]FDOPA PET/MRI in a patient with Parkinsonian syndrome. Normal structural MRI (T1-MPRAGE, left) and normal dopamine metabolism PET (right; middle: PET/MRI overlay) rendering this patient as without evidence of neurodegenerative course of disease. Clinical follow-up confirmed essential tremor

correction approaches in patients with PS revealed that the PET accuracy is clinically viable (Jena et al. 2014; Werner et al. 2016b). Similar to [^{18}F]FDG, the clinical standard visual dopamine transporter availability determination by [^{18}F]FP-CIT PET/MRI was reported to not being affected by the suboptimal attenuation correction used in the first years of PET/MRI, but may affect the absolute quantification of PET data (Choi et al. 2014; Kwon et al. 2016). Choi et al. recently published results on one of the first studies on hybrid [^{18}F]FP-CIT PET/MRI in 23 PS patients, assessing the simultaneous multimodal PET and MRI data delivery: Here, the surrogate PET readout of dopaminergic degeneration was obtained for different striatal compartments and related to the regional cortical atrophy as determined by voxel-based morphometry of T1-MR images. Based on these initial results, the authors reported an association between both parameters which differed in its direction and degree for different striatal sub-regions (Choi et al. 2016).

Our group recently started utilizing [^{18}F] FDOPA PET/MRI in patients with PS (Fig. 7.6) with the aim, among others, to explore whether online motion tracking during the PET acquisition by means of special MR sequences (Chun et al. 2012) and subsequent movement correction of the acquired PET data has the potential to improve diagnosis in these movement disorders.

7.5 Future Developments

There is still a considerable lack of PET/MRI studies investigating the potential of this hybrid multimodal imaging approach in patients with Huntington's disease or prion disorders, which is mainly caused by the fact that respective disease-specific PET tracers still await their development. However, it may be helpful to study more unspecific parameters in these disorders, like neurotransmitter deficiencies, neuroinflammation or apoptosis, as was shown for ALS in recent studies. The utilization of the novel glial activation marker [^{11}C]PBR28 for PET/MRI demonstrated that neuroinflammation was increased in the motor cortices and corticospinal tracts of ALS patients. Areas of neuroinflammation as determined by PET correlated with areas of reduced structural connectivity as determined by diffusion tensor MR imaging or cortical degeneration as determined by T1 morphological MRI (Alshikho et al. 2016; Zürcher et al. 2015).

Recent studies proposed hybrid amyloid PET/ MRI as a first-line "one-stop shop" biomarker delivery tool instead of the currently established sequential approach (Drzezga et al. 2014). Prospective clinical studies on hybrid amyloid PET/MRI will be required to clarify the acceptance of this "one-stop-shop" procedure by the established dementia diagnostics community.

Another, currently ongoing research project bears a highly interesting potential for early diagnosis with regard to future use of PET/MRI in dementia disorders: New PET probes targeting tau aggregates, another histopathological hallmark of AD, are currently undergo first in human testing (Holtzman et al. 2016). Provided the success of this testing, these tracers might further stimulate the use of the hybrid technology for multi-biomarker delivery in AD. The same holds true for some novel MR techniques, whereby especially Fe mapping by quantitative susceptibility mapping (QSM) seems to be of interest for potential AD diagnosis (Acosta-Cabronero et al. 2013), as Fe accumulates in amyloid plaques.

It needs to be mentioned that the full potential of hybrid PET/MRI has not been fully exploited in imaging neurodegeneration. Showing improved convenience to the parties involved can only be the first step in this regard. Thus, it will be the task of future studies to identify scenarios in which imaging-based diagnoses in suspected neurodegenerative disorders will benefit from improved quality of the hybrid image data and/or the fact that the data are acquired at the same time.

7.6   Summary and Conclusions

Integrated PET/MRI has been successfully introduced in the last years into clinical imaging of neurodegenerative disorders. This especially refers to dementia disorders, but also to Parkinsonian syndromes. By that, proof of concept for multi-biomarker delivery was demonstrated with improved convenience to the patients, their caregivers, the investigating, and the referring doctors. It will be the task of the next years to come to test hybrid PET/MRI also in other neurodegenerative disorders, and to answer the questions of whether the possibility to acquire the PET and MRI data at the same time will lead to new clinical applications and/or improved quality of early and differential neurodegeneration diagnosis.

Acknowledgements The acquisition of the Department of Nuclear Medicine, Leipzig University (Leipzig, Germany) PET/MRI system was co-funded by the German Research Foundation (grant number SA 669/9-1) and the German Max Planck Society.

Conflicts of Interest H.B. and O.S. received research support, speaker honoraria and well as travel expenses from Piramal Imaging (Berlin, Germany) related to amyloid PET imaging.

References

Acosta-Cabronero J, Williams GB, Cardenas-Blanco A, Arnold RJ, Lupson V, Nestor PJ. In vivo quantitative susceptibility mapping (QSM) in Alzheimer's disease. PLoS One. 2013;8(11):e81093.

Alshikho MJ, Zürcher NR, Loggia ML, Cernasov P, Chonde DB, Izquierdo Garcia D, Yasek JE, Akeju O, Catana C, Rosen BR, Cudkowicz ME, Hooker JM, Atassi N. Glial activation colocalizes with structural abnormalities in amyotrophic lateral sclerosis. Neurology. 2016;87(24):2554–61.

Barthel H, Gertz HJ, Dresel S, Peters O, Bartenstein P, Buerger K, Hiemeyer F, Wittemer-Rump SM, Seibyl J, Reininger C, Sabri O, Florbetaben Study Group. Cerebral amyloid-β PET with florbetaben (18F) in patients with Alzheimer's disease and healthy controls: a multicentre phase 2 diagnostic study. Lancet Neurol. 2011;10(5):424–35.

Choi H, Cheon GJ, Kim HJ, Choi SH, Lee JS, Kim YI, Kang KW, Chung JK, Kim EE, Lee DS. Segmentation-based MR attenuation correction including bones also affects quantitation in brain studies: an initial result of 18F-FP-CIT PET/MR for patients with parkinsonism. J Nucl Med. 2014;55(10):1617–22.

Choi H, Cheon GJ, Kim HJ, Choi SH, Kim YI, Kang KW, Chung JK, Kim EE, Lee DS. Gray matter correlates of dopaminergic degeneration in Parkinson's disease: a hybrid PET/MR study using (18) F-FP-CIT. Hum Brain Mapp. 2016;37(5):1710–21.

Chun SY, Reese TG, Ouyang J, Guerin B, Catana C, Zhu X, Alpert NM, El Fakhri G. MRI-based nonrigid motion correction in simultaneous PET/MRI. J Nucl Med. 2012;53(8):1284–91.

Drzezga A, Barthel H, Minoshima S, Sabri O. Potential clinical applications of PET/MR imaging in neurodegenerative diseases. J Nucl Med. 2014;55(Suppl 2):47S–55S.

Hitz S, Habekost C, Fürst S, Delso G, Förster S, Ziegler S, Nekolla SG, Souvatzoglou M, Beer AJ, Grimmer T, Eiber M, Schwaiger M, Drzezga A. Systematic comparison of the performance of integrated whole-body PET/MR imaging to conventional PET/CT for ^{18}F-FDG brain imaging in patients examined for suspected dementia. J Nucl Med. 2014;55(6):923–31.

Holtzman DM, Carrillo MC, Hendrix JA, Bain LJ, Catafau AM, Gault LM, Goedert M, Mandelkow E, Mandelkow EM, Miller DS, Ostrowitzki S, Polydoro M, Smith S, Wittmann M, Hutton M. Tau: From research to clinical development. Alzheimers Dement. 2016;12(10):1033–9.

Jena A, Taneja S, Goel R, Renjen P, Negi P. Reliability of semiquantitative ^{18}F-FDG PET parameters derived from simultaneous brain PET/MRI: a feasibility study. Eur J Radiol. 2014;83(7):1269–74.

Jochimsen TH, Schulz J, Busse H, Werner P, Schaudinn A, Zeisig V, Kurch L, Seese A, Barthel H, Sattler B, Sabri O. Lean body mass correction of standardized uptake value in simultaneous whole-body positron emission tomography and magnetic resonance imaging. Phys Med Biol. 2015;60(12):4651–64.

Jochimsen TH, Zeisig V, Schulz J, Werner P, Patt M, Patt J, Dreyer AY, Boltze J, Barthel H, Sabri O, Sattler B. Fully automated calculation of image-derived input function in simultaneous PET/MRI in a sheep model. EJNMMI Phys. 2016;3(1):2. https://doi.org/10.1186/s40658-016-0139-2.

Kwon S, Chun K, Kong E, Cho I. Comparison of the performances of (18)F-FP-CIT brain PET/MR and simultaneous PET/CT: a preliminary study. Nucl Med Mol Imaging. 2016;50(3):219–27.

Ladefoged CN, Law I, Anazodo U, St Lawrence K, Izquierdo-Garcia D, Catana C, Burgos N, Cardoso MJ, Ourselin S, Hutton B, Mérida I, Costes N, Hammers A, Benoit D, Holm S, Juttukonda M, An H, Cabello J, Lukas M, Nekolla S, Ziegler S, Fenchel M, Jakoby B, Casey ME, Benzinger T, Højgaard L, Hansen AE, Andersen FL. A multi-centre evaluation of eleven clinically feasible brain PET/MRI attenuation correction techniques using a large cohort of patients. NeuroImage. 2017;147:346–59.

Matías-Guiu JA, Cabrera-Martín MN, Oreja-Guevara C, Carreras JL, Matías-Guiu J. Pittsburgh compound B and other amyloid positron emission tomography tracers for the study of white matter and multiple sclerosis. Ann Neurol. 2016;80(1):166. https://doi.org/10.1002/ana.24666.

McKhann GM, Knopman DS, Chertkow H, Hyman BT, Jack CR Jr, Kawas CH, Klunk WE, Koroshetz WJ, Manly JJ, Mayeux R, Mohs RC, Morris JC, Rossor MN, Scheltens P, Carrillo MC, Thies B, Weintraub S, Phelps CH. The diagnosis of dementia due to Alzheimer's disease: recommendations from the National Institute on Aging-Alzheimer's Association workgroups on diagnostic guidelines for Alzheimer's disease. Alzheimers Dement 2011;7(3):263–269.

Moodley KK, Perani D, Minati L, Della Rosa PA, Pennycook F, Dickson JC, Barnes A, Contarino VE, Michopoulou S, D'Incerti L, Good C, Fallanca F, Vanoli EG, Ell PJ, Chan D. Simultaneous PET-MRI studies of the concordance of atrophy and hypometabolism in syndromic variants of Alzheimer's disease and frontotemporal dementia: an extended case series. J Alzheimers Dis. 2015;46(3):639–53.

Sabri O, Sabbagh MN, Seibyl J, Barthel H, Akatsu H, Ouchi Y, Senda K, Murayama S, Ishii K, Takao M, Beach TG, Rowe CC, Leverenz JB, Ghetti B, Ironside JW, Catafau AM, Stephens AW, Mueller A, Koglin N, Hoffmann A, Roth K, Reininger C, Schulz-Schaeffer WJ, Florbetaben Phase 3 Study Group. Florbetaben PET imaging to detect amyloid beta plaques in Alzheimer's disease: phase 3 study. Alzheimers Dement. 2015;11(8):964–74.

Schütz L, Lobsien D, Fritzsch D, Tiepolt S, Werner P, Schroeter ML, Berrouschot J, Saur D, Hesse S, Jochimsen T, Rullmann M, Sattler B, Patt M, Gertz HJ, Villringer A, Claßen J, Hoffmann KT, Sabri O, Barthel H. Feasibility and acceptance of simultaneous amyloid PET/MRI. Eur J Nucl Med Mol Imaging. 2016;43(12):2236–43.

Schwenzer NF, Stegger L, Bisdas S, Schraml C, Kolb A, Boss A, Müller M, Reimold M, Ernemann U, Claussen CD, Pfannenberg C, Schmidt H. Simultaneous PET/MR imaging in a human brain PET/MR system in 50 patients – current state of image quality. Eur J Radiol. 2012;81(11):3472–8.

Su Y, Rubin BB, McConathy J, Laforest R, Qi J, Sharma A, Priatna A, Benzinger TL. Impact of MR-based attenuation correction on neurologic PET studies. J Nucl Med. 2016;57(6):913–7.

Tahmasian M, Pasquini L, Scherr M, Meng C, Förster S, Mulej Bratec S, Shi K, Yakushev I, Schwaiger M, Grimmer T, Diehl-Schmid J, Riedl V, Sorg C, Drzezga A. The lower hippocampus global connectivity, the higher its local metabolism in Alzheimer disease. Neurology. 2015 May 12;84(19):1956–63.

Tahmasian M, Shao J, Meng C, Grimmer T, Diehl-Schmid J, Yousefi BH, Förster S, Riedl V, Drzezga A, Sorg C. Based on the network degeneration hypothesis: separating individual patients with different neurodegenerative syndromes in a preliminary hybrid PET/MR study. J Nucl Med. 2016;57(3):410–5.

Teipel S, Drzezga A, Grothe MJ, Barthel H, Chételat G, Schuff N, Skudlarski P, Cavedo E, Frisoni GB, Hoffmann W, Thyrian JR, Fox C, Minoshima S, Sabri O, Fellgiebel A. Multimodal imaging in Alzheimer's disease: validity and usefulness for early detection. Lancet Neurol. 2015;14(10):1037–53.

Tiepolt S, Hesse S, Patt M, Luthardt J, Schroeter ML, Hoffmann KT, Weise D, Gertz HJ, Sabri O, Barthel H. Early [(18)F]florbetaben and [(11)C]PiB PET images are a surrogate biomarker of neuronal injury in Alzheimer's disease. Eur J Nucl Med Mol Imaging. 2016;43(9):1700–9.

Tolosa E, Wenning G, Poewe W. The diagnosis of Parkinson's disease. Lancet Neurol. 2006;5(1):75–86.

Werner P, Saur D, Mildner T, Möller H, Classen J, Sabri O, Hoffmann KT, Barthel H. Combined PET/MRI: multimodality insights into acute stroke hemodynamics. Neurology. 2016a;86(20):1926–7.

Werner P, Rullmann M, Bresch A, Tiepolt S, Jochimsen T, Lobsien D, Schroeter ML, Sabri O, Barthel H. Impact of attenuation correction on clinical [(18)F]FDG brain PET in combined PET/MRI. EJNMMI Res. 2016b Dec;6(1):47. https://doi.org/10.1186/s13550-016-0200-0.

Zürcher NR, Loggia ML, Lawson R, Chonde DB, Izquierdo-Garcia D, Yasek JE, Akeju O, Catana C, Rosen BR, Cudkowicz ME, Hooker JM, Atassi N. Increased in vivo glial activation in patients with amyotrophic lateral sclerosis: assessed with [(11)C]-PBR28. Neuroimage Clin. 2015;7:409–14.

Cardiac PET/MRI

8

Kai Nassenstein, Felix Nensa,
and Christoph Rischpler

Magnetic resonance imaging (MRI) and positron emission tomography (PET) have been used for the assessment of diverse cardiac pathologies for decades.

Since cardiac MRI (CMR) offers a broad range of imaging possibilities ranging from functional imaging to quantitative tissue characterisation, it has become the standard of reference for a variety of cardiovascular applications including the quantification of left and right ventricular function, assessment of global and regional wall motion, tissue characterisation (scar, fat and oedema) as well as quantitative analysis of valve function.

Cardiac PET, on the other hand, allows absolute quantification of myocardial perfusion and coronary flow reserve as well as visualization and quantification of specific processes at a molecular level, such as metabolism, inflammation, or innervation (Hendel et al. 2009).

With cardiac MRI providing information on an anatomic level and PET imaging offering information on a molecular biological level, the two imaging modalities have to be considered as complementary, even though overlapping diagnostic information appear. Based on the conviction, that the complementary information derived from cardiac MRI and cardiac PET allow to improve diagnostic accuracy of cardiac imaging, hybrid cardiac PET/MR imaging using either sequential or integrated scanner platforms have been performed within the last few years either in individual cases or within clinical studies in various cardiac pathologies ranging from ischaemic heart disease to cardiac tumours (Hundley et al. 2010).

The following chapter provides a summary of the current scientific research in hybrid cardiac PET/MRI, and outlines potential new future applications.

8.1 Technical Aspects

Many technical aspects of cardiac PET/MRI are common to most applications of PET/MRI and are already discussed in great detail in a separate chapter of this book. In the following paragraphs we will outline some more or less specific technical aspects of cardiac PET/MRI.

8.1.1 Motion Correction

The assignment of MR or PET imaging data to a specific cardiac phase is normally performed using ECG-based triggering or gating. However, ECG signals can be significantly distorted by the

K. Nassenstein (✉) • F. Nensa
Institute of Diagnostic and Interventional Radiology
and Neuroradiology, University Hospital Essen,
Essen, Germany
e-mail: Kai.Nassenstein@uk-essen.de

C. Rischpler
Department of Nuclear Medicine, Technical
University Munich, München, Germany

© Springer International Publishing AG 2018
L. Umutlu, K. Herrmann (eds.), *PET/MR Imaging: Current and Emerging Applications*,
https://doi.org/10.1007/978-3-319-69641-6_8

magnetic field and radio frequency pulses of the MR device. Therefore, special caution should be exercised when attaching the electrodes and monitoring the signal. The comparatively long cumulative acquisition times of most cardiac MR protocols allow for a significantly extended parallel acquisition of PET signals in the cardiac bed position, which more than compensates for the loss of data occurring during ECG gating, and which then results in reconstructed PET images with high signal to noise ratio (Nensa et al. 2013).

A particularly promising, but still experimental, technical development of integrated PET/MRI is based on the detection of cardiac motion with ultrafast ("real-time") 3D MR acquisition and tagging techniques. This allows for the MR-based estimation of cardiac motion with vector fields in parallel to the acquisition of PET signals. These motion vector fields can then be used for motion compensation of the PET data, which improves the effective spatial resolution of PET and motion-related inaccuracies in PET quantification. Recent advances in this area suggest a relevant utility of this technology for simultaneous PET/MR cardiac imaging.

8.1.2 Reading and Post-Processing Software

Various commercial and/or free software packages offer semi-automatic or automatic processing of cardiac imaging data. However, software that allows for an integrated and quantitative reading of both modalities is still rare. Most products are dedicated to the use of either modality alone, and thus one cannot take full advantage of the spatial and temporal coherence of simultaneous image acquisition. Also several products with generic image fusion capabilities, like oncologic reading software, are available. However, these typically do not include the desired workflows for the reading of cardiac imaging studies, like the assessment of cardiac function and flow or the creation of parametric polar map displays. Some software packages such as "OsiriX" (OsiriX Foundation, Geneva, Switzerland), "MunichHeart" (TU München, Munich, Germany) and "syngo.via" (Siemens

Healthineers, Erlangen, Germany) utilize both cardiac PET and cardiac MRI data. However, software solutions for fully integrated cardiac PET/MRI analyses are still missing. Recently, a solution for the integrated reading of cardiac PET and MRI data using co-registered bully's eye plots has been proposed, which is based on a mutual segmentation of myocardial boundaries in MR images and thus provides robust segmentation and inherent co-registration (Nensa et al. 2017a, b).

8.1.3 Dietary Patient Preparation for Cardiac FDG PET/MRI

2-deoxy-2-(18F)fluoro-D-glucose (FDG) is by far the most widely used tracer for cardiac PET imaging. Normal myocardium is an insulin-sensitive tissue. Under uncontrolled metabolic conditions the myocardium uses a variable mixture of glucose, lactate, ketone bodies and free fatty-acids, with a preference for fatty-acids. Depending on the clinical question (inflammation/ tumor vs. viability), the myocardial metabolism must either be switched to free fatty acid or glucose utilization using a particular dietary preparation. Therefore, careful patient preparation is of great importance. It is strongly recommended to conduct detailed patient discussions on compliance with the dietary protocol. This is typically done by a nuclear medicine specialist before the injection of the radiotracer. In cases of incompliance with the protocol, the PET/MR scan can be postponed or certain countermeasures (e.g. insulin injection, unfractionated heparin injection, fatty acid loading) may be taken. In addition to pre-examination patient consultations, it is advisable to carry out blood tests of the glucose level.

For cardiac PET imaging of inflammation, infiltration and tumors with FDG, it is important to suppress the physiological glucose uptake by normal cardiomyocytes by low insulin levels and high fatty acid levels to distinguish between inflammatory infiltrates or tumor tissue and normal myocardium. This can be accomplished by a number of techniques including long fasting, high-fat, low-carbohydrate diet, fatty acid loading, and additional injection of unfractionated heparin (Ishida et al. 2014; Williams and Kolodny 2008; Manabe et al. 2016). However, fasting has been found to be an important cause of patient discomfort, potentially contributing to increased cancellation rates of cardiac PET/MR scans by patients (Nensa et al. 2013). In a recent study, a high-fat low-carbohydrate protein-permitted diet without fasting was described, that yields an 84% success rate regarding suppression of normal myocardial glucose uptake. Cancellation rate was less than 3% and thus comparable to routine CMR scans (Nensa et al. 2013).

For PET imaging of myocardial viability with FDG it is important to significantly increase insulin levels in order to favor the physiological uptake of glucose by normal cardiomyocytes. In principal, several techniques are available including hyperinsulinemic-euglycemic clamping, administration of hypolipidemic agents (e.g. Acipimox) and oral glucose loading. In our experience, the following protocol for oral glucose loading has been proven to be reliable, simple to perform and well received by patients: Patients fast before the scan, which usually means to skip breakfast in the morning. The glucose level of diabetics should be below 150 mg/dl (8.3 mmol/l). Prior to FDG injection, patients receive 75 g of glucose orally in a preparation commercially available for glucose tolerance tests. In problematic groups of patients suffering from e.g. diabetes or severe left ventricular dysfunction, however, studies indicate that the hyperinsulinemic-euglycemic technique may result in superior PET image quality (Vitale et al. 2001).

8.2 Ischemic Heart Disease

8.2.1 Coronary Heart Disease

Stable coronary heart disease, one of the most important issues in daily cardiological routine due to its high prevalence (Sanchis-Gomar et al. 2016), is the consequence of the increasing narrowing of the coronary artery lumen due to atherosclerosis.

Coronary angiography has been routinely used over decades for the diagnosis of coronary heart disease even though nowadays non-invasive techniques such as coronary CT angiography are increasingly practiced for the assessment of coronary arteriosclerosis (Montalescot et al. 2013). Unfortunately, the assessment of the morphologic severity of an epicardial stenosis either by coronary angiography or by CT angiography has been shown to provide only a poor prognostic value. Instead, the hemodynamic relevance of a coronary stenosis or the presence of myocardial perfusion defect is crucial, since these are prognostic for clinical outcome after coronary revascularization (De Bruyne et al. 2012).

Despite some promising recent approaches in non-invasive CT-based assessment of coronary fractional flow reserve, which is defined as the pressure distal to a stenosis relative to the pressure proximal to the stenosis, and which is considered the hallmark of hemodynamic significance, myocardial perfusion imaging either by MRI, SPECT or PET is currently used in clinical routine to assess the relevance of coronary stenosis.

Although cardiac MRI is widely used for myocardial perfusion imaging, PET in fact is considered to be the reference standard for non-invasive quantitative assessment of myocardial perfusion (Hagemann et al. 2015; Sciagra et al. 2016). Most myocardial perfusion tracers used in PET have to be produced onsite in cyclotrons due to their short half-lives, e.g. ^{13}N–NH$_3$ (T½ $\approx$ 10 min) or H$_2$^{15}O (T½ $\approx$ 2 min), which limits their broad application. Even though, with ^{82}Rb a generator-based PET perfusion tracer have become available, the current design and the high running expenses of such a generator do not allow an easy and cost-effective workflow for ^{82}Rb on PET/MRI systems (Rischpler et al. 2014). Novel ^{18}F–labeled perfusion tracers with a low positron range, a half-life of around 2 hours allowing distribution to sites without an on-site cyclotron, a high first-pass extraction, and a nearly linear flow-related uptake have been recently introduced (Sherif et al. 2011; Vermeltfoort et al. 2011) but these tracers are currently not broadly available and still evaluated in clinical Phase 3 trials.

Due to technical challenges concerning simultaneous PET/MRI perfusion such as the short half-life, simultaneous injection of radiotracer and MR contrast media while stressing the patient inside the scanner current publications on this topic are limited to few case reports and abstracts. Hence further research involving larger patient cohort studies on this topic is needed to investigate the value of PET perfusion imaging on hybrid PET/MR imaging systems in patients with stable coronary heart disease (Zhang et al. 2012).

8.2.2 Myocardial Infarction

Cardiac MR imaging has been well established for the assessment of myocardial infarction for more than a decade. Beside the analysis of global and regional left ventricular (LV) dysfunction caused by myocardial infarction, and the direct visualization of the area of infarction by late gadolinium enhancement (LGE), cardiac magnetic resonance imaging enables a unique insight into myocardial alterations associated with acute myocardial infarction like myocardial oedema, microvascular obstruction and intramyocardial haemorrhage. Beyond that, cardiac MRI also allows to assess involvement of the right ventricle, which is of high prognostic relevance.

PET imaging is an alternative method to assess myocardial infarction, since FDG PET imaging enables the analysis of metabolic myocardial alterations caused by myocardial infarction, as well as visualization of inflammatory response in areas of acute myocardial infarction (Kandler et al. 2014; Grothoff et al. 2012; Stillman et al. 2011).

Initial hybrid PET/MRI studies focused on the assessment of the infarct size, since the infarct size is considered a major predictor of outcome after myocardial infarction. These case reports and clinical studies demonstrated a moderate to good agreement between myocardial segments showing LGE and reduced FDG uptake after myocardial infarction (Nensa et al. 2013; Schlosser et al. 2013; Rischpler et al. 2015) but the agreement was far from perfect: While in some cases the area of reduced FDG uptake was smaller than the area of LGE, in other cases the opposite was observed. In cases of smaller infarct size in PET compared to LGE, this could be

explained by the higher spatial resolution of MRI with consecutive detection of even small areas of subendocardial infarction invisible for PET. In cases of a smaller area of LGE compared to the area of reduced FDG-uptake, this difference cannot be explained by technical differences. Interestingly, in one of the pilot studies on this topic, a patient with a short symptom-to-reperfusion time of 3 h did not show any infarction in LGE images but an area of reduced FDG uptake, which matched with the area of myocardial oedema in T2-weighted images within the perfusion territory of the culprit vessel. Therefore, it was hypothesized, that in reperfused acute infarction a reduced FDG uptake could represent the area-at-risk of infarction instead the area of myocardial necrosis. This hypothesis was confirmed by two further studies: In 25 patients with reperfused myocardial infarction the area with reduced myocardial FDG uptake was larger than the infarct size, and showed a good correlation with the area-at-risk of infarction as determined by the endocardial surface area (ESA), which is the projection of the LGE on the entire myocardial wall based on the "wave-front phenomenon" of irreversible injury during coronary artery occlusion (Nensa et al. 2015a). In a second study with 21 patients with ST-segment-elevation infarction the area of reduced FDG uptake was compared to the area of myocardial oedema in T2 mapping, which is another estimation parameter of the area-at-risk. This study found that the area with reduced FDG uptake closely matched the area-at-risk as determined by T2 mapping (Bulluck et al. 2016). Since the area with reduced FDG uptake represents the area-at-risk in patients with acute infarction, FDG PET/MRI has the potential for retrospective assessment of myocardial salvage in patients with reperfused acute myocardial infarction, which can be used for the evaluation of strategies to reduce infarct size, such as pre- and post- or remote conditioning.

In a further study the value of PET/MRI for the prediction of functional recovery in reperfused myocardial infarction was assessed, and 28 patients with acute myocardial infarction were examined 5–6 days after percutaneous coronary intervention (PCI). According to this study myocardial segments were rated as viable in PET images when the FDG uptake was greater than 50% compared with remote myocardium, and as viable in MR images, when a LGE transmurality less than 50% was present (Rischpler et al. 2015). While in 82% of LV segments an agreement between LGE transmurality and FDG uptake was observed, discrepant findings were found in 18% of the dysfunctional left ventricular segments ("PET non-viable" but "MR viable"). Interestingly, at follow-up 6 month later, only 41% of the "PET non-viable / MR viable" segments improved the regional wall motion, and the functional recovery of these segments was low and comparable to concordant "PET non-viable/MRI non-viable" segments, indicating that in these segments, FDG PET may be a superior predictor for functional recovery compared to MRI.

As initially mentioned, PET imaging allows additional investigation of the inflammatory response within the area of acute myocardial infarction (Fig. 8.1). In an initial study 49 patients received a low-carbohydrate diet the day before imaging followed by a 12-h fasting period to suppress physiological myocardial FDG uptake (Rischpler et al. 2016a). An increased tracer uptake was observed in an area that nicely matched the area of infarction. Additionally, in a subgroup of the study population the area at risk was assessed by myocardial perfusion scintigraphy with radiotracer injection (^{99m}Tc-sestamibi) prior to revascularization. The area at risk matched the area of FDG accumulation indicating that the inflammatory myocardial response exceeds the infarct zone. Moreover, this study showed that the FDG uptake within reperfused myocardial infarction, which did not show any association with levels of peripheral inflammatory blood cells (such as leukocytes or monocyte subsets), is correlated inversely with functional recovery. The authors concluded, that this imaging approach may offer additional prognostic information about adverse functional outcome, and that this approach might be helpful to monitor and guide novel immune modulatory therapies in patients with acute infarction. As FDG PET imaging reflects glucose metabolism, the FDG signal is not specific for inflammatory processes and may also indicate processes other than inflammation (e.g. ischemic memory of the myocardium after ischemia). Consequently, there is an unmet clinical need for tracers that are (more) specific for inflammation. One such example is ^{68}Ga-pentixafor, a radiotracer that binds with nanomolar affinity to the chemokine receptor 4 (CXCR4; Fig. 8.2). CXCR4 is involved in a variety of mechanisms in the body including neoangiogenesis, metastatic spread of malignant tumors and wound healing. First studies indicate that this tracer may be promising to image the post-ischemic inflammatory response after myocardial infarction (Rischpler et al. 2016b; Thackeray et al. 2015; Lapa et al. 2015) - however larger, prospective studies to evaluate the prognostic value of this approach are needed.

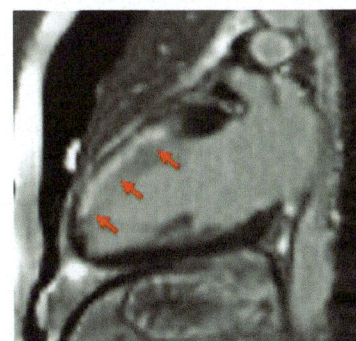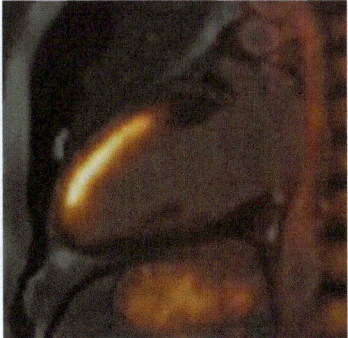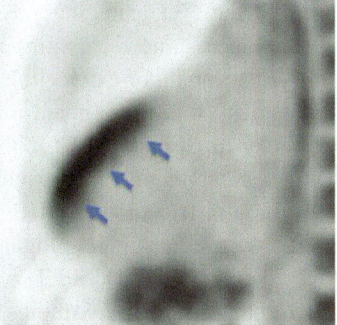

Fig. 8.1 'Fasted' FDG PET/MR images (2-chamber views: MRI only [left], FDG PET only [right] and overlay [middle]) of a patient who suffered from acute STEMI a few days before: Note subendocardial late gadolinium enhancement of the anterior wall on MR images (red arrows) with intense FDG accumulation on PET images (blue arrows) indicating intense post-ischemic inflammation in the infarcted area

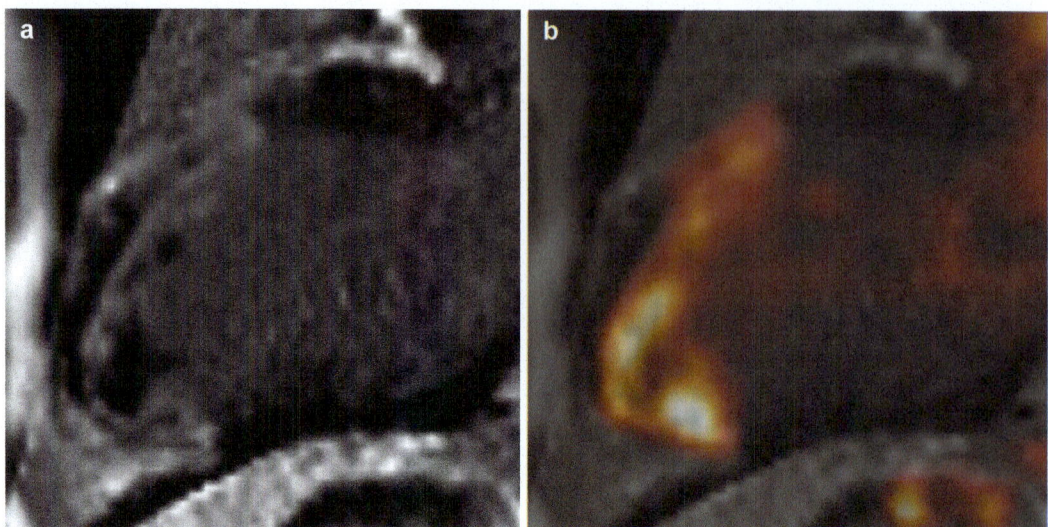

Fig. 8.2 ^{68}Ga-penixafor PET/MRI of a patient with large myocardial infarction. The images show an intense CXCR4-expression in the area of infarction and around the left ventricular thrombus in the apex

8.3   Inflammatory Heart Disease

The detection of cardiac inflammation either of the myocardium, the endocardium or the pericardium is of great clinical interest.

Within the last years cardiac MRI has become an established imaging modality for the noninvasive assessment of inflammation of the myocardium and pericardium, due to the fact that cardiac MRI enables the detection of even small areas of myocardial inflammation, the detection of regional and global wall motion abnormalities, the assessment of myocardial oedema and hyperaemia as well as pericardial effusion. Despite these encouraging possibilities of cardiac MRI and new emerging approaches like T1-/ T2-mapping or extracellular volume (ECV) assessment, it must be noted that the diagnostic accuracy of cardiac MRI for the assessment of cardiac inflammation is far from perfect.

In contrast to cardiac MRI which predominantly focuses on morphologic changes caused by inflammation, FDG-PET focuses on metabolic changes, and many studies showed the great potential of PET imaging for the detection and monitoring of inflammation. Furthermore, a number of non-FDG tracers targeting different aspects of inflammation ranging from chemokine expression over cellular involvement to changes in the myocardial tissue composition may add significant value to cardiac PET/MRI in future (Wu et al. 2013).

Therefore, a combination of multi-parametric MRI with the high sensitivity and outstanding quantification capabilities of ^{18}F–FDG-PET could represent a powerful imaging modality for cardiac inflammation.

8.3.1   Myocarditis

Myocarditis, also known as inflammatory cardiomyopathy, is the inflammation of the myocardium most often due to viral infections, even though other causes exists including bacterial infections, certain medications, toxins, autoimmune disorders or even physical agents. The symptoms of myocarditis can include shortness of breath, chest pain, decreased ability to exercise, and an irregular heartbeat. In most cases the symptoms of myocarditis are mild; however infarction like symptoms as well as rapid progressive heart failure can occur. Due to the often unspecific clinical symptoms myocarditis is not correctly diagnosed in many cases, leaving the true incidence of myocarditis unknown.

In a first feasibility study on PET/MRI 65 consecutive patients with suspected acute myocarditis according to the diagnostic criteria of the European Society of cardiology (ESC) were included (Nensa et al. 2016). Integrated PET/MRI with FDG was performed after preparing the patients with a high-fat and low-carbohydrate diet. While 42% of patients demonstrated typical MRI findings of myocarditis, pathological FDG uptake was found in 33%. Six patients showed pathological MR findings in the absence of pathological FDG uptake, whereas one patient showed a pathological FDG uptake in absence of pathological MR findings. Overall, a moderate spatial correlation was found between the areas of increased FDG uptake and the areas of pathological MR findings ($\kappa = 0.73$). Although this pilot study has demonstrated the feasibility of hybrid FDG PET/MRI in a medium-sized study population, further studies are needed to demonstrate the added value of integrated PET/MRI in the diagnostic work-up of patients with suspected myocarditis compared to MRI alone.

A case report (Fig. 8.3) has demonstrated the use of FDG-PET/MRI in a case of myocarditis caused by parvovirus B19 (Nensa et al. 2014). In this report, focal subepicardial LGE was closely matched by intense FDG uptake and accompanied by myocardial edema and hyperemia. While MRI would have been sufficient for the detection

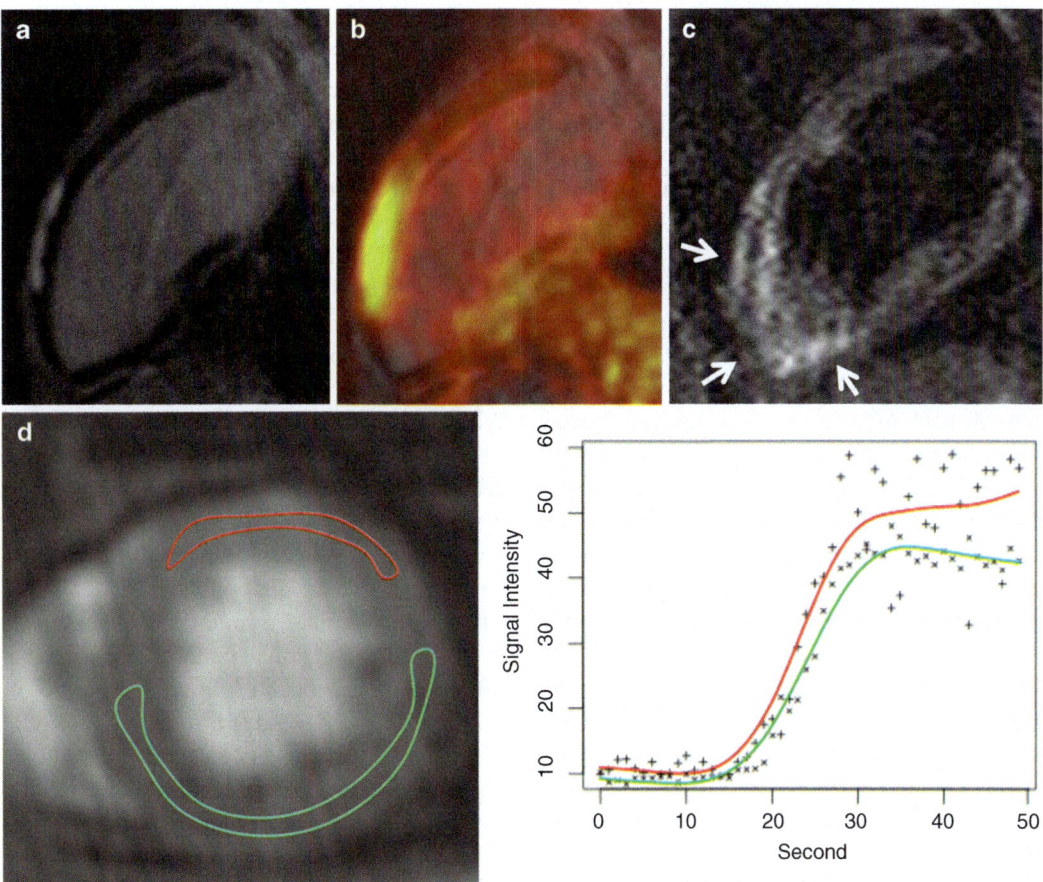

Fig. 8.3 FDG PET/MRI in a patient with acute viral myocarditis caused by parvovirus B19. Subepicardial late gadolinium enhancement (**a**) was found in the LV anterior wall that was in excellent agreement with increased FDG uptake (**b**). T2-weighted images revealed an edema in the LV anterior wall (**c**). Dynamic perfusion imaging revealed hyperemia in the LV anterior wall (**d**) [with kind permission from Ref. (Nensa et al. 2014)]

and diagnosis of myocarditis in this case, it highlights the ability of PET to quantify inflammatory activity, particularly with respect to disease monitoring. A similar case was reported involving a patient with myocarditis due to Epstein Barr Virus infection with diffuse FDG uptake in the lateral wall that again closely matched LGE and myocardial edema (von Olshausen et al. 2014). Besides monitoring of disease activity, integrated assessment using PET/MRI could increase diagnostic accuracy in cases with ambiguous MRI findings or improve differentiation between acute and chronic/persistent myocarditis. Inflammatory cells can utilize a high amount of glucose and, thus, might express high levels of glucose transporters and increase hexokinase activity, leading to increased FDG uptake in inflammatory infiltrates. As such, FDG uptake is truly complementary to LGE (necrosis and edema), T2-weighted MRI (edema) and early gadolinium enhancement (hyperemia) and could be useful to extend the well-known "Lake Louise Criteria" in the noninvasive assessment of myocardial inflammation in patients with suspected myocarditis ()

8.3.2　Cardiac Sarcoidosis

Sarcoidosis is a non-caseating granulomatous disease of unknown etiology that occurs throughout the world in all races with an average incidence of 16.5 per 100,000 in men and 19 per 100,000 in women. Sarcoidosis is most common in Northern Europe and the highest annual incidence of 60 per 100,000 has been reported for Sweden and Iceland. In the United States African American individuals, particularly women, have a three- to fourfold greater risk for sarcoidosis when compared to the Caucasian individuals. In most cases (70%) sarcoidosis occurs in young and middle aged adults (25–45 years), however, in Europe and Japan there is a second peak in women older than 50 years. Even though the exact cause of sarcoidosis remains unresolved, the current working hypothesis is, that in genetically susceptible individuals infectious (Mycobacterium tuberculosis, Mycoplasma species, Corynebacteria spe-

cies, spirochetes) or environmental (aluminium, pollen, clay, talc) agents trigger primarily the helper-inducer T cells leading to the formation of non-caseating granuloma lesions. Albeit the lung being the most common organ affected by sarcoidosis, sarcoidosis may also involve the heart. While cardiac involvement occurs in at least 25% of patients with sarcoidosis in the United States, and accounts for 13–25% of deaths from sarcoidosis in the US, cardiac sarcoidosis is more common in Japan and is responsible for approximately 85% of deaths from sarcoidosis. The granulomas may involve the pericardium, myocardium, and endocardium, with myocardium being the most frequently involved tissue. Despite the fact, that autopsy studies showed a high prevalence of cardiac involvement of up to 30%, clinical symptoms occur in only 5% of patients. The clinical manifestations of cardiac sarcoidosis range from asymptomatic conduction abnormalities to fatal ventricular arrhythmias and heart failure, depending upon the location, extent, and activity of the granulomatous inflammation. Since early therapy of cardiac involvement (immunosuppression, heart failure therapy, antiarrhythmic therapy and—if necessary—ICD implementation) improves patients' outcome, an early detection of cardiac sarcoidosis is of great clinical interest (Birnie et al. 2014; Doughan and Williams 2006; Costabel et al. 2014).

Several studies showed, that CMR allows the detection of cardiac involvement in sarcoidosis in symptomatic as well as asymptomatic patients. Cardiac sarcoidosis can result in different functional or structural abnormalities in CMR: In cine images cardiac sarcoidosis may demarcate as zones of myocardial thinning and regional wall motion abnormalities in terms of hypo- or akinesia. In T2-weighted images areas of increased signal intensity can be observed as a result of focal myocardial edema due to granulomatous inflammation. In late gadolinium enhancement (LGE) images focal areas of contrast enhancement can be observed due to an increased intercellular space and focal myocardial necrosis in the area of non-caseating granulomatous inflammation. Although areas of LGE predominantly manifest in the mid portion of the myocardium and epicardium, and not in the endocardium, no specific pattern of LGE exists in cardiac sarcoidosis, and cardiac sarcoidosis can even imitate myocardial infarction. Therefore, images must be interpreted in the context of the patient's history and by a cardiologist or radiologist with specific expertise. Despite the challenges in CMR reading, a high sensitivity (100%) and specificity (78%) has been reported for CMR for the diagnosis of cardiac sarcoidosis (Smedema et al. 2005). Moreover, it was shown, that the presence of LGE is associated with death and other adverse events in patients with sarcoidosis (Greulich et al. 2013). As LGE has been shown to diminish in size and intensity after corticosteroid treatment with a strong correlation to clinical improvement, CMR may be utilized for therapy monitoring in cardiac sarcoidosis (Doughan and Williams 2006). Despite all these encouraging facts, it must mentioned, that the differentiation between active inflammation and post-inflammatory residua is difficult in CMR in clinical routine.

Lymphocytes and macrophages are known to be components of non-caseating granulomas in sarcoidosis, revealing high levels of glucose transporters and hexokinase activity, facilitating the utilization of FDG PET as another imaging modality to test for cardiac involvement in sarcoidosis. A meta-analysis comprising 7 studies with an overall of 164 patients yielded a sensitivity of 89% and specificity of 78% for FDG-PET in the detection of cardiac involvement in sarcoidosis.

Therefore, CMR, just as FDG PET are recommended in international guidelines for the non-invasive cardiac assessment of patients with sarcoidosis and cardiac abnormalities (cardiac symptoms like significant palpitations, abnormal ECG, abnormal echocardiogram).

Given that CMR assesses functional and structural changes, while FDG PET assesses metabolic changes due to cardiac sarcoidosis, CMR and FDG PET have to be considered as complementary, synergistic tests, and, therefore, it is expected that a combination of the two features may exhibit a higher diagnostic accuracy when compared to each method alone. Particularly,

the imperfection of CMR in the differentiation between active inflammation and post-inflammatory residua may be compensated for by FDG PET. Several case reports (Fig. 8.4) demonstrated the feasibility of integrated FDG PET/MRI in the detection and therapy monitoring of cardiac sarcoidosis (White et al. 2013; Nensa et al. 2015b; Schneider et al. 2014) and a larger study recently confirmed an improved diagnostic accuracy of integrated PET/MRI. Wicks et al. reported sensitivity rates of 89% for integrated PET/MRI, whereas FDG PET alone yielded a sensitivity of only 65%, and CMR alone of 60% in 51 patients with biopsy-proven or clinically suspected cardiac sarcoidosis (Wicks et al. 2014). Interestingly only poor agreement between the location of increased FDG uptake and LGE was found in this study, which may reflect the circumstance that FDG PET detects active inflammatory, while CMR visualizes additional post-inflammatory residua.

Due to these promising initial results for hybrid PET/MRI and the importance of early diagnosis of cardiac involvement in sarcoidosis it can be expected, that hybrid PET/MRI will move into clinical routine for the diagnosis of cardiac sarcoidosis. Moreover, it is to be expected that hybrid PET/MRI will gain importance in therapy monitoring in cardiac sarcoidosis since FDG PET enables quantitative analysis of inflammation in contrast to CMR.

8.3.3 Infective Endocarditis

Infective endocarditis has an estimated annual incidence of 3 to 9 cases per 100,000 persons in industrialized countries. The highest rates are observed among patients with prosthetic valves, intracardiac devices, or unrepaired cyanotic congenital heart diseases, even though 50% of the cases are shown in patients without a history of valve disease. Risk factors for endocarditis involve age-related degenerative valvular lesions, chronic rheumatic heart disease, hemodialysis, as well as coexisting conditions like diabetes, immunodeficiency, or intravenous drug use (Hoen and Duval 2013).

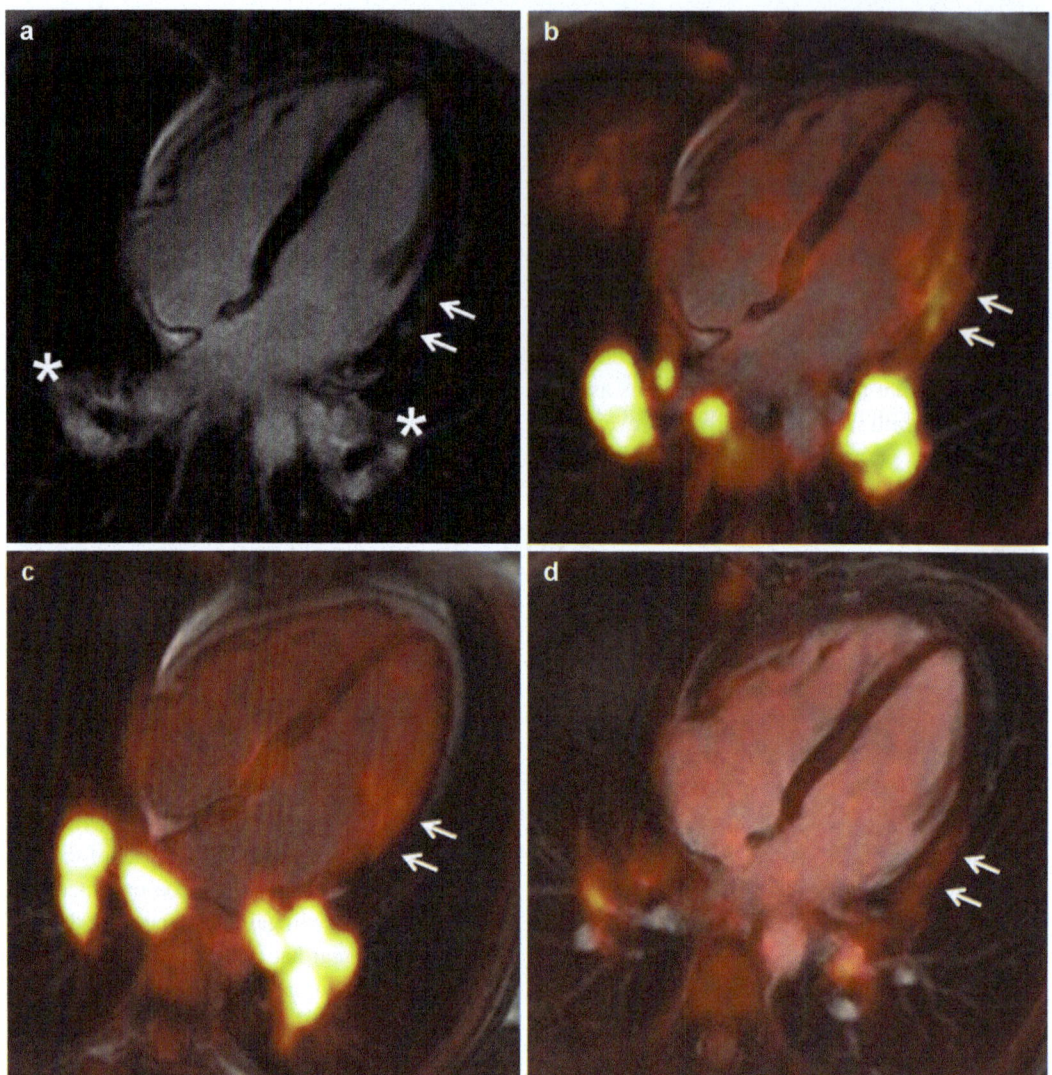

Fig. 8.4 FDG PET/MRI in a patient with general mal-aise, acute retrosternal chest pain, and palpitations. Baseline examination (**a, b**) showed bihilar lymphade-nopathy (**a**, stars) and focal late gadolinium enhancement in the lateral left ventricular wall (**a**, arrows) with corre-sponding intense FDG uptake, supporting the diagnosis of sarcoidosis with myocardial involvement (**b**). After 4 weeks of treatment, PET images (**c**) still demonstrated increased lymphonodular and myocardial (**c**, arrows) FDG uptake, whereas FDG uptake was significantly reduced after 4 months of treatment (**d**). In contrast to FDG uptake, myocardial late gadolinium enhancement remained constant in all three examinations and thus was not an indicator of treatment response [With kind permis-sion from Ref. (Nensa et al. 2015b)]

MRI allows the direct visualization of the valve, as well as the detection and quantification of valve insufficiency caused by endocarditis (Pham et al. 2012). Unfortunately, the diagnostic accuracy of cardiac MRI is relatively low for the detection of valvular vegetations. In a recent study in 16 patients with preliminary diagnosis of infective endocarditis and without valve replace-ment, multi-parametric cardiac MRI was limited to the identification of only 11 patients valvular vegetations (Dursun et al. 2015). Moreover, in case of prosthetic valves cardiac MRI is limited by severe artifacts caused by the prosthetic valve itself.

FDG-PET, on the other hand, allows the direct visualisation of the inflammation due to the fact that active inflammatory cells like lymphocytes and macrophages incorporate FDG, and a recent PET/CT study showed high sensitivity (87%) and specificity (92.1%) for the detection of infectious endocarditis in patients with suspected prosthetic valve endocarditis. Moreover, since PET allows quantitative analyses this imaging modality may also be utilized to monitor therapy response after the initiation of antimicrobial treatment.

Given that cardiac MRI and PET feature complementary information in endocarditis, hybrid PET/MRI seems to be promising in case of native valve endocarditis, but difficult in case of prosthetic valve infection due to metal artefact in MRI as well as in attenuation-corrected PET images (Buchbender et al. 2013). Nevertheless, up to current status, no dedicated studies on the diagnostic value of hybrid PET/MRI in infective endocarditis have been published.

8.4 Cardiac Masses

Cardiac masses can be broadly categorized as either neoplastic or non-neoplastic. While non-neoplastic masses notably in terms of thrombi are frequent findings in clinical routine, neoplastic cardiac masses are exceedingly rare with a reported prevalence of 0.001 to 0.03% based on autopsy observations. Neoplastic cardiac masses can be grouped into primary cardiac tumors, which are tumors that originate from the heart, and into secondary cardiac tumors, which are metastases involving the heart via direct invasion or hematologic spread. While cardiac metastases are uncommon findings in clinical routine, they are reported to be 20–40 times more common than primary cardiac tumors. Approximately 75% of all primary cardiac tumors are benign comprising myxomas, lipomas, fibroelastomas and hemangiomas among the most common ones in adult patients, and rhabdomyoma and fibroma in infants. Albeit their benign biology, these tumors can cause significant clinical effects primarily in dependency of their exact localization within the heart and their extent by altering the

hemodynamics, by embolization or by causing cardiac arrhythmias. The remaining 25% of primary cardiac tumors are malignant, whereas the vast majority (95%) of these entail sarcomas notably angiosarcomas in adults and rhabdomyosarcomas in infants (Motwani et al. 2013).

Due to its wide availability, low costs, lack of contrast material or radiation exposure, its dynamic assessment of cardiac masses in relation to the surrounding chambers, valves, and pericardium, echocardiography is considered the first-line diagnostic test in case of cardiac masses. Moreover, it must be noted, that many cardiac masses are incidental findings in routine echocardiography performed for other indications. Apart from its important diagnostic value as a first-line diagnostic test for cardiac masses, echocardiography has several limitations such as operator dependency, a restricted field of view particularly in patients with pulmonary disease or a large body habitus, and limited imaging of the right heart and mediastinal and extra-cardiac structures. Therefore, in many cases echocardiography either transthoracic or transesophageal does not allow the assessment of cardiac masses with sufficient accuracy. Computed tomography allows further assessment of cardiac masses and offers information regarding anatomical localization, extent, vascularity by means of contrast enhancement, presence of calcification or fat, as well as information about functional consequences in regard to hemodynamics. However, computed tomography has several intrinsic limitations including radiation exposure, necessity of contrast media, lower temporal resolution compared to echocardiography, and lower soft-tissue contrast compared to magnetic resonance imaging, which restrict CT only as a second-line diagnostic modality for the assessment of cardiac tumors. As cardiac MRI features a large field of view, versatility in imaging planes, good temporal resolution, sophisticated possibilities to analyze the tissue composition of a cardiac mass and to assess the tumor's vascularization, cardiac MRI has become the primary imaging technique in the work-up of cardiac masses (Motwani et al. 2013). In a study of 55 patients with cardiac masses a multiparametric MR imaging protocol

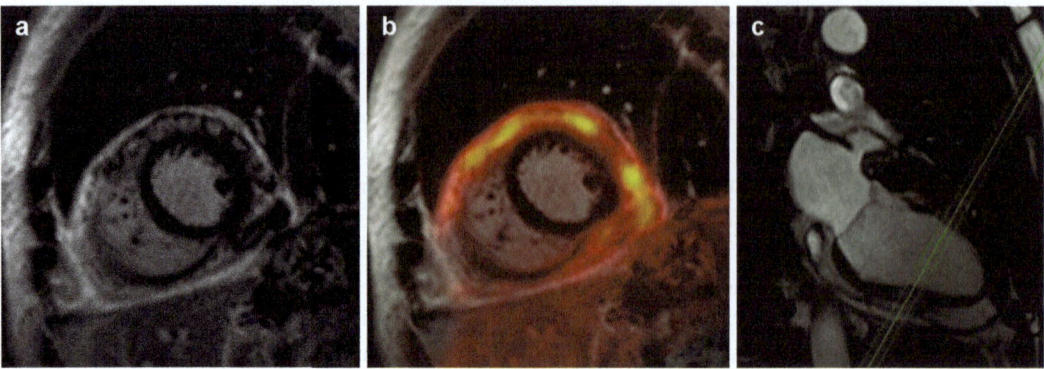

Fig. 8.5 FDG PET/MRI in a patient with pericardial carcinomatosis due to advanced adenocarcinoma of the lung. The short-axis LGE image (**a**) demonstrated multiple pericardial metastases with intense FDG uptake (**b**) involving nearly the entire circumference of the heart. Cine imaging demonstrated the beginning pericardial tamponade due to malignant pericardial effusion (**c**)

comprising analyses of signal properties, morphologic characteristics (location, size, infiltrative nature, presence of pericardial effusions) and contrast enhancement showed a diagnostic accuracy of 0.92 for determining a cardiac mass to be malignant or benign (Hoffmann et al. 2003). However, despite the excellent performance of cardiac MRI, the exact classification of a cardiac mass can remain difficult in individual cases in clinical routine. FDG-PET is a different approach to determine the biology (begin vs. malignant) of a tumor, and innumerous oncological studies demonstrated the usefulness of this approach. A recent pilot study evaluated the diagnostic potential of hybrid FDG-PET MRI (Fig. 8.5) for the assessment of cardiac masses (Nensa et al. 2015c): Twenty patients, involving 16 patients with cardiac masses of unknown identity and 4 patients with cardiac sarcoma after surgical therapy, were prospectively examined using integrated cardiac FDG PET/MR imaging comprising a multiparametric MR imaging protocol (cine imaging, T2-weighted images, T1-weighted images before and after contrast administration). Significantly higher maximum standardized uptake values (SUVmax) were found in malignant masses compared to benign and, when a threshold of 5.2 or greater was used, the SUVmax yielded 100% sensitivity and 92% specificity for the differentiation between malignant and benign cases. Cardiac MRI alone showed 100% sensitivity and 92% specificity or the differentiation

between malignant und benign tumors. Combined reading of MRI and PET improved sensitivity and specificity to 100%. Even though this pilot study demonstrated that hybrid FDG PET/MR imaging is convenient for the diagnostic work-up of cardiac masses, this study confirmed the excellent diagnostic performance of cardiac MRI alone, so that hybrid PET/MR imaging seems to be reserved for selected cases in which cardiac MRI is non-conclusive.

8.5 Rare Cardiomyopathies

Cardiomyopathies are a heterogeneous group of diseases, elicited by numerous etiologies, commonly based on some kind of genetic origin, and often part of a systemic disease (Maron et al. 2006). While common features of cardiomyopathies such as myocardial hypertrophy or dilatation can regularly be visualized using diagnostic imaging, the underlying pathomechanisms often remain unclear.

Up to current status publications on FDG-PET/MRI in cardiomyopathies are mainly restricted to case reports and small patient cohort studies. A case report has shown the use of FDG PET/MRI in a patient with stress-induced transient mid ventricular ballooning syndrome, a variant of Takotsubo cardiomyopathy (Ibrahim et al. 2012). The patient was prepared with a low-fat, low-carbohydrate diet before the examination. An increased glucose metabolism within the dysfunctional mid ventricular segments was observed, whereas the FDG uptake was suppressed in the normal myocardium. Using cine MRI sequences a left ventricular mid ventricular dysfunction was observed, while late gadolinium-enhancement MRI did not depict any myocardial hyper enhancement. The combined information allowed for the delineation of neurogenic myocardial stunning. The authors concluded that cardiac PET/MRI may provide further insight into the underlying pathophysiology of stress-induced cardiomyopathy.

Another case report showed the use of FDG PET/MRI after oral glucose loading in a patient with non-obstructive hypertrophic cardiomyopathy (HCM) (Kong et al. 2013). First pass MR perfusion imaging showed reduced myocardial blood flow in the hypertrophic septum, that corresponded to contrast-enhancement in LGE images and patchy FDG uptake defects in PET images. This was interpreted as myocardial fibrosis. Based on the results of an animal study the authors speculate, that the reduction of glucose uptake in progressive HCM over time could precede its progression to heart failure (Handa et al. 2007). They concluded that cardiac FDG PET/MRI could be helpful in the differential diagnosis of LGE and risk stratification of HCM.

Anderson-Fabry disease is an x-linked lysosomal storage disease which is known to cause characteristic basal inferolateral wall fibrosis. A PET/MRI study of 13 patients with FDG revealed that all patients showed increased myocardial tracer uptake, but only few showed corresponding late gadolinium-enhancement on MR images (Nappi et al. 2015). The authors conclude, that further studies evaluating the role of hybrid PET/MR in disease management and monitoring the effect of enzyme replacement therapy in larger patient populations are needed.

Loeffler's endocarditis is a rare restrictive cardiomyopathy characterized by hypereosinophilia and fibrous thickening of the endocardium, with usually large thrombi attached to the ventricular walls that can cause cardiovascular complications such as heart failure and thromboembolism. One case report described FDG PET/MRI in a patient with Loeffler's endocarditis (Langwieser

et al. 2014). While cardiac MRI revealed late gadolinium enhanced (LGE) circumferentially to the endocardium within the apical region of both ventricles, as well as apical thrombotic masses, PET revealed the presence of active inflammation not only in the areas of LGE but also within the apical masses, demonstrating the complementary information facilitated by CMR and PET.

8.6 Summary

Several studies demonstrated, that hybrid cardiac PET/MRI is feasible with a robust and high image quality of the MR as well as PET images. Moreover, it was demonstrated that the MR image quality is not compromised by the PET component and that the MR-based attenuation-correction provides sufficient accuracy for most clinical applications.

Several case reports and initial pilot studies demonstrated, that hybrid PET/MRI is promising for the application in various pathologies including myocardial infarction, inflammatory heart diseases such as myocarditis and cardiac sarcoidosis as well as cardiac tumors. However, larger studies are necessary to demonstrate its potential to provide clinically relevant added value in comparison to current standards of care.

Emerging technical improvements such as MR-based PET motion correction will lead to higher spatial and temporal resolution, possibly enabling advanced applications such as imaging of coronary atherosclerosis. Beyond that, the translation of already existing PET tracers from preclinical imaging into clinical routine will open up further new possibilities for PET/MR cardiac imaging.

References

Ahmadian A, Pawar S, Govender P, Berman J, Ruberg FL, Miller EJ. The response of FDG uptake to immuno-suppressive treatment on FDG PET/CT imaging for cardiac sarcoidosis. J Nucl Cardiol. 2016;
Birnie DH, Sauer WH, Bogun F, et al. HRS expert consensus statement on the diagnosis and management of arrhythmias associated with cardiac sarcoidosis. Heart Rhythm. 2014;11:1305–23.

Buchbender C, Hartung-Knemeyer V, Forsting M, Antoch G, Heusner TA. Positron emission tomography (PET) attenuation correction artefacts in PET/CT and PET/MRI. Br J Radiol. 2013;86:20120570.

Bulluck H, White SK, Frohlich GM, et al. Quantifying the area at risk in reperfused ST-segment-elevation myocardial infarction patients using hybrid cardiac positron emission tomography-magnetic resonance imaging. Circ Cardiovasc Imaging. 2016:9.

Costabel U, Skowasch D, Pabst S, et al. Konsensuspapier der Deutschen Gesellschaft für Pneumologie und Beatmungsmedizin (DGP) und der Deutschen Gesellschaft für Kardiologie – Herz und Kreislaufforschung (DGK) zur Diagnostik und Therapie der kardialen Sarkoidose. Kardiologe. 2014;8:13–25.

De Bruyne B, Pijls NH, Kalesan B, et al. Fractional flow reserve-guided PCI versus medical therapy in stable coronary disease. N Engl J Med. 2012;367:991–1001.

Doughan AR, Williams BR. Cardiac sarcoidosis. Heart. 2006;92:282–8.

Dursun M, Yilmaz S, Yilmaz E, et al. The utility of cardiac MRI in diagnosis of infective endocarditis: preliminary results. Diagn Interv Radiol. 2015;21:28–33.

Friedrich MG, Sechtem U, Schulz-Menger J, et al. Cardiovascular magnetic resonance in myocarditis: a JACC White Paper. J Am Coll Cardiol. 2009;53:1475–87.

Greulich S, Deluigi CC, Gloekler S, et al. CMR imaging predicts death and other adverse events in suspected cardiac sarcoidosis. JACC Cardiovasc Imaging. 2013;6:501–11.

Grothoff M, Elpert C, Hoffmann J, et al. Right ventricular injury in ST-elevation myocardial infarction: risk stratification by visualization of wall motion, edema, and delayed-enhancement cardiac magnetic resonance. Circ Cardiovasc Imaging. 2012;5:60–8.

Hagemann CE, Ghotbi AA, Kjaer A, Hasbak P. Quantitative myocardial blood flow with Rubidium-82 PET: a clinical perspective. Am J Nucl Med Mol Imaging. 2015;5:457–68.

Handa N, Magata Y, Mukai T, Nishina T, Konishi J, Komeda M. Quantitative FDG-uptake by positron emission tomography in progressive hypertrophy of rat hearts in vivo. Ann Nucl Med. 2007;21:569–76.

Hendel RC, Berman DS, Di Carli MF, et al. ACCF/ASNC/ACR/AHA/ASE/SCCT/SCMR/SNM 2009 Appropriate Use Criteria for Cardiac Radionuclide Imaging A Report of the American College of Cardiology Foundation Appropriate Use Criteria Task Force, the American Society of Nuclear Cardiology, the American College of Radiology, the American Heart Association, the American Society of Echocardiography, the Society of Cardiovascular Computed Tomography, the Society for Cardiovascular Magnetic Resonance, and the Society of Nuclear Medicine Endorsed by the American College of Emergency Physicians. J Am Coll Cardiol. 2009;53:2201–29.

Hoen B, Duval X. Clinical practice. Infective endocarditis. N Engl J Med. 2013;368:1425–33.

Hoffmann U, Globits S, Schima W, et al. Usefulness of magnetic resonance imaging of cardiac and paracardiac masses. Am J Cardiol. 2003;92:890–5.

Hundley WG, Bluemke DA, Finn JP, et al. ACCF/ACR/AHA/NASCI/SCMR 2010 Expert consensus document on cardiovascular magnetic resonance: a report of the American College of Cardiology Foundation Task Force on Expert Consensus Documents. Circulation. 2010;121:2462–508.

Ibrahim T, Nekolla SG, Langwieser N, et al. Simultaneous positron emission tomography/magnetic resonance imaging identifies sustained regional abnormalities in cardiac metabolism and function in stress-induced transient midventricular ballooning syndrome: a variant of Takotsubo cardiomyopathy. Circulation. 2012;126:e324–6.

Ishida Y, Yoshinaga K, Miyagawa M, et al. Recommendations for (18)F-fluorodeoxyglucose positron emission tomography imaging for cardiac sarcoidosis: Japanese Society of Nuclear Cardiology recommendations. Ann Nucl Med. 2014;28:393–403.

Kandler D, Lucke C, Grothoff M, et al. The relation between hypointense core, microvascular obstruction and intramyocardial haemorrhage in acute reperfused myocardial infarction assessed by cardiac magnetic resonance imaging. Eur Radiol. 2014;24:3277–88.

Kong EJ, Lee SH, Cho IH. Myocardial fibrosis in hypertrophic cardiomyopathy demonstrated by integrated cardiac F-18 FDG PET/MR. Nucl Med Mol Imaging. 2013;47:196–200.

Langwieser N, von Olshausen G, Rischpler C, Ibrahim T. Confirmation of diagnosis and graduation of inflammatory activity of Loeffler endocarditis by hybrid positron emission tomography/magnetic resonance imaging. Eur Heart J. 2014;35:2496.

Lapa C, Reiter T, Werner RA, et al. [(68)Ga]pentixafor-PET/CT for imaging of chemokine receptor 4 expression after myocardial infarction. JACC Cardiovasc Imaging. 2015;8:1466–8.

Manabe O, Yoshinaga K, Ohira H, et al. The effects of 18-h fasting with low-carbohydrate diet preparation on suppressed physiological myocardial (18)F-fluorodeoxyglucose (FDG) uptake and possible minimal effects of unfractionated heparin use in patients with suspected cardiac involvement sarcoidosis. J Nucl Cardiol. 2016;23:244–52.

Montalescot G, Sechtem U, Achenbach S, et al. 2013 ESC guidelines on the management of stable coronary artery disease: the Task Force on the management of stable coronary artery disease of the European Society of Cardiology. Eur Heart J. 2013;34:2949–3003.

Maron BJ, Towbin JA, Thiene G, et al. Contemporary definitions and classification of the cardiomyopathies: an American Heart Association Scientific Statement from the Council on Clinical Cardiology, Heart Failure and Transplantation Committee; Quality of Care and Outcomes Research and Functional

Genomics and Translational Biology Interdisciplinary Working Groups; and Council on Epidemiology and Prevention. Circulation. 2006;113:1807–16.

Motwani M, Kidambi A, Herzog BA, Uddin A, Greenwood JP, Plein S. MR imaging of cardiac tumors and masses: a review of methods and clinical applications. Radiology. 2013;268:26–43.

Nappi C, Altiero M, Imbriaco M, et al. First experience of simultaneous PET/MRI for the early detection of cardiac involvement in patients with Anderson-Fabry disease. Eur J Nucl Med Mol Imaging. 2015;42:1025–31.

Nensa F, Poeppel TD, Beiderwellen K, et al. Hybrid PET/MR imaging of the heart: feasibility and initial results. Radiology. 2013;268:366–73.

Nensa F, Poeppel TD, Krings P, Schlosser T. Multiparametric assessment of myocarditis using simultaneous positron emission tomography/magnetic resonance imaging. Eur Heart J. 2014;35:2173.

Nensa F, Poeppel T, Tezgah E, et al. Integrated FDG PET/MR imaging for the assessment of myocardial salvage in reperfused acute myocardial infarction. Radiology. 2015a;276:400–7.

Nensa F, Tezgah E, Poeppel T, Nassenstein K, Schlosser T. Diagnosis and treatment response evaluation of cardiac sarcoidosis using positron emission tomography/magnetic resonance imaging. Eur Heart J. 2015b;36:550.

Nensa F, Tezgah E, Poeppel TD, et al. Integrated 18F-FDG PET/MR imaging in the assessment of cardiac masses: a pilot study. J Nucl Med. 2015c;56:255–60.

Nensa F, Kloth J, Tezgah E, Poeppel TD, et al. Feasibility of FDGPET in myocarditis: Comparison to CMR using integrated PET/MRI. J Nucl Cardiol. 2016. [Epub ahead of print] PubMed PMID: 27638745.

Nensa F, Tezgah E, Schweins K, et al. Evaluation of a low-carbohydrate diet-based preparation protocol without fasting for cardiac PET/MR imaging. J Nucl Cardiol. 2017a;24(3):980–88. doi: 10.1007/s12350-016-0443-1. Epub 2016 Mar 18. PubMed PMID: 26993494.

Nensa F, Poeppel TD, Tezgah E, et al. Integrated assessment of cardiac PET/MRI: co-registered PET and MRI polar plots by mutual MR-based segmentation of the left ventricular myocardium. World J Cardiovasc Dis. 2017b;7:91–104.

von Olshausen G, Hyafil F, Langwieser N, Laugwitz KL, Schwaiger M, Ibrahim T. Detection of acute inflammatory myocarditis in Epstein Barr virus infection using hybrid 18F-fluoro-deoxyglucose-positron emission tomography/magnetic resonance imaging. Circulation. 2014;130:925–6.

Petibon Y, Ouyang J, Zhu X, et al. Cardiac motion compensation and resolution modeling in simultaneous PET-MR: a cardiac lesion detection study. Phys Med Biol. 2013;58:2085–102.

Pham N, Zaitoun H, Mohammed TL, et al. Complications of aortic valve surgery: manifestations at CT and MR imaging. Radiographics. 2012;32:1873–92.

Rischpler C, Higuchi T, Nekolla SG. Current and Future Status of PET Myocardial Perfusion Tracers. Curr Cardiovasc Imaging Rep. 2014;8:9303.

Rischpler C, Langwieser N, Souvatzoglou M, et al. PET/MRI early after myocardial infarction: evaluation of viability with late gadolinium enhancement transmurality vs. 18F-FDG uptake. Eur Heart J Cardiovasc Imaging. 2015;16:661–9.

Rischpler C, Dirschinger RJ, Nekolla SG, et al. Prospective evaluation of 18F-fluorodeoxyglucose uptake in postischemic myocardium by simultaneous positron emission tomography/magnetic resonance imaging as a prognostic marker of functional outcome. Circ Cardiovasc Imaging. 2016a;9:e004316.

Rischpler C, Nekolla SG, Kossmann H, et al. Upregulated myocardial CXCR4-expression after myocardial infarction assessed by simultaneous GA-68 pentixafor PET/MRI. J Nucl Cardiol. 2016b;23:131–3.

Sanchis-Gomar F, Perez-Quilis C, Leischik R, Lucia A. Epidemiology of coronary heart disease and acute coronary syndrome. Ann Transl Med. 2016;4:256.

Schlosser T, Nensa F, Mahabadi AA, Poeppel TD. Hybrid MRI/PET of the heart: a new complementary imaging technique for simultaneous acquisition of MRI and PET data. Heart. 2013;99:351–2.

Schneider S, Batrice A, Rischpler C, Eiber M, Ibrahim T, Nekolla SG. Utility of multimodal cardiac imaging with PET/MRI in cardiac sarcoidosis: implications for diagnosis, monitoring and treatment. Eur Heart J. 2014;35:312.

Sciagra R, Passeri A, Bucerius J, et al. Clinical use of quantitative cardiac perfusion PET: rationale, modalities and possible indications. Position paper of the Cardiovascular Committee of the European Association of Nuclear Medicine (EANM). Eur J Nucl Med Mol Imaging. 2016;43:1530–45.

Sherif HM, Nekolla SG, Saraste A, et al. Simplified quantification of myocardial flow reserve with flurpiridaz F 18: validation with microspheres in a pig model. J Nucl Med. 2011;52:617–24.

Smedema JP, Snoep G, van Kroonenburgh MP, et al. Evaluation of the accuracy of gadolinium-enhanced cardiovascular magnetic resonance in the diagnosis of cardiac sarcoidosis. J Am Coll Cardiol. 2005;45:1683–90.

Stillman AE, Oudkerk M, Bluemke D, et al. Assessment of acute myocardial infarction: current status and recommendations from the North American society for Cardiovascular Imaging and the European Society of Cardiac Radiology. Int J Cardiovasc Imaging. 2011;27:7–24.

Task Force M, Montalescot G, Sechtem U, et al. 2013 ESC guidelines on the management of stable coronary artery disease: the Task Force on the management of stable coronary artery disease of the European Society of Cardiology. Eur Heart J. 2013;34:2949–3003.

Thackeray JT, Derlin T, Haghikia A, et al. Molecular imaging of the chemokine receptor CXCR4 after acute myocardial infarction. JACC Cardiovasc Imaging. 2015;8:1417–26.

Vermeltfoort IA, Raijmakers PG, Lubberink M, et al. Feasibility of subendocardial and subepicardial myocardial perfusion measurements in healthy normals with (15)O-labeled water and positron emission tomography. J Nucl Cardiol. 2011;18:650–6.

Vitale GD, deKemp RA, Ruddy TD, Williams K, Beanlands RS. Myocardial glucose utilization and optimization of (18)F-FDG PET imaging in patients with non-insulin-dependent diabetes mellitus, coronary artery disease, and left ventricular dysfunction. J Nucl Med. 2001;42:1730–6.

White JA, Rajchl M, Butler J, Thompson RT, Prato FS, Wisenberg G. Active cardiac sarcoidosis: first clinical experience of simultaneous positron emission tomography--magnetic resonance imaging for the diagnosis of cardiac disease. Circulation. 2013;127: e639–41.

Wicks E, Menezes L, Pantazis A, et al. Novel hybrid positron emission tomography magnetic resonance (Pet-Mr) multi-modality inflammatory imaging has improved diagnostic accuracy for detecting cardiac sarcoidosis. Heart. 2014;100:A80.

Williams G, Kolodny GM. Suppression of myocardial 18F-FDG uptake by preparing patients with a high-fat, low-carbohydrate diet. AJR Am J Roentgenol. 2008;190:W151–6.

Wu C, Li F, Niu G, Chen X. PET imaging of inflammation biomarkers. Theranostics. 2013;3:448–66.

Zhang SH, Rischpler C, Souvatzoglou M, et al. First simultaneous measurement of myocardial perfusion on whole-body PET/MR. J Nucl Med Meeting Abstr. 2012;53:29.

PET/MRI in Inflammatory Diseases

9

Onofrio Antonio Catalano, Aoife Kilcoyne,
Chiara Lauri, and Alberto Signore

Abbreviations

DWI	Diffusion weighted imaging
GE	Gradient echo
HASTE	Half Fourier single shot fast spin echo T2 weighted
MR	Magnetic resonance
PET	Positron emission tomography
SPECT	Single photon emission computerized tomography
STIR	Short tau inversion recovery
VIBE	Volume interpolated breath hold T1 weighted

9.1 Introduction

PET/MRI offers multiple potential advantages in the evaluation of patients affected by benign conditions, such as inflammatory diseases, where

O.A. Catalano, M.D. (✉)
A. Kilcoyne, M.B. B.Ch. B.A.O.
Department of Radiology, Massachusetts General Hospital, Harvard University Medical School, Boston, MA, USA
e-mail: ocatalano@mgh.harvard.edu

C. Lauri, M.D. • A. Signore, M.D., Ph.D.
Nuclear Medicine Unit, Department of Medical-Surgical Sciences and of Translational Medicine, Faculty of Medicine and Psychology, Sapienza University Rome, Rome, Italy

patients may require serial imaging studies and in cases where radiation exposure is of great concern. The most clinically relevant advantages of PET/MRI compared to PET/CT include reduction in radiation exposure, higher soft tissue resolution and co-acquisition.

For equivalent injected activity, PET/MRI allows a 20% reduction in radiation exposure compared to PET/CT, if attenuation correction only is used, or up to 60–73% when both attenuation correction and diagnostic quality CT studies are acquired with PET-CT (Atkinson et al. 2016; Schafer et al. 2014). The peculiar geometry of PET components within PET/MRI scanners, with increased sensitivity in the center of the PET field of view (FOV), allows the administration of a theoretical activity of 35% and a clinical activity of 50% of that required for comparable PET quality from PET/CT (Queiroz et al. 2015).

Moreover, the potential to extend PET data counting over the entire MR acquisition time, improving the quality of the PET images, allows the injected activity to be reduced in an inversely proportional manner. In a phantom study, it has been shown that increasing bed position time by a factor of 8 provides the same signal to contrast with just 12.5% of the activity (Oehmigen et al. 2014). The superior soft tissue contrast of MRI compared to CT allows a better anatomic layout that provides for a more detailed assessment of soft tissues, bones, joints, vessels, and bowel loop lesions. This is also likely to improve the

L. Umutlu, K. Herrmann (eds.), *PET/MR Imaging: Current and Emerging Applications*,
https://doi.org/10.1007/978-3-319-69641-6_9

characterization of incidentally discovered indeterminate findings seen on whole body imaging, as already demonstrated in the oncology population (Catalano et al. 2013). Finally, and as described in greater detail in the paragraphs below, PET/MRI allows co-acquisition of PET and MR data. This may be of value in demonstrating anatomic correlates of PET findings and in allowing matching of biomarkers produced by PET and MRI that might be helpful to investigate, for example the dominant histology of strictures in Crohn's disease or to evaluate the risk of non-stenotic carotid plaques (Catalano et al. 2016; Hyafil et al. 2016).

The combination of reduced ionizing radiation exposure, superior soft tissue resolution and multiple quantitative biomarkers leverages PET/MRI to a highly promising modality for imaging of inflammatory diseases.

9.2   Vascular Pathology

Cardiovascular diseases (CVDs) encompass a wide spectrum of multifactorial pathologic entities, including, but not limited to, transient ischemic attacks, stroke, peripheral arterial disease, angina, and myocardial infarction, that affect >68% of women and >69% of men between the ages of 60 and 79. CVDs are also the leading cause of death worldwide (Benjamin et al. 2017). Inflammatory processes underlie the vast majority of CVDs. Inflammatory cells are involved in each step of plaque pathology, from initiation of plaque formation, to progression, promotion of smooth muscle proliferation, neo-vessel formation, intra-plaque hemorrhage, and even plaque rupture (Amsallem et al. 2016). Several treatment options are available for clinically significant CVDs. However, prevention and early detection are often deemed ineffective, as they are predominantly focused on addressing risk factors and on screening for clinical symptoms and morphologic correlates of overt vascular pathology, at which point CVDs is at an advanced stage.

In this context, there is a clinical need for noninvasive imaging of the inflammatory components of CVDs to aid early detection, quantification of severity, prediction of high risk cases, guide to treatment and monitoring of treatments (Amsallem et al. 2016). PET/MRI may be the ideal imaging technology to address previously encountered shortcomings given its inherent advantages when compared to PET/CT such as co-acquisition of PET and MR data, better metabolic-anatomic matching, lower radiation exposure, higher soft tissue resolution and added functional capabilities (Fig. 9.1).

MRI, even without gadolinium injection, can provide high-quality images of the vascular anatomy, differentiate lumen from the vessels wall, better delineate plaques, and provide insights into their composition, including evaluation of the lipid core and assessment of the plaque cap. Moreover MRI can detect inflammatory changes, including edema and increased vascular permeability, displayed by T2 weighted hyperintensity and early contrast enhancement after Gadolinium injection (Amsallem et al. 2016; LaForest et al. 2016). However, both T2 weighted hyperintensity and the early gadolinium enhancement are difficult to quantitate, being strongly influenced by a plethora of factors, including, but not limited to, B0 strength, sequence specifics and signal processing (Jacobs et al. 2007). As a result, they are considered insufficient as valid quantitative biomarkers.

For these reasons, PET, as an intrinsically quantitative imaging modality, is more appropriate. PET has been shown to allow for the assessment of the inflammatory component of CVDs with common radiopharmaceuticals, like fluorodeoxyglucose (FDG), while other more specific drugs that interact with very selective inflammatory molecules are under investigation, such as 2-fluoropropionyl labeled PEGylated dimeric RGD peptide (FPPRGD2), which targets $\alpha\nu\beta3$-integrin-positive macrophages and neovessels (Amsallem et al. 2016). Maximum standardized uptake value (SUVmax) and maximum target to blood pool ratio (TBRmax) have been successfully used to quantify plaque inflammation, both in PET/CT and in PET/MRI. However due to different attenuation correction methods applied in PET/MRI and PET/CT technology, discrepancies

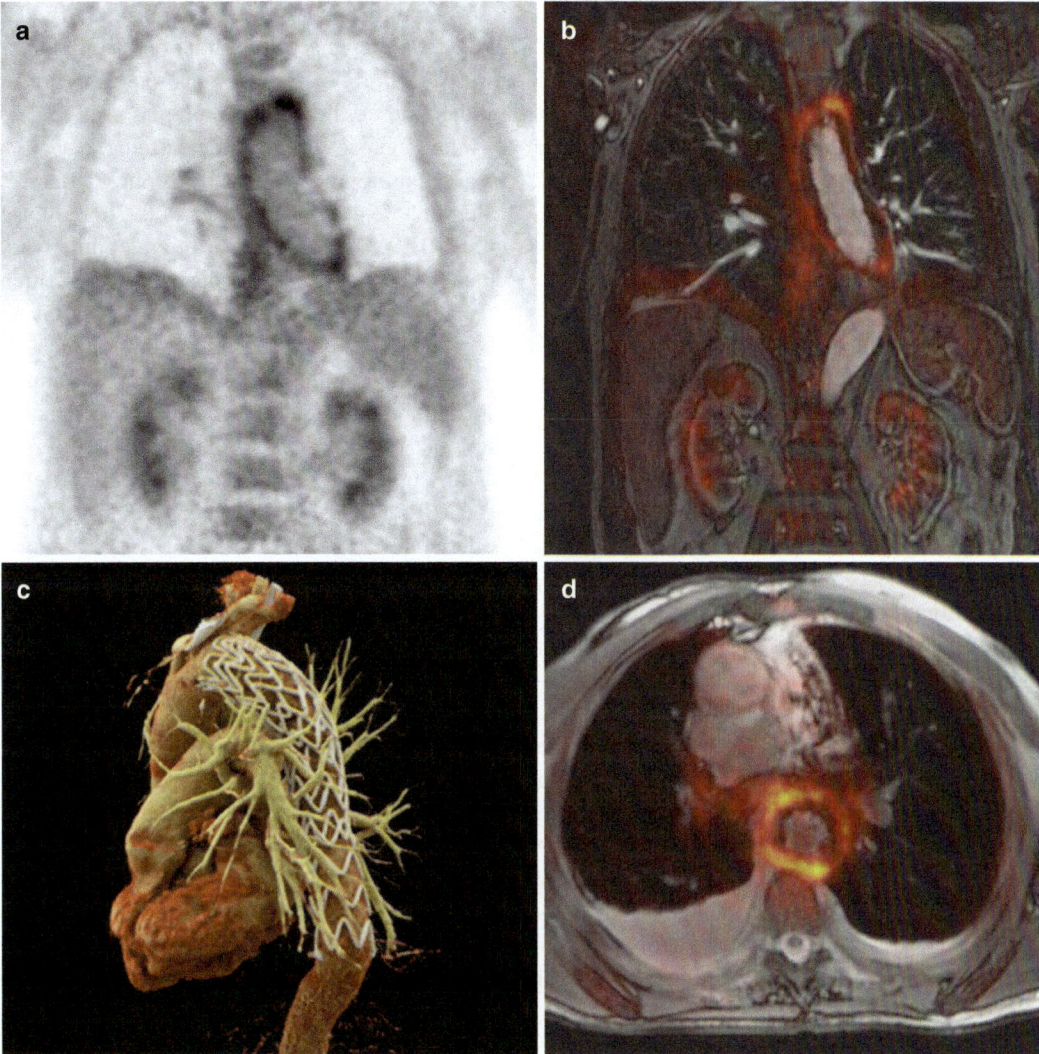

Fig. 9.1 Images of a 82 year old patient with acute inflammation of the aorta after stent graft implantation after acute aortic dissection. The acute aortitis is displayed by pathologic tracer uptake shown in the PET (**a**) and fused images (**b**, **d**). Image (**c**) shows cinematic rendering of the stent graft. Courtesy of Dr. Felix Nensa, Department of Diagnostic and Interventional Radiology and Neuroradiology, University Hospital Essen

between PET/CT and PET/MRI based values exist. In patients undergoing PET/CT followed by PET/MRI, SUVmax of carotid artery plaques were lower on PET/MRI compared to the previously acquired PET/CT, although the values were significantly correlated (Spearman's $r = 0.67$, $P < 0.01$). Conversely, no statistically significant differences were observed between TBRmax as measured on PET/CT and PET/MRI (Li et al. 2016).

In a recent study on ischemic stroke patients classified as cryptogenic and demonstrating non-stenotic carotid plaques, PET/MRI documented higher prevalence (40%) of MR morphologic features of high-risk in non-stenotic plaques in the same carotid territory as that of the stroke. In addition, these high-risk plaques exhibited higher FDG uptake values, facilitating their identification, despite being non-stenotic (Hyafil et al. 2016). As stressed by the authors, the simultaneous evaluation of plaque morphology and metabolism was made possible by the co-acquisition of PET and MR and by the high soft tissue contrast of MR. These factors also permitted localization of FDG uptake to the vessel walls, thereby excluding perivascular structures (Hyafil et al. 2016). Alternative non-invasive imaging techniques have not been shown to be capable of obtaining this information.

9.3 Chronic Inflammatory Bowel Disease

Crohn's disease (CD), along with ulcerative colitis (UC), are responsible for the vast majority of inflammatory bowel disease (IBD) affecting children and adolescents in the developed world. IBD has important epidemiological implications due to its high incidence (10 per 100.000 children in the USA and Canada) and prevalence (100–200 per 100.000 in the USA) in the pediatric population (Rosen et al. 2015). While ulcerative colitis is a long-term condition that results in inflammation and ulcers of the colon and rectum based on continuous involvement of (sub)mucosal wall tissue, CD is characterized by a chronic/relapsing course, the tendency to involve any segment of the gastrointestinal tract and by asymmetric transmural inflammation of the bowel wall (Sleisenger et al. 2010; Ford et al. 2013).

Imaging can assist in establishing the diagnosis, assessing disease extent, determining activity, as well as detecting and characterizing complications, including abscesses, fistulae, and strictures (Anupindi et al. 2014). It also assists with the phenotyping of CD into inflammatory, penetrating, and stricturing variants (Baumgart and Sandborn 2012). While abscesses and fistulae can be confidently evaluated using several imaging modalities, strictures present a greater challenge (Panes et al. 2013). They occur in >10% of patients at diagnosis of CD, with prevalence increasing over time, and constitute a common cause of acute clinical symptoms (Sleisenger et al. 2010; Rieder et al. 2013; Speca et al. 2012). Strictures can be caused by acute transmural inflammation or chronic fibrosis, or a combina-

tion of both (Rieder and Fiocchi 2009; Rieder et al. 2013). Precise differentiation of inflammatory from fibrotic strictures has relevant clinical implications, with medical therapies used in case of inflammatory strictures and surgical resection or dilatation in case of fibrotic strictures (Sleisenger et al. 2010; Rieder et al. 2013; Lenze et al. 2012). However this differentiation is very challenging, with endoscopic techniques often incapable of evaluating the bowel wall layers deep to the mucosa where fibrosis mainly occurs. Therefore, several clinical, laboratory and imaging biomarkers, with variable degrees of accuracy and clinical success, have been employed for this purpose (Sleisenger et al. 2010; Rieder et al. 2013; Lenze et al. 2012; Gee et al. 2011; Adler et al. 2012).

Hybrid imaging, in terms of PET/CT and especially PET/MRI, bears the potential to address both the basic clinical imaging needs for UC and CD patients, including assessment of disease extent and therapy response, as well as distinguishing inflammatory from fibrotic strictures. Despite these benefits, their role in clinical practice remains controversial (Panes et al. 2013; Glaudemans et al. 2010)

^{18}F-FDG PET/CT has been demonstrated to be of benefit in determining the location and severity of disease activity in many inflammatory disorders (Bettenworth et al. 2013; Treglia et al. 2013). Particularly SUV_{max}, and $PVC\text{-}SUV_{mean}$ (partial volume-corrected SUV_{mean}) have been demonstrated to correlate significantly with CDEIS (Crohns Disease Endoscopy Index) subscores ($p < 0.05$) (Saboury et al. 2014). Hence, PET also has a potential role in the assessment of stricturing disease in this context. In particular, the ability of PET to detect active inflammation in strictured segments of bowel could aid in the differentiation of such regions from fibrotic strictures. PET/MRI offers advantages over PET/CT in these clinical context due to the improved anatomic detail and soft tissue contrast of MR, additional functional capabilities of MR, including diffusion weighted imaging (DWI) and apparent diffusion coefficient (ADC) maps, and the simultaneous acquisition of PET data and MR images (Maccioni et al. 2012) (Fig. 9.2). The latter may

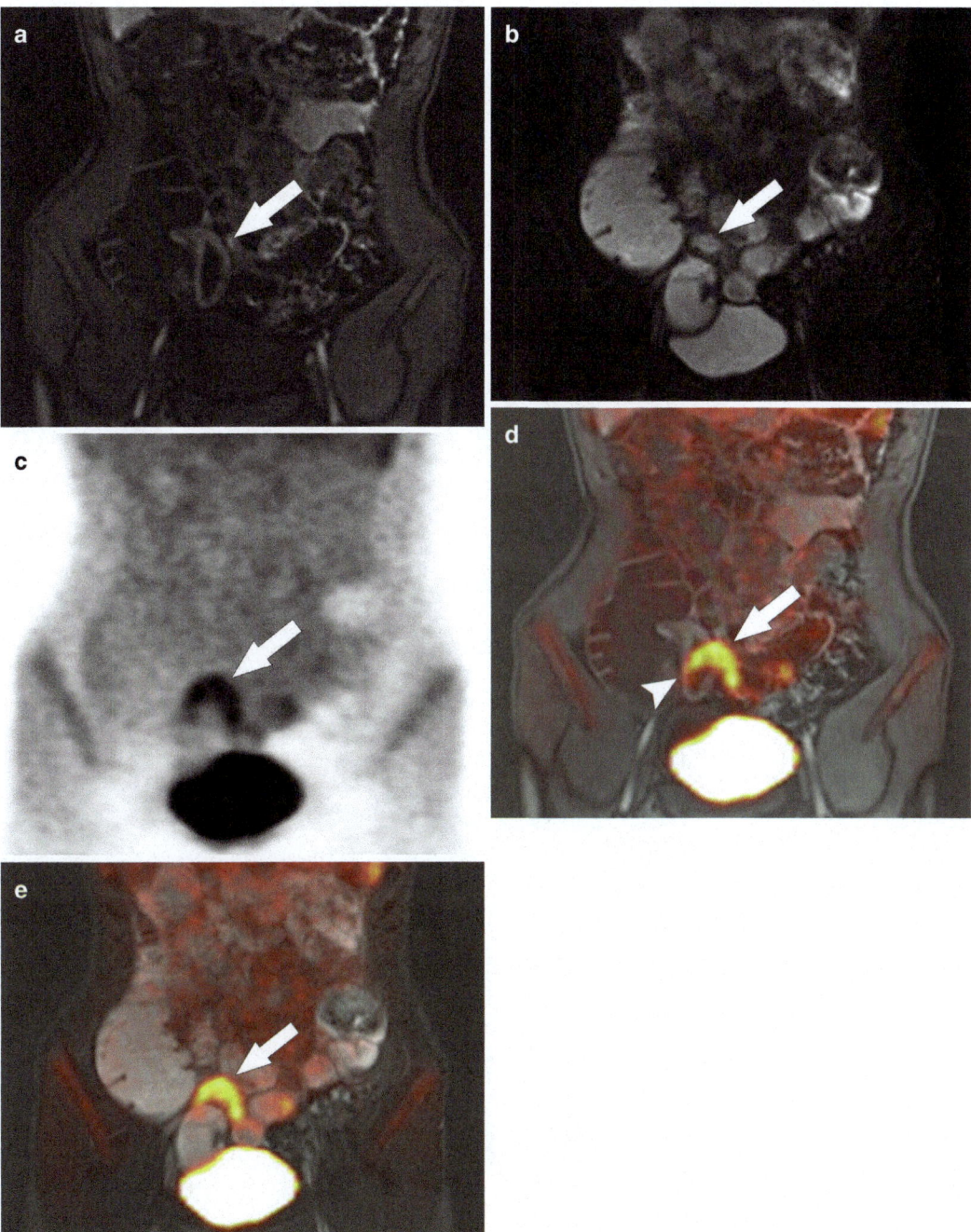

Fig. 9.2 Importance of simultaneous acquisition (co-acquisition) of PET and MR data in evaluating bowel loops in Crohn disease. Coronal portal venouos phase contrast enhanced VIBE acquired after PET (**a**), coronal STIR co-acquired with PET (**b**), coronal PET (**c**), fused coronal portal venous phase VIBE/PET (**d**), fused coronal STIR/PET (**e**). The inflamed last ileal loop (*arrow*) demonstrates wall thickening, increased enhancement, edema, and marked FDG uptake. In (**d**), the morphologic abnormalities as seen on the post-acquired portal venouos phase VIBE do not match with the metabolic abnormalities depicted in the previously acquired PET. On the other hand, a superb match of morphologic and metabolic abnormalities is achieved using co-acquired PET and MR data as in (**e**)

Fig. 9.3 Concordance of MR and PET in demonstrating acute findings of Crohn disease affecting the last ileal loop. Coronal portal venous phase contrast enhanced VIBE (**a**), coronal STIR (**b**), coronal PET (**c**), and fused coronal PET/STIR (**d**). Affected bowel loop (arrow) demonstrate thickened wall, edema, marked contrast enhancement, vascular engorgement, and pronounced FDG uptake

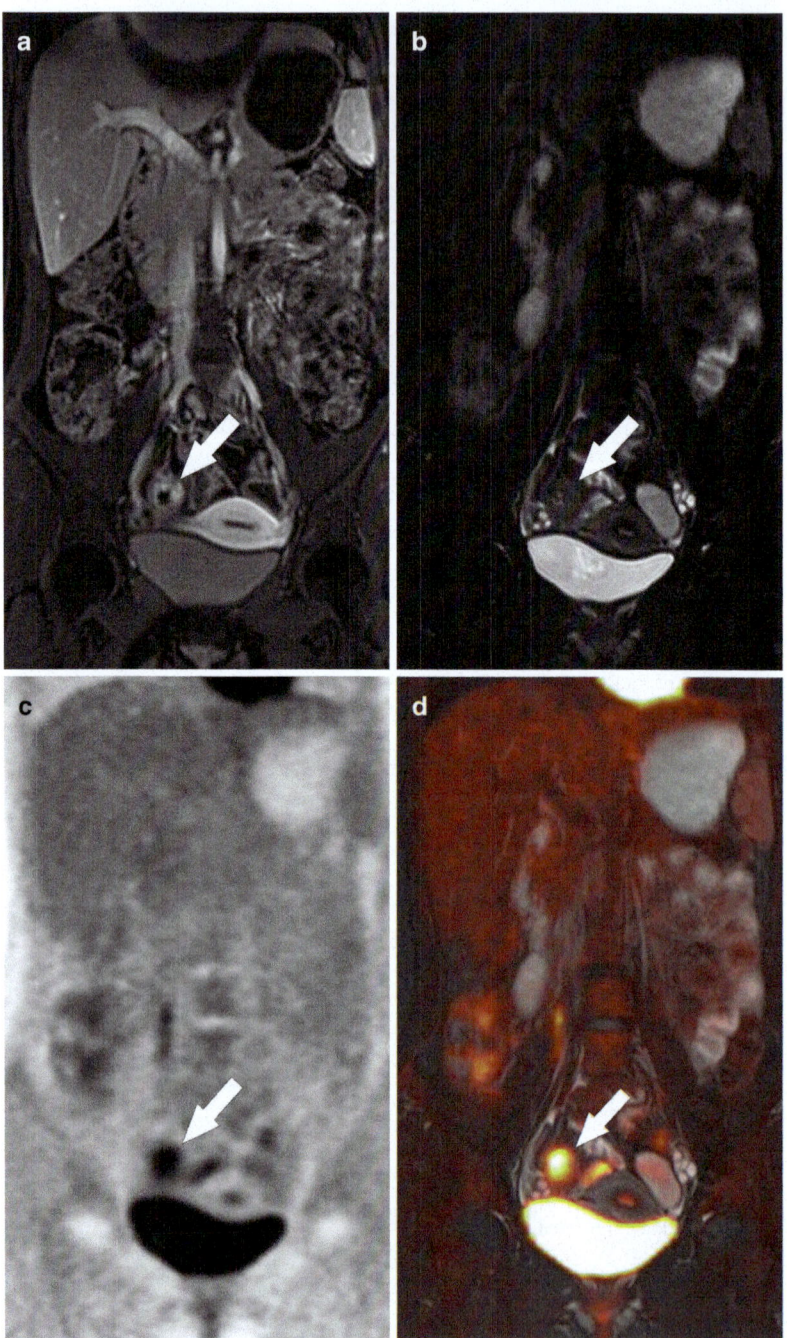

allow an ideal co-registration and fusion of the PET data over the simultaneously acquired MR anatomic layout of the bowel segments, overcoming the challenges imposed by bowel peristalsis that may affect the asynchronously acquired PET/CT data (Fig. 9.3).

Whole body PET/MRI has been shown to offer a significant dose reduction (73%) compared with PET/CT (Schafer et al. 2014). Given the high incidence of CD in the pediatric population, radiation dose and exposure is of significant concern. Several studies have attempted to quantify radiation dose. In a study of over 300 patients with CD in Ireland, CT was identified to account for 77.2% of diagnostic radiation exposure (Desmond et al. 2008). In many of these patients PET/MRI is a now a viable alternative.

Despite the extreme paucity of literature on PET/MRI of Crohn's disease, this new hybrid technique is promising (Catalano et al. 2016; Pellino et al. 2016; Beiderwellen et al. 2016). Therefore we have described our personal experience as well as reviewing the limited available PET/MRI literature, selecting also stand-alone MR and PET research.

9.4 Author's Experience

At our institutions, patients fast for at least 6 hours before imaging to ensure blood glucose levels <140 mg/ml. About two hours before being scanned, patients start drinking two liters of a diluted polyethylene-glycol solution, at the rate of 125 ml every 5 minutes, to be followed by as much as possible of further two liters of the same solution. Eighty to ninety minutes before being scanned, [18]fluorodeoxyglucose (FDG), at an activity level of 40% of that suggested by EANM guidelines, is injected. Five minutes before the start of the PET/MRI-Enterography (PET/MR-E) acquisition, 20 mg of Joscine N-butilbromure (Buscopan; Boehringer Ingelheim, Milan, Italy), or 0.5–1 mg of Glucagon, are injected intravenously. PET/MR-E images are acquired with a Biograph mMR imaging unit (Siemens Healthcare, Erlangen, Germany) by using two 12-channel body coils combined to form a multichannel abdominal and pelvic coil by using total imaging matrix technology. PET/MR-E imaging typically begins 80 minutes after the FDG injection on average. Acquisitions begin from the mid-thigh and move upward to the diaphragm with co-acquired PET and MR sequences, namely coronal short tau inversion recovery (STIR), axial T2w half-Fourier acquisition single shot turbo spin echo (HASTE), coronal T1w Dixon and axial diffusion weighted imaging (DWI), to ensure temporal and spatial matching of the respective data. Thereafter stand-alone breath-hold MR sequences, namely coronal

T2w HASTE, axial T1w dual gradient echo (GE) and dynamic contrast enhanced T1w volume interpolated breath-hold (VIBE) are obtained. Both co-acquired and post-PET-acquired MR images are co-registered and fused with PET.

PET, STIR, and portal venous phase contrast enhanced VIBE are evaluated, both stand-alone and after having been co-registered and fused with PET, to ascertain the quality of the acquisition, identify possible areas of active disease, evaluate disease extent and severity, and rule out false positives. After this preliminary assessment, all the other MR sequences are evaluated on both a stand-alone basis and after fusion with PET. The co-performed portion of the protocol ensures temporal and spatial matching of the MR and PET information, a feature unique to PET/MRI imaging (Catalano et al. 2016).

Overall, actively inflamed bowel loops demonstrate variable degrees of wall thickening (usually >3 mm), mural edema, engorgement of the vasa recta, contrast enhancement, and increased FDG uptake, with high SUV_{max} (> 4), as per stand-alone MR and PET images (Toriihara et al. 2011; Allen and Leyendecker 2014; Dillman et al. 2016; Grand et al. 2015) (Fig. 9.4). High SUV values with associated bowel loops tethering, fixation and distortion are also encountered in case of fistulae.

Inactive sequelae of CD, typically demonstrating less FDG avidity, might be more difficult to detect on stand-alone PET (Lenze et al. 2012; Jacene et al. 2009). In these cases, MR is capable of demonstrating lipomatous hypertrophy, bowel wall thickening, absence of intramural edema and reduced signal on T2w images, as well as focal, slow and progressive contrast enhancement. However MR accuracy in distinguishing active from inactive CD is questionable. For example the target sign (bowel wall thickening and stratified mural enhancement) that is observed in 75% of fibrotic strictures also correlates positively with active inflammation (Steward et al. 2012; Al-Hawary et al. 2014). In our unpublished PET/MRI experience, non-increased FDG avidity (SUV_{max} < 4) may facilitate this distinction.

Strictures, regardless of their histology, are heralded by upstream bowel dilatation that improves

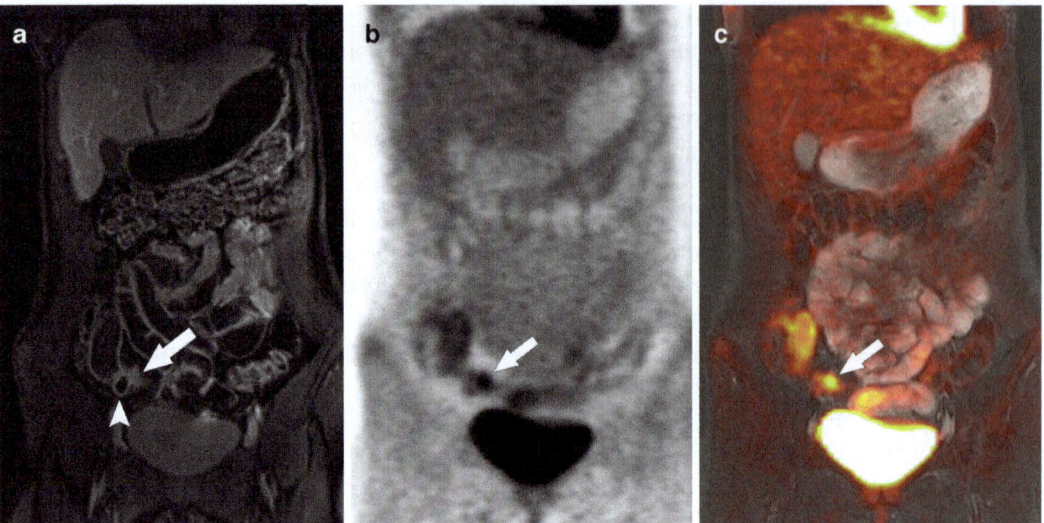

Fig. 9.4 Acute relapse in chronic Crohn's disease in the ileum. Coronal portal venous phase contrast enhanced VIBE (**a**), fused PET/MRI (**b**), Coronal PET (**c**). A pseudo-sacculation (arrowed) is clearly depicted in (**a**) and (**b**) demon- strating the chronicity of the process. On the other side, high FDG uptake (**b**, **c**), with mild thickening and enhancement on the mesenteric border (arrow) of the same affected bowel loop, superimposed, demonstrates an active lesion

detection. Endoscopy or endoscopic biopsy is limited for this purpose (Gee et al. 2011; Burke et al. 2007). Even computed tomography enterography (CT-E) and MR-E, despite the ability to evaluate the entire gastrointestinal tract, and, in case of MR-E, to enable a multiparametric investigation (including reduced T2w signal intensity, lack of early mucosal enhancement, slow and progressive contrast enhancement of the submucosa and muscularis) have moderate accuracy in distinguishing inflammatory from fibrotic strictures (Lenze et al. 2012; Gee et al. 2011; Adler et al. 2012; Lee et al. 2009; Siddiki et al. 2009). Different PET biomarkers, including the ratio between SUVmax of the stricture and SUV median of the liver (SUVmax Stricture/SUVmedLiver), and SUV maximum lean standardized uptake value (SULmax), have been used for the same purpose with varying results. SULmax correlated positively with the intensity of inflammation (8.2 ± 2.8 in severe inflammation versus 4.7 ± 2.5 in mild to moderate inflammation), and was <8 in predominantly fibrotic strictures. However, while sensitivity and specificity were 60% and 100% respectively in detecting active inflammation, SULmax was not capable of differentiating fibrosis or hypertrophy from inflammation. Similarly, another PET/CT bio-

marker, SUVmaxStricture/SUVmedLiver, demonstrated lower values in fibrotic (2.1–4.3) than in mixed (1.8–5.4) or inflammatory (1.7–10.6) strictures, correctly differentiating 53% of strictures, although these results were not statistically significant (Lenze et al. 2012; Jacene et al. 2009).

In a recent study that investigated the performance of PET/MRI in distinguishing active versus fibrotic strictures, with surgical pathology serving as standard of reference, a new hybrid PET/MRI biomarker (ADC*SUV_{max}) that takes into account both the diffusion of water molecules in the intercellular space (apparent diffusion coefficient or ADC) and the FDG uptake, proved useful for this purpose. ADC*SUV_{max} cutoff <3000, was the best discriminator between fibrosis and active inflammation with a mean sensitivity of 67%, mean specificity of 73%, and mean accuracy of 71%, with associated statistical significance (Catalano et al. 2016).

9.5   Spondylodiscitis

Spondylodiscitis (SD) is a particular form of osteomyelitis that specifically involves the intervertebral disk. It is often caused by surgical spine procedures and, less frequently, by hematogenous spread of infectious microorganisms. This infectious disease may destroy the disc, extend to nearby bone tissue causing low back pain, spine deformities and, in serious cases, neurological deficit (Jain 2010; Jutte and van Loenhout-Rooyackers 2006; Hadjipavlou et al. 2000). The incidence of SD is 1:250,000 (about 5% of all cases of osteomyelitis) and it mainly affects men in the fifth to seventh decades (Pigrau et al. 2005).

Radiography is typically one of the first steps in the identification of SD, however it lacks specificity and sensitivity, especially in the initial stages of the disease when bone abnormalities are not present yet. In these situations CT can be useful in order to guide biopsy for a definitive diagnosis (Leone et al. 2012). For its properties to image bone marrow and soft tissue abnormalities, MR is the preferred imaging modality when SD is suspected as it is able to promptly identify one of the first signs of infection: the increase in extracellular fluid of the vertebral body that appears as a reduced signal intensity at T1-weighted and increased signal intensity in T2 weighted sequences (Tins et al. 2007; Tohtz et al. 2010; Tins and Cassar-Pullicino 2004). MR with gadolinium is also crucial for the differentiation between an epidural abscess, that requires surgical drainage, and phlegmon, which represents granulation tissue and is treated with a conservative approach.

While MRI is considered the gold standard in the diagnosis of primary / untreated SD, a recent meta-analysis performed by the Infection/Inflammation Committee of the European Association of Nuclear Medicine (EANM) in conjunction with the European Society of Neuroradiology revealed that the diagnostic accuracy of MR and FDG-PET/CT is similar in case of haematogenous SD, but FDG is superior in case of post-surgical SD (unpublished data). Indeed, the role of [18F]FDG PET/CT in the diagnosis of infection and inflammation is well established (Jamar et al. 2013; Glaudemans et al. 2013) and in this specific situation [18F]FDG PET/CT represents the nuclear medicine modality of choice as it provides a higher diagnostic accuracy than white blood cell scintigraphy

(Turpin and Lambert 2001). In 2013 Hungenbach et al. proposed a five point visual scale for FDG pattern uptake in order to define the severity of the disease (Hungenbach et al. 2013). This classification is used in several centers in the diagnostic setting and for follow-up. Several groups have explored the feasibility of [18F]FDG PET/CT over MR in the diagnosis of SD and in the evaluation of treatments. In a population of nine patients affected by SD, Nakahara and co-authors demonstrated that FDG demonstrates higher sensitivity and specificity than MRI (100% and 79% vs. 76% and 42%). They identified an SUVmax of 4.2 as a threshold for defining the infection (Nakahara et al. 2015). Similarly, Smids et al. demonstrated a superior diagnostic value of [18F]FDG in the earlier phases of the disease (within 2 weeks) and a similar performance after 2 weeks (Smids et al. 2017). Fuster et al. suggest to use [18F]FDG PET/CT as a first line imaging modality and they also proposed the combination of both modalities in order to improve the diagnostic accuracy (Fuster et al. 2015). These studies and their respective results indicate the high diagnostic potential of integrated PET/MRI for assessment of SD, as integrated PET/MRI combines the functional information provided by PET with the high resolution contrast for soft tissue of MR, bearing the potential to significantly improve hybrid imaging when high soft-tissue contrast is desired, e.g. in the diagnostic workup of SD, Fahnert et al. studied 34 consecutive patients with a suspected SD with combined [18F]FDG-PET/MRI using both visual and semiquantitative analyses (SUVmax, SUVmean, SUV ratios between affected and unaffected disk). The results were compared with histopathological findings based on biopsy or surgery (Fahnert et al. 2016). They demonstrated high sensitivity, specificity, PPV and NPV (100%, 88%, 86% and 100% respectively) when PET was fused to MR (Figs. 9.5 and 9.6). The absence of false negative cases in their series enforces the hypothesis that PET/MRI should be used in patients with suspected SD, particularly when MR findings are inconclusive.

However, more studies with larger patient cohorts are necessary to reinforce these results.

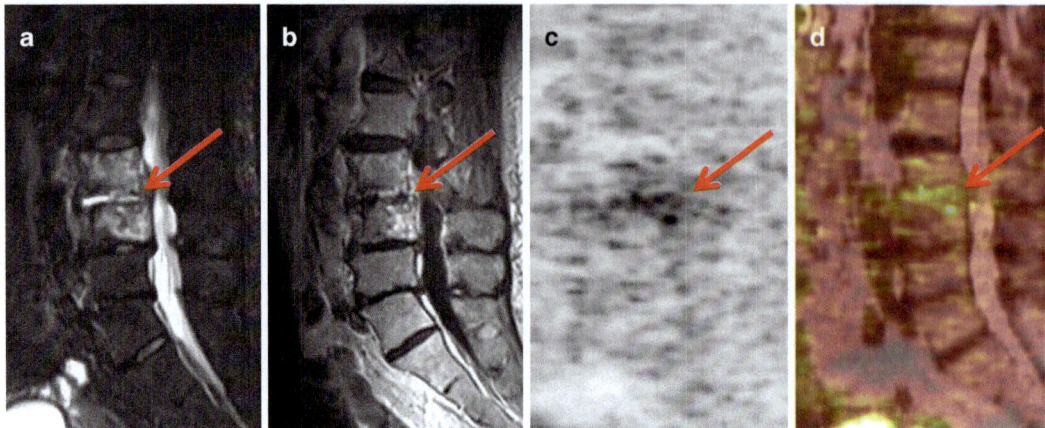

Fig. 9.5 Simultaneous ^{18}F-FDG PET/MRI in a 71-year-old female patient with final diagnosis of spondylodiscitis. MRI was inconclusive: (**a**) TIRM (turbo inversion recovery magnitude) with typical hyperintense signal alterations in the intervertebral disc level L4/5 (arrow) and a moderate post-contrast MRI T1-WI signal (**b**). ^{18}F-FDG PET and combined ^{18}F-FDG PET/MRI (**c**, **d**) show a focally elevated uptake in the affected disc (arrow) as a sign of active inflammation. Courtesy of Dr. Jeanette Fahnert, Department of Diagnostic and Interventional Radiology, University Hospital Leipzig

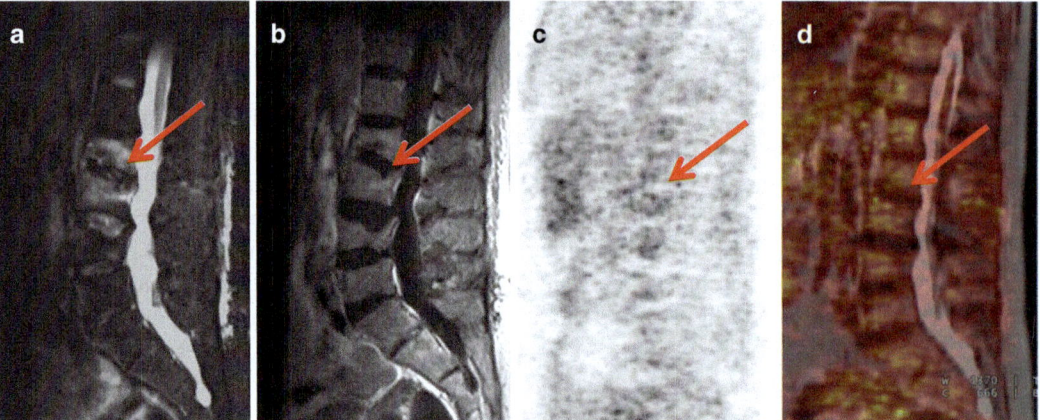

Fig. 9.6 Simultaneous ^{18}F-FDG PET/MRI in a 59-year-old female patient with suspected spondylodiscitis in level L2/3 and final diagnosis of "no spondylodiscitis" but post-fracture changes. Single MRI was inconclusive: MRI, TIRM (turbo inversion recovery magnitude) (**a**) with typical hyperintense signal alterations in intervertebral disc level L2/3 (arrow) but poor post-contrast signal in MRI T1-weighted (**b**). ^{18}F-FDG PET and fused ^{18}F-FDG PET/MRI (**c**, **d**) show no elevated tracer uptake in the suspected disc (arrow), thus active inflammation was excluded. Courtesy of Dr. Jeanette Fahnert, Department of Diagnostic and Interventional Radiology, University Hospital Leipzig

Conclusions

PET/MRI is a versatile and innovative hybrid imaging technique that combines the metabolic information of PET with the high soft tissue resolution, fine anatomic detailing and tissue characterization of MR (Glaudemans et al. 2012). Simultaneous PET/MRI improves co-registration of PET and MR and benefits from the complementarity of the techniques. This makes PET/MRI suitable for all the applications for which MR or PET are currently used in patients with several inflammatory/infective diseases and has demonstrated promising potential in assessing active inflammatory disease and distinguish from fibrotic lesions or scars (e.g. in CD or SD).

In the future, we foresee the use of many other radiopharmaceuticals, in addition to FDG, which have already been successfully applied by SPECT or PET/CT (D'Alessandria et al. 2007), or adapted from other chronic inflammatory diseases. These may ultimately be labelled with positron emitters (such as 18F, 68Ga or 64Cu or 69Zr) for PET/MRI investigations (Nie et al. 2016; Pedersen et al. 2015; Bucerius et al. 2017).

Acknowledgements Authors wish to thank the Nuclear Medicine Discovery association for help provided in bibliographic search. Aoife Kilcoyne would like to acknowledge the support of the Mac Erlaine scholarship from the Academic Radiology Research Trust, St. Vincent's Radiology Group Dublin, Ireland and the Higher Degree Bursary from the Faculty of Radiologists at the Royal College of Surgeons in Ireland.

References

Adler J, Punglia DR, Dillman JR, et al. Computed tomography enterography findings correlate with tissue inflammation, not fibrosis in resected small bowel Crohn's disease. Inflamm Bowel Dis. 2012;18: 849–56.

Al-Hawary MM, Zimmermann EM, Hussain HK. MR imaging of the small bowel in Crohn disease. Magn Reson Imaging Clin N Am. 2014;22:13–22.

Allen BC, Leyendecker JR. MR enterography for assessment and management of small bowel Crohn disease. Radiol Clin N Am. 2014;52:799–810.

Amsallem M, Saito T, Tada Y, Dash R, McConnell MV. Magnetic resonance imaging and positron emission tomography approaches to imaging vascular and cardiac inflammation. Circ J. 2016;80:1269–77.

Anupindi SA, Grossman AB, Nimkin K, Mamula P, Gee MS. Imaging in the evaluation of the young patient with inflammatory bowel disease: what the gastroenterologist needs to know. J Pediatr Gastroenterol Nutr. 2014;59:429–39.

Atkinson W, Catana C, Abramson JS, et al. Hybrid FDG-PET/MRI compared to FDG-PET/CT in adult lymphoma patients. Abdom Radiol. 2016;41:1338–48.

Baumgart DC, Sandborn WJ. Crohn's disease. Lancet. 2012;380:1590–605.

Beiderwellen K, Kinner S, Gomez B, Lenga L, Bellendorf A, Heusch P, Umutlu L, Langhorst J, Ruenzi M, Gerken G, Bockisch A, Lauenstein TC. Hybrid imaging of the bowel using PET/MR enterography: feasibility and first results. Eur J Radiol. 2016;85(2):414–21. https://doi.org/10.1016/j.ejrad.2015.12.008. Epub 2015 Dec 17

Benjamin EJ, Blaha MJ, Chiuve SE, et al. Heart disease and stroke statistics-2017 update: a report from the American Heart Association. Circulation. 2017;135: e146–603.

Bettenworth D, Reuter S, Hermann S, et al. Translational 18F-FDG PET/CT imaging to monitor lesion activity in intestinal inflammation. J Nucl Med. 2013;54: 748–55.

Bucerius J, Barthel H, Tiepolt S, et al. Feasibility of in vivo 18F-florbetaben PET/MRI imaging of human carotid amyloid-beta. Eur J Nucl Med Mol Imaging. 2017;44:1119–28.

Burke JP, Mulsow JJ, O'Keane C, Docherty NG, Watson RW, O'Connell PR. Fibrogenesis in Crohn"s disease. Am J Gastroenterol. 2007;102:439–48.

Catalano OA, Rosen BR, Sahani DV, et al. Clinical impact of PET/MRI imaging in patients with cancer undergoing same-day PET/CT: initial experience in 134 patients--a hypothesis-generating exploratory study. Radiology. 2013;269:857–69.

Catalano OA, Gee MS, Nicolai E, et al. Evaluation of quantitative PET/MRI enterography biomarkers for discrimination of inflammatory strictures from fibrotic strictures in Crohn disease. Radiology. 2016;278:792–800.

D'Alessandria C, Malviya G, Viscido A, et al. Use of a 99mTc labeled anti-TNFalpha monoclonal antibody in Crohn's disease: in vitro and in vivo studies. Q J Nucl Med Mol Imaging. 2007;51:334–42.

Desmond AN, O'Regan K, Curran C, et al. Crohn's disease: factors associated with exposure to high levels of diagnostic radiation. Gut. 2008;57:1524–9.

Dillman JR, Trout AT, Smith EA. MR enterography: how to deliver added value. Pediatr Radiol. 2016;46:829–37.

Fahnert J, Purz S, Jarvers JS, et al. Use of Simultaneous 18F-FDG PET/MRII for the detection of spondylodiskitis. J Nucl Med. 2016;57:1396–401.

Ford AC, Moayyedi P, Hanauer SB. Ulcerative colitis. BMJ. 2013;346:f432. https://doi.org/10.1136/bmj.f432.

Fuster D, Tomas X, Mayoral M, et al. Prospective comparison of whole-body (18)F-FDG PET/CT and MRI of the spine in the diagnosis of haematogenous spondylodiscitis. Eur J Nucl Med Mol Imaging. 2015;42:264–71.

Gee MS, Nimkin K, Hsu M, et al. Prospective evaluation of MR enterography as the primary imaging modality for pediatric Crohn disease assessment. AJR Am J Roentgenol. 2011;197:224–31.

Glaudemans AW, Maccioni F, Mansi L, Dierckx RA, Signore A. Imaging of cell trafficking in Crohn's disease. J Cell Physiol. 2010;223:562–71.

Glaudemans AW, Quintero AM, Signore A. PET/MRII in infectious and inflammatory diseases: will it be a useful improvement? Eur J Nucl Med Mol Imaging. 2012;39:745–9.

Glaudemans AW, de Vries EF, Galli F, Dierckx RA, Slart RH, Signore A. The use of (18)F-FDG-PET/CT for diagnosis and treatment monitoring of inflammatory and infectious diseases. Clin Dev Immunol. 2013;2013:623036.

Grand DJ, Guglielmo FF, Al-Hawary MM. MR enterography in Crohn's disease: current consensus on optimal imaging technique and future advances from the SAR Crohn's disease-focused panel. Abdom Imaging. 2015;40:953–64.

Hadjipavlou AG, Mader JT, Necessary JT, Muffoletto AJ. Hematogenous pyogenic spinal infections and their surgical management. Spine (Phila PA 1976). 2000;25:1668–79.

Hungenbach S, Delank KS, Dietlein M, Eysel P, Drzezga A, Schmidt MC. 18F-fluorodeoxyglucose uptake pattern in patients with suspected spondylodiscitis. Nucl Med Commun. 2013;34:1068–74.

Hyafil F, Schindler A, Sepp D, et al. High-risk plaque features can be detected in non-stenotic carotid plaques of patients with ischaemic stroke classified as cryptogenic using combined (18)F-FDG PET/MRI imaging. Eur J Nucl Med Mol Imaging. 2016;43:270–9.

Jacene HA, Ginsburg P, Kwon J, et al. Prediction of the need for surgical intervention in obstructive Crohn's disease by 18F-FDG PET/CT. J Nucl Med. 2009;50:1751–9.

Jacobs MA, Ibrahim TS, Ouwerkerk RAAPM. RSNA physics tutorials for residents: MR imaging: brief overview and emerging applications. Radiographics. 2007;27:1213–9.

Jain AK. Tuberculosis of the spine: a fresh look at an old disease. J Bone Joint Surg Br. 2010;92:905–13.

Jamar F, Buscombe J, Chiti A, et al. EANM/SNMMI guideline for 18F-FDG use in inflammation and infection. J Nucl Med. 2013;54:647–58.

Jutte PC, van Loenhout-Rooyackers JH. Routine surgery in addition to chemotherapy for treating spinal tuberculosis. Cochrane Database Syst Rev. 2006:CD004532.

LaForest R, Woodard PK, Gropler RJ, Cardiovascular PET. MRII: challenges and opportunities. Cardiol Clin. 2016;34:25–35.

Lee SS, Kim AY, Yang SK, et al. Crohn disease of the small bowel: comparison of CT enterography, MR enterography, and small-bowel follow-through as diagnostic techniques. Radiology. 2009;251:751–61.

Lenze F, Wessling J, Bremer J, et al. Detection and differentiation of inflammatory versus fibromatous Crohn's disease strictures: prospective comparison of 18F-FDG-PET/CT, MR-enteroclysis, and transabdominal ultrasound versus endoscopic/histologic evaluation. Inflamm Bowel Dis. 2012;18:2252–60.

Leone A, Dell'Atti C, Magarelli N, et al. Imaging of spondylodiscitis. Eur Rev Med Pharmacol Sci. 2012;16(Suppl 2):8–19.

Li X, Heber D, Rausch I, et al. Quantitative assessment of atherosclerotic plaques on (18)F-FDG PET/MRII: comparison with a PET/CT hybrid system. Eur J Nucl Med Mol Imaging. 2016;43:1503–12.

Maccioni F, Patak MA, Signore A, Laghi A. New frontiers of MRI in Crohn's disease: motility imaging, diffusion-weighted imaging, perfusion MRI, MR spectroscopy, molecular imaging, and hybrid imaging (PET/MRII). Abdom Imaging. 2012;37:974–82.

Nakahara M, Ito M, Hattori N, et al. 18F-FDG-PET/CT better localizes active spinal infection than MRI for successful minimally invasive surgery. Acta Radiol. 2015;56:829–36.

Nie X, Laforest R, Elvington A, et al. PET/MRII of hypoxic atherosclerosis using 64Cu-ATSM in a rabbit model. J Nucl Med. 2016;57:2006–11.

Oehmigen M, Ziegler S, Jakoby BW, Georgi JC, Paulus DH, Quick HH. Radiotracer dose reduction in integrated PET/MRI: implications from national electrical manufacturers association phantom studies. J Nucl Med. 2014;55:1361–7.

Panes J, Bouhnik Y, Reinisch W, et al. Imaging techniques for assessment of inflammatory bowel disease: joint ECCO and ESGAR evidence-based consensus guidelines. J Crohns Colitis. 2013;7:556–85.

Pedersen SF, Sandholt BV, Keller SH, et al. 64Cu-DOTATATE PET/MRII for detection of activated macrophages in carotid atherosclerotic plaques: studies in patients undergoing endarterectomy. Arterioscler Thromb Vasc Biol. 2015;35:1696–703.

Pellino G, Nicolai E, Catalano OA, et al. PET/MRI Versus PET/CT imaging: impact on the clinical management of small-bowel Crohn's disease. J Crohns Colitis. 2016;10:277–85.

Pigrau C, Almirante B, Flores X, et al. Spontaneous pyogenic vertebral osteomyelitis and endocarditis: incidence, risk factors, and outcome. Am J Med. 2005;118:1287.

Queiroz MA, Delso G, Wollenweber S, et al. Dose optimization in TOF-PET/MRI compared to TOF-PET/CT. PLoS One. 2015;10:e0128842.

Rieder F, Fiocchi C. Intestinal fibrosis in IBD--a dynamic, multifactorial process. Nat Rev Gastroenterol Hepatol. 2009;6:228–35.

Rieder F, Zimmermann EM, Remzi FH, Sandborn WJ. Crohn's disease complicated by strictures: a systematic review. Gut. 2013;62:1072–84.

Rosen MJ, Dhawan A, Saeed SA. Inflammatory bowel disease in children and adolescents. JAMA Pediatr. 2015;169:1053–60.

Saboury B, Salavati A, Brothers A, et al. FDG PET/CT in Crohn's disease: correlation of quantitative FDG PET/CT parameters with clinical and endoscopic surrogate markers of disease activity. Eur J Nucl Med Mol Imaging. 2014;41:605–14.

Schafer JF, Gatidis S, Schmidt H, et al. Simultaneous whole-body PET/MRI imaging in comparison to PET/CT in pediatric oncology: initial results. Radiology. 2014;273:220–31.

Siddiki HA, Fidler JL, Fletcher JG, et al. Prospective comparison of state-of-the-art MR enterography and CT enterography in small-bowel Crohn's disease. AJR Am J Roentgenol. 2009;193:113–21.

Sleisenger MH, Feldman M, Friedman LS, Brandt LJ. Sleisenger and Fordtran's gastrointestinal and liver disease : pathophysiology, diagnosis, management. 9th ed. Philadelphia, PA: Saunders/Elsevier; 2010.

Smids C, Kouijzer IJ, Vos FJ, et al. A comparison of the diagnostic value of MRI and 18F-FDG-PET/CT in suspected spondylodiscitis. Infection. 2017;45:41–9.

Speca S, Giusti I, Rieder F, Latella G. Cellular and molecular mechanisms of intestinal fibrosis. World J Gastroenterol. 2012;18:3635–61.

Steward MJ, Punwani S, Proctor I, et al. Non-perforating small bowel Crohn's disease assessed by MRI enterography: derivation and histopathological validation of an MR-based activity index. Eur J Radiol. 2012;81:2080–8.

Tins BJ, Cassar-Pullicino VN. MR imaging of spinal infection. Semin Musculoskelet Radiol. 2004;8:215–29.

Tins BJ, Cassar-Pullicino VN, Lalam RK. Magnetic resonance imaging of spinal infection. Top Magn Reson Imaging. 2007;18:213–22.

Tohtz SW, Rogalla P, Taupitz M, Perka C, Winkler T, Putzier M. Inter- and intraobserver variability in the postoperative evaluation of transpedicular stabilization: computed tomography versus magnetic resonance imaging. Spine J. 2010;10:285–90.

Toriihara A, Yoshida K, Umehara I, Shibuya H. Normal variants of bowel FDG uptake in dual-time-point PET/CT imaging. Ann Nucl Med. 2011;25:173–8.

Treglia G, Quartuccio N, Sadeghi R, et al. Diagnostic performance of Fluorine-18-Fluorodeoxyglucose positron emission tomography in patients with chronic inflammatory bowel disease: a systematic review and a meta-analysis. J Crohns Colitis. 2013;7:345–54.

Turpin S, Lambert R. Role of scintigraphy in musculoskeletal and spinal infections. Radiol Clin N Am. 2001;39:169–89.

Pediatric Imaging

10

Sergios Gatidis, Konstantin Nikolaou, and Jürgen F. Schäfer

10.1 Introduction

Pediatric imaging has been identified as a key application of combined PET/MRI (Gatidis et al. 2017). Both single modalities, MRI and PET, are well-established diagnostic tools in pediatric radiology for a variety of indications.

MRI can be considered as the most versatile and comprehensive single imaging modality for children due to a number of properties. The most obvious advantage specifically for its use in children is the lack of radiation exposure in contrast to alternative imaging techniques like X-ray, CT or scintigraphy. In addition, the superior soft tissue contrast and the ability of MRI to depict functional tissue properties allow for comprehensive local and whole-body assessment of pathologies in a single examination (Goo et al. 2005). Thus, numerous studies have shown the value of MRI particularly for imaging of pediatric oncologic, inflammatory, neurologic and musculoskeletal disorders. In the context of pediatric oncology, MRI displays a high sensitivity for the detection of tumor lesions (Pfluger et al. 2012).

In the clinical context PET is nowadays widely used as a part of hybrid imaging modalities, mostly in combination with CT. The distinct diagnostic strength of PET is given by its potential of depicting metabolic, molecular and functional information through the use of a variety of available PET tracers. The main indication for the use of PET in children is imaging of solid tumors for primary evaluation, assessment of therapy response and in follow-up after therapy, mainly using the PET tracer 18F-FDG. Especially in a post-therapeutic situation, 18F–FDG-PET has been shown to increase specificity for the evaluation of tumor vitality compared to morphological imaging by MRI only (Pfluger et al. 2012).

From a diagnostic point of view, the combination of the high morphologic sensitivity of MRI with the high specificity of PET in combined PET/MRI thus promises to constitute a comprehensive and precise whole-body imaging modality for pediatric patients (Gatidis et al. 2016a; Schafer et al. 2014).

A specific aspect of medical imaging in children is the minimization of diagnostic radiation exposure. In contrast to adults, children have a significantly higher susceptibility to potential adverse long-term effects caused by ionizing radiation. Furthermore, childhood cancer is fortunately associated with an overall high cure rate (Robison et al. 2005), however, this may result in long-term follow-up by repeated imaging studies (Rathore et al. 2012). Apart from secondary cancer risk from therapeutically induced radiation exposure there

S. Gatidis (✉) • K. Nikolaou • J.F. Schäfer
Radiologische Klinik, Diagnostische
und Interventionelle Radiologie,
Universitätsklinikum Tübingen, Tübingen, Germany
e-mail: Sergios.Gatidis@med.uni-tuebingen.de

© Springer International Publishing AG 2018
L. Umutlu, K. Herrmann (eds.), *PET/MR Imaging: Current and Emerging Applications*,
https://doi.org/10.1007/978-3-319-69641-6_10

are also concerns about the effect of radiation exposure caused by diagnostic imaging. Thus, the cumulative radiation exposure especially of pediatric cancer patients undergoing PET/CT studies can be substantial (Chawla et al. 2010). In comparison, PET/MRI allows for a reduction in radiation dose by replacing CT with MRI, making it particularly suitable for pediatric applications.

10.2 Technical Aspects

Due to specific anatomic and physiological characteristics of children, certain technological aspects of PET/MRI have to be considered. MR-based PET attenuation correction is affected by the smaller body size and lower body weight as well as the anatomical distribution of cortical bone and fat tissue (Gatidis et al. 2016a; Schafer et al. 2014). In segmentation-based PET/MR attenuation correction, tissue classes (water, fat, lung, air) are segmented based on a dual-echo MR sequence for chemical shift fat/water separation. Subsequently, known attenuation coefficients for these tissues are applied. Attenuation caused by cortical bone can be additionally addressed using dedicated atlases in the so-called atlas-based attenuation correction (Bezrukov et al. 2013). These methods include image processing and segmentation steps that have to be tailored to patient size and anatomy. Especially for atlas-based attenuation correction, a children-specific underlying atlas is necessary to ensure correct localization of bone structures and to avoid artifacts caused by attenuation correction (Bezrukov et al. 2015).

Apart from effects on PET attenuation correction, MRI and PET as such are also affected by children's physiology. Higher respiratory frequency and heart rate in children require adaptation of MR imaging parameters, especially respiratory and cardiac trigger parameters and breath hold duration. Also, in both, PET and MRI, a higher spatial resolution may be required in small children compared to adults. Concerning MR acquisition times, delays in measurement time due to higher specific absorption rates also need to be considered.

10.3 Preparation, Imaging Protocol and Data Analysis

PET/MRI is a complex imaging modality that requires thorough preparation and careful planning, especially with respect to pediatric examinations (Stauss et al. 2008).

The indication for a pediatric PET/MR examination should be established in close collaboration between imaging experts (pediatric radiologist and nuclear medicine physician) and specialized pediatricians and anesthesiologists. Potential contraindications against MRI and the potential necessity for patient sedation should be discussed. Patients and legal guardians should be informed as early as possible about the course of the examination, especially about relatively long examination times and necessary preparation. The necessity for patient sedation has to be evaluated beforehand, depending on patient age and ability to cooperate.

Children-specific aspects have to be considered prior to the examination. Appropriate preparation for the respective tracer application is indispensable. When using the tracer 18-FDG, patients should fast for at least 4–6 h in order to ensure good sensitivity. Blood glucose levels should be determined prior to the examination. If possible, FDG PET/MR-examinations should be scheduled during the morning hours as the tolerance for necessary fasting is reduced in children. In addition, activated brown adipose tissue has a high prevalence in children and can deteriorate diagnostic PET information. In order to avoid activation of brown adipose tissue, patients should be kept in a warm environment and if possible the application of a beta blocker is recommended. Finally, in patients with tumors adjacent to the genitourinary tract the administration of diuretic medication after FDG-injection and transurethral catheterization can be discussed.

The course of a typical oncologic whole-body FDG PET/MR examination is shown in Fig. 10.1. After informed consent of patients/legal guardians, the tracer is injected and uptake time is spent outside the scanner. In principle, tracer uptake time could already be used for acquisition of MR-only measurements. However, from a perspective of

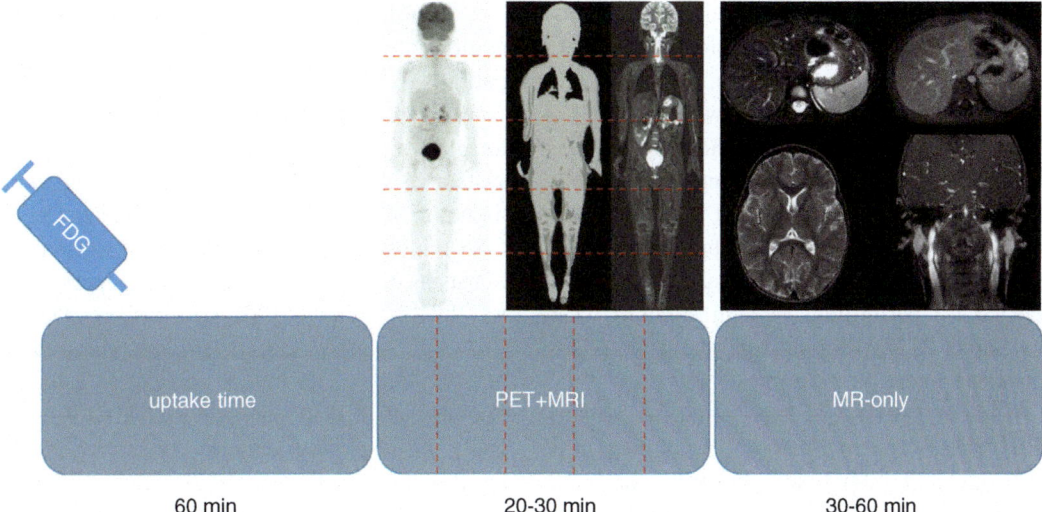

Fig. 10.1 Typical course of a whole-body FDG-PET/MRI examination. PET acquisition is initiated 1 hour after tracer administration and performed simultaneously to whole-body MR measurements. Subsequently, additional local MR sequences are acquired

optimizing PET image quality and reducing local radiation dose, it seems preferable to allow the patient to void the tracer-containing bladder after the FDG uptake time, directly prior to the examination.

Whole body PET/MRI in pediatric examinations consists of two parts which can be planned independently—simultaneous PET/MRI acquisition and MR-only measurements. During simultaneous PET/MRI, image data are acquired in a bed-per-bed manner following the typical PET acquisition pattern. Simultaneously acquired MRI mostly consists of a dedicated sequence for MR-based PET attenuation correction, a coronal STIR sequence and potentially whole-body diffusion-weighted MR imaging. Typical PET measurement times per bed position depend on the duration of parallel MR sequences and are in the range of 3–6 min. Depending on patient size and required scan field, this part of the examination thus takes approximately 20–30 min. If needed, subsequent MR-only examinations (e.g. additional dedicated local imaging, e.g. liver imaging) and contrast-enhanced MRI can be added depending on the clinical question. The duration of this part of the examination is variable and is typically in a range of 30–60 min. Initial studies on fast PET/MR protocols, including T2 weighted, diffusion-weighted MRI and post-contrast VIBE imaging, demonstrated its diagnostic potential for whole-body imaging applications and may be of high clinical importance for pediatric applications (Kircher et al. 2017).

The multiparametric nature of combined PET/MR examinations results in a high output of image data that require competent analysis. Importantly, dedicated software is of crucial importance in order to enable efficient management of this image load. Due to the technical complexity of the modality and the often complex clinical questions, reading should be performed in a multidisciplinary approach, involving experts in pediatric radiology and nuclear medicine, as well as pediatricians. Findings should be reported in a combined report considering the information provided by PET and MRI in the process of the diagnostic decision.

10.4 Indications

Recent literature on PET/MRI in children and adults supports the diagnostic equivalence of PET derived from PET/MRI and PET/CT with respect to detection of PET-positive findings and—using atlas-based attenuation correction—also with respect to quantification of PET standardized uptake values. Hence, PET/MRI is in general indicated in children whenever PET is indicated and no MR contraindications are present. Although PET/MRI as a combined modality has been available for over half a decade (Delso et al. 2011), the clinical availability is still very limited. Thus, despite being the modality of choice for performing PET in children where available, PET/MRI still cannot be regarded as a standard modality.

The largest field of application for pediatric PET/MRI is imaging of solid tumors. First clinical data of PET/MRI have shown the diagnostic equivalence with PET/CT for pediatric cancer and suggest potential benefits concerning anatomical allocation of focal PET uptake and characterization of PET-equivocal lesions due to the high soft-tissue contrast of MRI (Gatidis et al. 2016a; Schafer et al. 2014).

Pediatric lymphoma is a prime example for the use of FDG-PET/CT in pediatric oncology for the purpose of staging and assessment of therapy response (Depas et al. 2005). Especially in Hodgkin's disease, tumor vitality after chemotherapy as defined by FDG-PET has a direct impact upon therapy management regarding the necessity of radiation therapy. MRI can potentially add additional information in cases of low or unknown FDG-avidity and when assessing changes in FDG-avid organs like the kidneys.

The diagnostic value of MRI for local and whole-body assessment of pediatric soft-tissue tumors, specifically sarcomas, is well-established. With respect to therapy planning and assessment of therapy response, PET can add metabolic information, increasing specificity for the detection of vital tumor lesions with impact particularly on local treatment (e.g., extent of surgical resection, Fig. 10.2) (Tzeng et al. 2007). Furthermore, FDG-PET has been shown to provide prognostic information based on the quantification of metabolic tumor volume (Byun et al. 2013). A potential limitation of PET/MRI specifically for the diagnostic work-up of pediatric sarcoma is the limited sensitivity of MRI for small pulmonary nodules (Rauscher et al. 2014). Thus, an additional chest CT may be indicated in these patients.

Another field of application for PET/MRI is imaging of primary tumors of the central nervous system (Bisdas et al. 2013). The excellent soft-tissue of MRI allows for precise localization of CNS tumors and further functional characterization using diffusion-weighted imaging, perfusion-weighted imaging and MR spectroscopy. On the PET side, amino acid tracers are preferred in order to depict vital tumor parts or to estimate tumor grade. Thus, combined PET/MRI is especially useful for the definition of biopsy targets and for the post-therapeutic detection of tumor recurrence.

In patients with Type I Neurofibromatosis, combined FDG-PET/MRI is an excellent modality for the early detection of potential malignant transformation of neurofibromata to malignant peripheral nerve sheet tumors. The high soft-tissue contrast of MRI allows for precise anatomic allocation of single lesions and assessment of changes in size, signal properties and diffusivity (Wasa et al. 2010), while elevated FDG-uptake is a good marker for malignant transformation (Bredella et al. 2007). In addition, associated pathologies in these patients such as optic nerve glioma can be precisely diagnosed in MRI.

Apart from oncologic applications, hybrid PET/MRI is also promising diagnostic tool for the assessment of metabolic dysfunction and inflammatory conditions. Especially for these non-oncologic indications, the relatively low radiation exposure of PET/MRI compared to PET/CT can potentially widen the use and lead to increased acceptance of the modality. With respect to pediatric central nervous system disorders, the combination of MRI and FDG-PET allows for comprehensive examination of patients with epileptic disorders by revealing structural and metabolic changes of the brain indicating epileptogenic foci (Fig. 10.3) (Gok et al. 2013). Regarding inflammatory conditions, FDG-PET is highly specific and sensitive for evaluating inflammatory activity; MRI on the other hand allows for precise depiction of

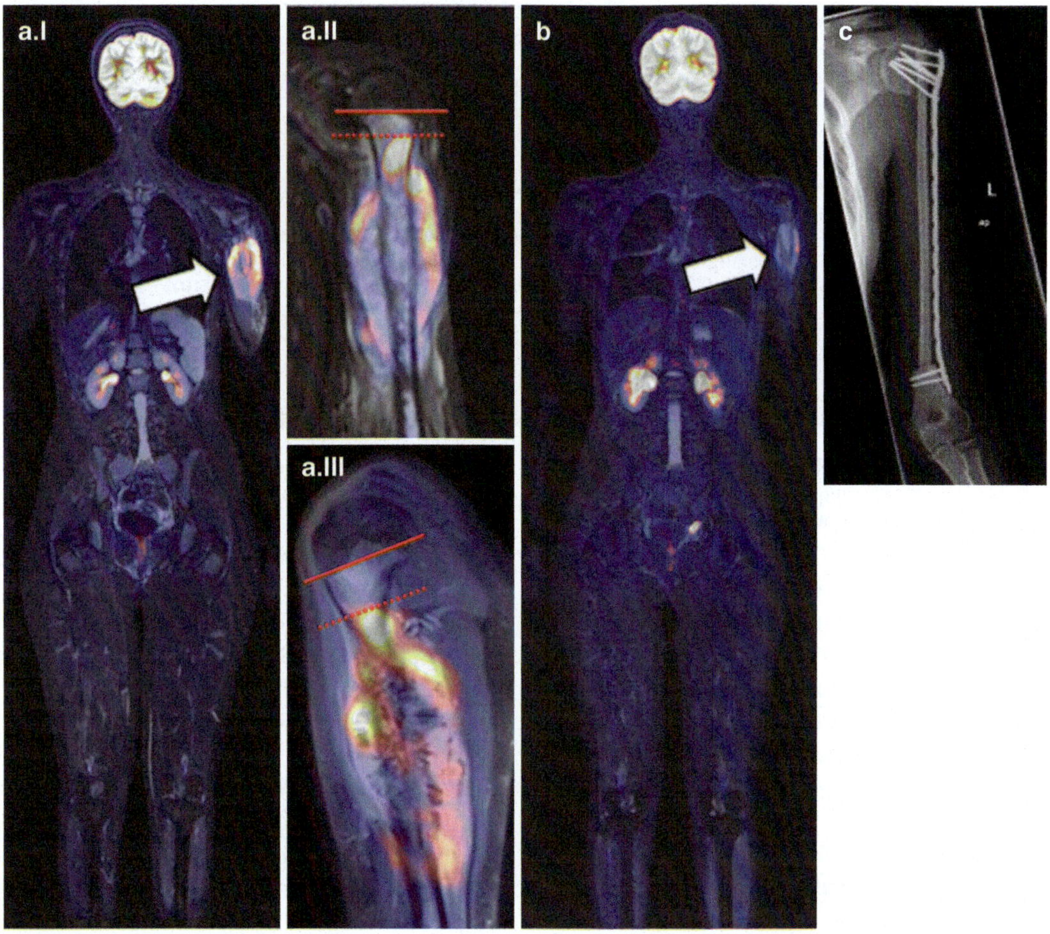

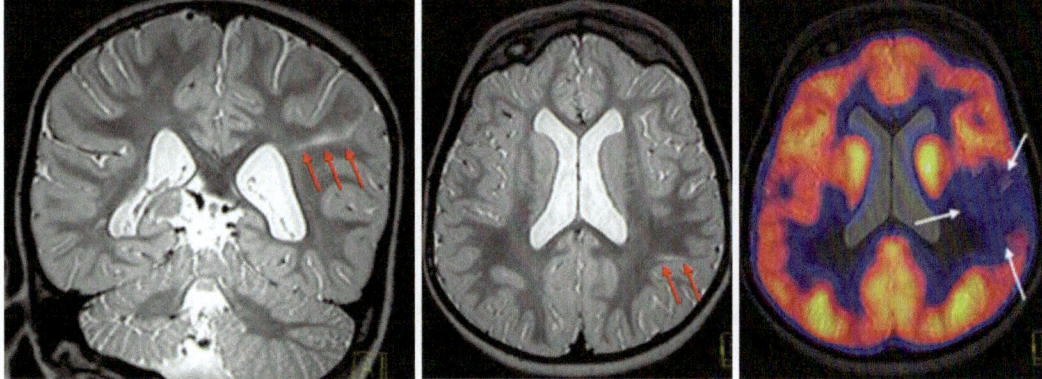

Fig. 10.2 Simultaneous whole-body and local staging using PET/MRI in a patient with osteosarcoma of the left humerus before (A) and after (B) chemotherapy. FDG-PET increases specificity for the assessment of the local tumor extent (A.II and A.III) compared to MRI enabling joint-preserving tumor resection (C). (from Gatidis et al. 2017)

Fig. 10.3 Combined FDG-PET/MRI in a patient with recurrent seizures reveals focal cortical dysplasia (red arrows) as the epileptogenic source with typical hypometabolism in FDG-PET (white arrows). (from Gatidis et al. 2017)

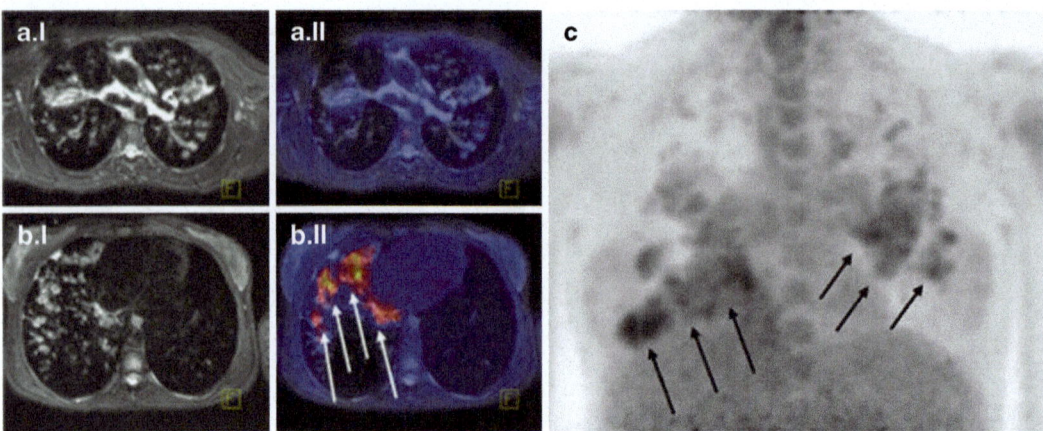

Fig. 10.4 FDG-PET/MRI for the assessment of active inflammation (arrows) in a patient with cystic fibrosis. A long PET acquisition time of 20 minutes in this patient allowed for a drastic reduction of administered FDG-activity to 1 MBq/kg. (from Gatidis et al. 2017)

associated morphologic changes in affected organs. Thus, combined FDG-PET/MRI has a high diagnostic potential in patients with rheumatoid disorders, chronic inflammatory bowel disease, graft-versus-host disease but also infectious states, e.g. in patients with cystic fibrosis or immunodeficiency (Fig. 10.4).

10.5 Patient Safety and Dose Aspects

In general, existing literature shows that PET/MRI is a safe imaging modality for pediatric patients (Guckel et al. 2015). The potential examination-related risks arise from MR contraindications (especially metal implants) and adverse reactions to MR contrast media. The overall risk profile is thus equal to MRI examinations that have been performed safely for several decades, also in pediatric patients. In a similar manner, patient compliance in PET/MRI mainly depends on the ability of patients to stay still for a longer period of time, to hold their breath, and to tolerate scanner noise, which are potential sources of discomfort.

Due to long examination times and the requirement for good patient compliance, sedation may be necessary in PET/MRI for pediatric patients up to an age of 6–8 years, in order to achieve diagnostically sufficient image quality. The same applies to alternative examinations including PET/CT and MRI. By offering comprehensive local and whole-body staging within a single examination, PET/MRI may help reduce the total number of necessary imaging studies and thus the number of necessary sedations. For this reason, patient safety may be improved and potential adverse long-term effects caused by sedation can be reduced using PET/MRI as a single and comprehensive modality.

As mentioned above, aspects of radiation dose reduction are of particular importance in pediatric patients. By replacing CT with MRI, diagnostic radiation exposure can already be markedly reduced by up to 50–80% in PET/MRI compared to PET/CT (Gatidis et al. 2016a; Schafer et al. 2014). In addition, the possibility of simultaneous PET and MRI acquisition—in contrast to sequential PET and CT acquisition in PET/CT—allows for longer PET measurement times without relevant increase in total examination time (Gatidis et al. 2016b). Thus, administered tracer activities can be further reduced in combined PET/MRI, maintaining high diagnostic PET image quality. For the examination of single organs (e.g. inflammatory changes of the lung), effective doses of PET in PET/MR can thus be reduced to values lower than 1 mSv (Fig. 10.4).

10.6 Outlook

The further development of hybrid PET/MRI strongly depends on the technical and clinical development of the single modalities.

With respect to PET, the development and clinical implementation of novel tracers will potentially give new diagnostic and pathophysiologic insight into the development of pediatric diseases. One of many examples is the development of PET tracers for imaging of neuroblastoma, such as 18F-MFBG or labeled anti-GD2 antibodies (Zhang et al. 2014). This development may then open the way for a theranostic approach using diagnostic PET markers as therapeutic agents.

The technical development of MRI on the other hand already allows for significant acceleration of examinations using novel sequence techniques combining parallel imaging, compressed sensing and improved scanner hardware. It can be expected that these techniques will be implemented also on PET/MR scanners in the near future, potentially leading to significantly reduced PET/MR examination times. Furthermore, new developments in sequence techniques allow for artifact-robust and motion-robust acquisition of MR data, yielding higher image quality and diagnostic confidence.

Finally, a main role of hybrid PET/MRI is to be seen in basic science, where the combination of specific PET tracers and multiparametric functional MRI parameters will potentially provide substantial information for a better understanding of pediatric diseases, (patho-)physiology and (tumor) biology, and thus help to improve patient care.

References

Bezrukov I, Mantlik F, Schmidt H, Scholkopf B, Pichler BJ. MR-Based PET attenuation correction for PET/MR imaging. Semin Nucl Med. 2013;43(1):45–59.

Bezrukov I, Schmidt H, Gatidis S, Mantlik F, Schafer JF, Schwenzer N, et al. Quantitative evaluation of segmentation- and atlas-based attenuation correction for PET/MR on pediatric patients. J Nucl Med. 2015;56(7):1067–74.

Bisdas S, Ritz R, Bender B, Braun C, Pfannenberg C, Reimold M, et al. Metabolic mapping of gliomas using hybrid MR-PET imaging: feasibility of the method and spatial distribution of metabolic changes. Investig Radiol. 2013;48(5):295–301.

Bredella MA, Torriani M, Hornicek F, Ouellette HA, Plamer WE, Williams Z, et al. Value of PET in the assessment of patients with neurofibromatosis type 1. AJR Am J Roentgenol. 2007;189(4):928–35.

Byun BH, Kong CB, Park J, Seo Y, Lim I, Choi CW, et al. Initial metabolic tumor volume measured by 18F-FDG PET/CT can predict the outcome of osteosarcoma of the extremities. J Nucl Med. 2013;54(10):1725–32.

Chawla SC, Federman N, Zhang D, Nagata K, Nuthakki S, McNitt-Gray M, et al. Estimated cumulative radiation dose from PET/CT in children with malignancies: a 5-year retrospective review. Pediatr Radiol. 2010;40(5):681–6.

Delso G, Furst S, Jakoby B, Ladebeck R, Ganter C, Nekolla SG, et al. Performance measurements of the Siemens mMR integrated whole-body PET/MR scanner. J Nucl Med. 2011;52(12):1914–22.

Depas G, De Barsy C, Jerusalem G, Hoyoux C, Dresse MF, Fassotte MF, et al. 18F-FDG PET in children with lymphomas. Eur J Nucl Med Mol Imaging. 2005;32(1):31–8.

Gatidis S, Bender B, Reimold M, Schafer JF. PET/MRI in children. Eur J Radiol. 2017;94:A64–A70. doi: 10.1016/j.ejrad.2017.01.018. Epub 2017 Jan 21.

Gatidis S, Schmidt H, Gucke B, Bezrukov I, Seitz G, Ebinger M, et al. Comprehensive oncologic imaging in infants and preschool children with substantially reduced radiation exposure using combined simultaneous (1)(8)F-fluorodeoxyglucose positron emission tomography/magnetic resonance imaging: a direct comparison to (1)(8)F-fluorodeoxyglucose positron emission tomography/computed tomography. Investig Radiol. 2016a;51(1):7–14.

Gatidis S, Schmidt H, la Fougere C, Nikolaou K, Schwenzer NF, Schafer JF. Defining optimal tracer activities in pediatric oncologic whole-body 18F-FDG-PET/MRI. Eur J Nucl Med Mol Imaging. 2016;43(13):2283–9. Epub 2016 Aug 26.

Gok B, Jallo G, Hayeri R, Wahl R, Aygun N. The evaluation of FDG-PET imaging for epileptogenic focus localization in patients with MRI positive and MRI negative temporal lobe epilepsy. Neuroradiology. 2013;55(5):541–50.

Goo HW, Choi SH, Ghim T, Moon HN, Seo JJ. Whole-body MRI of paediatric malignant tumours: comparison with conventional oncological imaging methods. Pediatr Radiol. 2005;35(8):766–73.

Guckel B, Gatidis S, Enck P, Schafer J, Bisdas S, Pfannenberg C, et al. Patient comfort during positron emission tomography/magnetic resonance and positron emission tomography/computed tomography examinations: subjective assessments with visual analog scales. Investig Radiol. 2015;50(10):726–32.

Kirchner J, et al. 18F-FDG PET/MRI in patients suffering from lymphoma: how much MRI information is really needed? EJNMMI. 2017. https://doi.org/10.1007/s00259-017-3635-2. [Epub ahead of print]

Pfluger T, Melzer HI, Mueller WP, Coppenrath E, Bartenstein P, Albert MH, et al. Diagnostic value of combined (1)(8)F-FDG PET/MRI for staging and restaging in paediatric oncology. Eur J Nucl Med Mol Imaging. 2012;39(11):1745–55.

Rathore N, Eissa HM, Margolin JF, Liu H, Wu MF, Horton T, et al. Pediatric Hodgkin lymphoma: are we over-scanning our patients? Pediatr Hematol Oncol. 2012;29(5):415–23.

Rauscher I, Eiber M, Furst S, Souvatzoglou M, Nekolla SG, Ziegler SI, et al. PET/MR imaging in the detection and characterization of pulmonary lesions: technical and diagnostic evaluation in comparison to PET/CT. J Nucl Med. 2014;55(5):724–9.

Robison LL, Green DM, Hudson M, Meadows AT, Mertens AC, Packer RJ, et al. Long-term outcomes of adult survivors of childhood cancer. Cancer. 2005;104(11 Suppl):2557–64.

Schafer JF, Gatidis S, Schmidt H, Guckel B, Bezrukov I, Pfannenberg CA, et al. Simultaneous whole-body PET/MR imaging in comparison to PET/CT in pediatric oncology: initial results. Radiology. 2014;273(1):220–31.

Stauss J, Franzius C, Pfluger T, Juergens KU, Biassoni L, Begent J, et al. Guidelines for 18F-FDG PET and PET-CT imaging in paediatric oncology. Eur J Nucl Med Mol Imaging. 2008;35(8):1581–8.

Tzeng CW, Smith JK, Heslin MJ. Soft tissue sarcoma: preoperative and postoperative imaging for staging. Surg Oncol Clin N Am. 2007;16(2):389–402.

Wasa J, Nishida Y, Tsukushi S, Shido Y, Sugiura H, Nakashima H, et al. MRI features in the differentiation of malignant peripheral nerve sheath tumors and neurofibromas. AJR Am J Roentgenol. 2010;194(6):1568–74.

Zhang H, Huang R, Cheung NK, Guo H, Zanzonico PB, Thaler HT, et al. Imaging the norepinephrine transporter in neuroblastoma: a comparison of [18F]-MFBG and 123I-MIBG. Clin Cancer Res. 2014;20(8):2182–91.

The manufacturer's authorised representative in the EU is Springer
Nature Customer Service Centre GmbH, Europaplatz 3, 69115 Heidelberg,
Germany. If you have any concerns regarding our products, please
contact ProductSafety@springernature.com

Printed and bound by CPI Group (UK) Ltd, Croydon, CR0 4YY
20/04/2026
02093312-0003